Richard Rudgley was born in Hampshire in 1961. After receiving a degree in social anthropology and religious studies at the University of London, he continued his studies in ethnology, museum ethnography and prehistory at the University of Oxford. In 1991 he became the first winner of the British Museum Prometheus Award which resulted in the publication of his first book, *The Alchemy of Culture: Intoxicants in Society*. He is also the author of *Lost Civilisations of the Stone Age* (Century, 1998) and *Wildest Dreams: An Anthology of Drug-Related Literature* (Little, Brown, 1999). He is married with a daughter and a son and lives in Notting Hill.

'Rare and unusual is an encyclopaedia that you can read from cover to cover without wanting to put it down ... Richard Rudgley's book is one of those rarities ... fascinating, funny, informative and provocative'
*Literary Review*

'A gold-leaf reference book'
*Attitude*

'A perfect psychonaut's guide to a strange galaxy ... a brilliant index to the weird and wonderful and a timely reminder that ours is not an unusually reckless age'
*Frank*

*Also by Richard Rudgley*

The Alchemy of Culture: Intoxicants in Society
Lost Civilisations of the Stone Age
Wildest Dreams: An Anthology of Drug-Related Literature

# THE ENCYCLOPAEDIA OF
# PSYCHOACTIVE SUBSTANCES

## Richard Rudgley

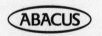

An *Abacus* Book

First published in Great Britain by Little, Brown and
Company 1998
This edition published by Abacus 1999

Copyright © Richard Rudgley 1998

The moral right of the author has been asserted.

A CIP catalogue record for this book is available from the
British Library.

ISBN 0 349 11127 8

Typeset by Solidus (Bristol) Ltd
Printed and bound in Great Britain by Clays Ltd, St Ives plc

Abacus
A Division of
Little, Brown and Company (UK)
Brettenham House
Lancaster Place
London WC2E 7EN

**To Andrew**

# CONTENTS

# ACKNOWLEDGEMENTS

I would like to thank all those who have helped in some way or another in bringing this book to fruition: in particular Dr Andrew Sherratt of the Ashmolean Museum, University of Oxford, for many fascinating (to me at least!) conversations on the Stone Age and later use of psychoactive plants. He has done much to convince me how deeply indebted the cultures of historical times are to their prehistoric forebears; my friend Michael Carmichael for introducing me to little understood aspects of the history of alchemy, particularly relating to psychoactive fauna, and for his constant enthusiasm and moral support; Professor Wendy James of the Institute of Social and Cultural Anthropology, University of Oxford, for alerting me to a very unusual article on the apparent hallucinogenic properties of the giraffe; Emeritus Professor William Emboden for his lively and informative correspondence on psychoactive water lilies, puffballs and sundry other matters; Barry Mason of the Psychedelic Shamanic Institute for valuable references to some works I was not previously aware of; Dr Oric Basirov of the School of Oriental and African Studies, University of London, and Dr Alona Yefimenko of the Palana Museum, Kamchatka, for translating material concerning the Siberian fly-agaric petroglyphs from the Russian; Paul Devereux for kindly sending me his paper on nutmeg-induced hallucinations; and Adrian Morgan for sending me his interesting book on toads and toadstools.

I would like to thank Leslie Du Cane for helping to put the manuscript into an intelligible form and I also look forward to reading his book on the history of Notting Hill, an area much loved by us both.

I would also like to thank Richard Beswick at Little, Brown for taking an interest in the book and publishing it.

Finally, I want to thank my wife, Robin, and my children, Rebecca and Benedict, for their understanding whilst I have spent many days and nights away in Oxford researching and writing this book. Robin has made it all possible.

# INTRODUCTION

In this book I have used the term psychoactive substances in preference to psychoactive drugs. Although this alternative would be equally correct I have nevertheless avoided it, since the word 'drugs' conjures up the wrong sort of picture for many people. For drugs are not just used by addicts and criminals but all kinds of people, and I mean *all* kinds. I define psychoactive substances as those that alter the state of consciousness of the user. These effects may range from the mild stimulation caused by a single cup of tea or coffee to the powerful mind-altering effects induced by hallucinogens such as LSD or certain mushrooms, in which profound changes may occur in the perception of time, space and self. This book is neither an assault on the use of psychoactive substances nor an extended eulogy extolling their use. The use of such substances is simply a fact of life; people have always used them and, no doubt, they always will. I have tried to give a balanced and, as far as is possible, impartial account.

Psychoactive substances are always in the news and the use of them (or rather the use of some of them) is widely considered to be a danger that threatens the very fabric of society. Therefore, many of those in authority have decided to wage a war on drugs in an attempt to eradicate them. Few of these zealots have ever considered the great antiquity of the human interaction with these psychoactive substances, for if they had they would realise that they are fighting a losing war. Psychoactive substances cannot be eradicated simply by outlawing them, as the failure of Prohibition to purge American society of alcohol demonstrates. Whether one likes these substances or not – and very few people are indifferent to them – the lesson of history is that they are here to stay. Like many of the War on Drugs persuasion, I do not condone the use of many of these substances and, like them, I believe that some are socially and individually destructive, but I do question the wisdom of such a war. Of course the modern world has created some problems which do not appear to have existed in the past. Advances in the science of chemistry have allowed many psychoactive alkaloids to be extracted from their plant sources and made into more concentrated forms than ever existed in nature. One can only speculate what even more potent substances await our descendants.

But what of our ancestors and their psychoactive substances; when did it all start? Although it is possible, even likely, that early man, experimenting with the plants around him, chanced upon psychoactive species in remote prehistory, there is not sufficient evidence one way or the other to say which, if any of such substances were used by the people of the Palaeolithic period (the Old Stone Age). By the Neolithic (New Stone Age) period they had most certainly begun to be employed. Cannabis, opium, betel, tobacco and even fermented alcoholic drinks were widely used at this time. In Europe, for example, opium and later cannabis were the substances of choice even before the arrival of alcohol from the Near East. When looked at in this longer time frame the sequence of events differs markedly from the widely held and wildly incorrect version of events that puts alcohol at the beginning and portrays cannabis and opium as late arrivals from the east. There is a growing body of evidence that suggests that man's exchange of the hunting way of life for the sedentary security of the farm was not undertaken solely in order to ensure a steady supply of staple crops. It has been suggested by the Oxford archaeologist Andrew Sherratt that the inhabitants of Neolithic Jericho (one of the world's first towns) traded in the readily portable medicinal and psychoactive drugs rather than the bulky and difficult to transport staple foodstuffs. There is also ethnographic evidence of recent hunting and gathering societies that disdained the labours of agriculture but yet compromised their foraging way of life to ensure a steady supply of psychoactive substances. Among the North American Indian peoples there are some who have tended only one crop, and that crop is tobacco. The Australian Aborigines walked great distances – sometimes hundreds of miles – to tend to their beloved *pituri*, another nicotine-bearing plant.

Having shown the antiquity and ubiquity of the use of psychoactive substances it is now necessary to discuss the many ways in which they are classified into types or groups. They can, of course, be classified according to their legal status, into illegal and legal substances. This tells us more about the society that so divides them than the actual nature of the substances themselves. For it cannot be readily assumed that the most dangerous, physically debilitating and addictive ones are illegal and the comparatively harmless ones are legal. We need not look to different places or times to see that this is not the case. Our own legal taxonomy provides all the evidence required to demonstrate this point. Neither tobacco nor alcohol can be considered harmless. Tobacco consumption is directly responsible for more deaths than all the other legal and illegal psychoactive substances put together. It is also extremely addictive. The problems caused by alcohol are more indirect; its excessive use leads to countless road accidents and violent incidents. It is sometimes said that if tobacco was introduced today as a new drug, then, with the medical knowledge we have now concerning its effects, it would never be made legal. This is almost certainly true. But it also shows the arbitrary nature of much legal taxonomy concerning such substances. What is legal in one era is illegal in another.

Psychoactive substances can also be classified according to their botanical identity (if they have one) and their chemical structures. They may also be placed in groups based upon their effects on their users. In this book I have kept the botanical and chemical details concerning the substances included in it to a minimum. For those with a particular interest in these fascinating aspects of the subject the relevant sources for each entry are given for the interested reader to follow up. The emphasis throughout the book is on the human side, what people do with the substances rather than the substances themselves. Wherever possible I have tried to let the sources speak for themselves and there are many first-hand accounts of drug experiences of all kinds in the book. The substances detailed in the various entries cover both naturally-occurring substances (most of them plants but a smaller number of animal origin) and synthetic drugs created in the laboratory. Most works that deal with drugs tend to concentrate on one or the other. I feel, however, that it is necessary to include numerous examples of both types in order to get a more complete understanding of the whole phenomenon of the human interaction with these substances. Some of the entries are generic and so cover numerous plants and substances under a single title (e.g. fungi, inhalants, stimulants, tropane alkaloids), most of the others cover a specific substance.

I have deliberately set out to describe the various methods by which people administer them both to themselves and, in certain circumstances, to others (e.g. in the communal drinking of a sacred hypnotic infusion such as kava, or in the forcible injection of unwilling subjects in dubious drug tests carried out by the CIA among others). Whilst the most popular means of taking these substances are drinking (e.g. tea, alcoholic drinks), smoking (e.g. tobacco, cannabis), sniffing or snuffing (e.g. cocaine, the *Anadenanthera* and *Virola* hallucinogenic snuffs of the Amazon, amphetamines or speed), chewing (e.g. tobacco, coca, betel, *pituri*) and simply swallowing (e.g. LSD, Ecstasy, Prozac) there are other less popular routes. Intramuscular and intravenous injections have been available since the invention of the hypodermic syringe in the middle of the last century and are common ways to take heroin and other narcotics. Psychoactive preparations in the form of massage oils and ointments have been used by the Aztecs, the European witches and the mountain peoples of Afghanistan. Enemas containing hallucinogens were quite widely used among Amazonian peoples and caffeine enemas have been made use of by professional bicyclists just before a race to give them that extra edge. Needless to say, many of these substances can be administered in many, if not all, of the ways detailed above.

Different societies not only have different psychoactive substances to those in use in our own but they also treat some of the same ones in radically different ways. In the Americas tobacco was considered to be a sacred plant and was only smoked on ceremonial occasions. The recreational use of hallucinogens in our own society would be unthinkable in other cultures who value these kinds of substances as gifts from the gods. Our largely secular use of psychoactive substances is something of an anomaly in the whole scheme of human history and that they could have some sacred function is inconceivable to many people in our society. I have not considered the most commonly used substances to automatically be the most important and have juxtaposed entries on the major plants and synthetic derivatives with entries dealing with obscure and esoteric preparations. Nor have I favoured our own contemporary society in this account of the myriad cultural uses to which the psychoactive substances have been put. Rather I have deliberately and consciously sought to draw evidence from all corners of the globe, from Alaska to the South Seas and from West Africa to Scotland. The same approach has been taken with the temporal aspect of their use. Evidence has been gleaned from prehistory, the ancient world, the medieval world and the modern world, with no particular bias towards a specific era.

In order to get away from stereotypical views of 'drug-takers', I have collected numerous reports of individuals and human types who would not, perhaps, be readily thought to be related to such activities. Thus there are stories and anecdotes concerning presidents and dictators on speed, popes and cardinals praising wine imbued with coca leaves (the plant source of cocaine), monarchs collecting magical mandrake roots, Japanese nuns accidentally consuming hallucinogenic mushrooms and seventeenth-century Eton schoolboys being whipped for forgetting to bring their tobacco pipes to school. Film stars such as Cary Grant and Judy Garland appear in cameo roles. Philosophers and academics are also included, Pythagoras and Michel Foucault among them. More predictably there are accounts of the use of psychoactive substances by shamans, witches, voodoo priests, occultists, tribal elders, poets, writers, musicians and hippies.

Psychoactive substances are, as I have said, integral rather than marginal in social life. Thus, they are inextricably linked with the major concerns of human beings, such as trade and war, love and religion. Again I have sought to provide a representative sample of these interactions. The reader will find information on the Aboriginal inter-tribal trade in a rare psychoactive plant, details of opium dealing in the Bronze Age and an account of the Colombian drug baron Pablo Escobar. Various military uses of psychoactive substances are given, ranging from their use in tribal conflicts, the deliberate poisoning of entire armies in antiquity with the aid of poisonous and intoxicating plants, the covert plans of the CIA to investigate LSD, hallucinogenic mushrooms and other hallucinogenic agents in order to develop new forms of chemical warfare, and the endemic abuse of morphine during the American Civil War and of amphetamines in the Second World War. Psychoactive substances with aphrodisiac effects have likewise been eagerly sought out down the ages. Therefore a considerable number of these have been detailed. Mandrake has been valued as an aphrodisiac since Biblical times and is cited as a fertility drug in the Old Testament. Wild erotic fantasies played a prominent role in the hallucinogenic flights of witches and in the visionary journeys of South American shamans under the influence of *ayahuasca*, 'the vine of the soul'. Spanish Fly (made from the wings of beetles), the bark of the *yohimbe* tree and the pearls of amyl nitrite have all been experimented with by those seeking prolonged sexual arousal.

Although stimulants such as tea, *qat* and coffee have been used by nuns, monks and clergymen of the Christian, Islamic and Buddhist faiths to maintain a state of alertness during meditation and prayer, it is the hallucinogens which have played the most prominent role in spiritual life. The use of sacred psychoactive substances, or entheogens as they are sometimes called, was widespread in prehistoric and ancient times and still is so in many tribal societies. There have been numerous finds of psychoactive plant remains and artefacts associated with their consumption at prehistoric sites in Europe, Asia and the Americas. There is also a wealth of information on the use of entheogens in the religious cults of the ancient world. Opium was used in such a way in Crete, Greece and Iran. Cannabis was consumed in the archaic rituals of the Middle East and Central Asia. The mysterious hallucinogen *soma*, once taken by the priesthoods of India and Iran, has been variously identified as the fly-agaric mushroom, Syrian rue and a mixture of opium, cannabis and *Ephedra*.

Some people are of the opinion that the origin of religion is to be found in the ingestion of psychoactive substances by pre-historic man. To me, this is clearly not the case. The use of sacred hallucinogens is only one of the ways that humans have used to gain spiritual awareness and experience altered states of con-sciousness, and there is no reason to suppose that it is the earliest. I also do not believe that the ritual use of hallucinogens and other psychoactive substances is a degenerate and decadent decline from a more ascetic path, as the historian of religion Mircea Eliade thought. There is no historical evidence for this belief either. What sets aside the shamanic use of hallucinogens from modern recreational drug taking is the highly ascetic nature of such practices. The ingestion of hallucinogens in these traditional settings is invariably preceded by a period of fasting (taking neither food nor water) and prolonged absence from sleep. By such privations the shaman distances himself from his animal needs (sexual abstinence is also a typical prelude to entering these states) and the mundane world and thus he becomes closer to the dead and to the spirits. Only certain shamans use psychoactive substances and, for example, in some parts of Siberia only those shamans who are considered weaker than their more austere counterparts consume the fly-agaric mushroom. Medicine men among the Woodland Cree of Canada know of hallucinogenic plants in their environment but choose not to use them because they are felt to have psychoactive effects that are difficult to control and therefore seen as of little use. It is clear that hallucinogens are simply one of a number of shamanic tools that are only made use of by a minority.

Even in a book of this length it is inevitable that there are omissions. A truly comprehensive account of all known psychoactive substances and their historical and contemporary uses would require a work of truly encyclopedic proportions, running into several thick volumes. There is only one psychoactive substance of major importance that has been deliberately left out, and that is alcohol. So prevalent and multi-faceted is the human interaction with drinking that it requires a work to be dedicated to it alone.

Finally it should be stated that this book is designed to provide historical and cultural information concerning psychoactive substances. It is not intended to be a guide to the use of drugs. Ingestion of some of these substances may be harmful or even fatal.

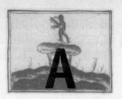

## ACONITE

Aconite is the name given to species of the genus *Aconitum* which are found in numerous parts of the world. It has been used since time immemorial as a hunting poison in areas of both the Old World and the New (in places as far apart as East Africa, India, Alaska and Japan). All species contain poisonous alkaloids and, in sufficient amounts, can be deadly. Its fearsome reputation as a poison made it sacred to Hecate, the Greek goddess of sorcery and witchcraft.

*Aconitum napellus,* commonly known as wolf's bane, friar's hat and monkshood, was used as a poison in Roman times and its cultivation was restricted for this very reason. As among the Greeks, aconite was venerated by the ancient Germanic peoples, who called it Thor's hat. Aconite was also used in European witchcraft and often features as an ingredient in the psychoactive drugs prepared by the descendants of Hecate (see **Witches' Ointments**). Although aconite does not seem to have genuine psychoactive properties, it can have marked physiological effects (such as reducing the rate of the heartbeat) and may thus have contributed to the overall effects of such ointments. It is also reported to cause the unusual feeling of having fur or feathers, which may well have been a highly desirable effect to witches seeking magical transformations into mammals and birds. This curious form of tactile hallucination may have been used in shamanic cultures who were aware of the various properties of aconite intoxication.

Outside Europe it was widely used for its medical properties. The Tibetans used it to treat heart complaints and the Chinese believed it to be an aphrodisiac capable of curing impotence. It also features as one of the ingredients of a Taoist preparation called 'five mineral powder', developed by one He Yan, who stated that: 'When a person takes the five mineral powder, not only are illnesses healed, but the mind is also aroused and opened to clarity.'

**Sources:** Rätsch 1992, Rudgley 1993, Sherratt 1996a, Turner 1568.

## ACORUS CALAMUS

An uncommon but widespread semi-aquatic plant found in temperate and subtemperate zones of both the Old and New Worlds. It has a branched and aromatic root or rhizome from which rise its long erect leaves. It is classified as belonging to the arum family *Araceae* but recent studies suggest that it should be placed in its own family. Both the leaves and rhizome are apparently psychoactive, due to the presence of asarones, which have mescaline-like hallucinogenic properties if taken in

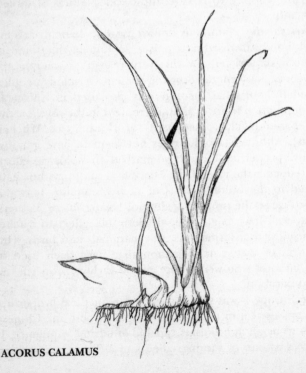

**ACORUS CALAMUS**

sufficient quantities. In lesser amounts it has stimulating and tonic effects. According to Arabic, Roman and later European folk botany, the plant is also an aphrodisiac.

It is commonly known as sweet flag, flag root and sweet calomel in Europe and was once dubbed the Tatar or Mongolian Poison by those peoples who were invaded and conquered by the Mongols, who used it for the innocent purpose of purifying water. It was used in the sacred incenses of both the Sumerians and the ancient Egyptians and remains of the plant were found in the tomb of Tutankhamun. It may also have had a similar use in Biblical times. In Exodus 30: 23,24,34, when God ordered Moses to make the Holy Oil, one of its constituents was an aromatic reed which some authorities have suggested might have been *Acorus calamus*. The plant is mentioned by many of the great classical writers on medicine, from Hippocrates (460–377 BC) and Theophrastus (371–287 BC) onwards. According to Dioscorides the smoke of *Acorus calamus*, if taken orally through a funnel, relieves a cough. Celsus records that the plant was readily available in the markets of India almost 2,000 years ago.

The aromatic leaves were placed on the floors of medieval churches and houses as effective air-fresheners and insecticides. The earliest record of its cultivation in a European garden seems to be that of the Austrian botanist Clusius in 1574. It was known in Germany by 1588 and the great herbalist Gerard tended it in England from 1596. In the doctrine of correspondences as expounded by the occult philosopher Henry Cornelius Agrippa, *Acorus calamus* is under the influence of the sun, although other sources give it a lunar attribution. It was also used as an additive to the hallucinogenic ointments of the witches (see **Witches' Ointments**). More innocently the root was made into a candied confection in Europe and was popular among settlers in the New World. Appreciation of the plant is by no means a thing of the past. The great American poet Walt Whitman dedicated no less than thirty-nine poems to the sweet flag: they are known as the 'Calamus poems' and are to be found in *Leaves of Grass*.

The use of *Acorus calamus* was, and still is, widespread among the native peoples of North America. It can justly be called the 'coca of the north', as it plays a similar role as a stimulant in medical and ritual life to its more famous southerly counterpart (see **Coca**). There is strong evidence that certain Indian peoples, including the Pawnee and the Sioux, planted it, as it is commonly found at old Indian village sites and camping grounds. This planting was probably undertaken not only to maintain a supply of it for medical use but also to provide the muskrat with its favourite food (hence the common Indian name for the sweet flag, 'muskrat root', or simply 'rat root') and thereby profit from a steady supply of furs. It was an important sacred plant to the Pawnee and in their ceremonial mysteries there are a number of songs eulogising it. It is still widely used among rural and urban Indians today, particularly to alleviate toothache.

Whilst the traditional use of sweet flag as a stimulant by many native North Americans is not contested, the purported use of it as a hallucinogen among the Cree of northern Alberta has been the source of much confusion. Hoffer and Osmond's 1967 account has been cited in many books since its publication as evidence of the plant's use as a native hallucinogen. In fact, Hoffer and Osmond clearly state that the two individuals who were their informants were both white. Both the male informant and his wife (who was a psychiatric nurse) had already tried LSD before consuming 10-inch pieces of rat root (a normal stimulant dose is about 2 inches) on five separate occasions. They reported LSD-like effects but did not state that any native people used the root in hallucinogenic doses. The idea that native Americans used the sweet flag as a hallucinogen could be rejected were it not for a passing but telling comment in a written account of a people of the Canadian far north. The anthropologist June Helm was told by a local Indian man that chewing a large piece of the root was done to 'have a good time'. It is also used in the introductory ceremonies of the hallucinogenic fly-agaric mushroom cult among the Ojibwa people of the Great Lakes (see **Fly-Agaric**), but because these rites are little known it cannot be said whether sweet flag is used in stimulant or hallucinogenic doses, although it does seem to have been used in this context as a ritual purgative. But since the Ojibwa use of the hallucinogenic fly-agaric was only discovered by western researchers about twenty years ago it is possible that the Ojibwa have kept secret their knowledge of the hallucinogenic properties of the muskrat root.

Among the Iai people of New Guinea the ceremonial eating of the rhizome of *Acorus calamus* is said to aid communication with the spirit world. The Chinese use of *Acorus calamus* has largely been for rather mundane purposes such as an insecticide. However, there is an interesting passage from a book written about

AD 370 by one Wang Chia which is quoted by Joseph Needham as follows: 'In Ying-chou [one of the isles of the Immortals] there is a herb called *yün miao*, in appearance like the rush [*Acorus calamus*], but if any man eats the leaves he becomes drunk, howbeit if he then eat of the root he will be made sober.' Is this a flight of pure fancy or a vague memory of a psychoactive plant? The ancient Chinese are also reported to have made a hallucinogenic substance out of sweet flag, cannabis and other ingredients. There are thus hints from both hemispheres that sweet flag's apparent hallucinogenic properties were made use of.

**Sources:** Agrippa 1651, De Smet 1985a and 1985b, Gunther 1959, Hoffer and Osmond 1967, Morgan 1980, Motley 1994, Needham SCC 6/1, Rätsch 1992, Schultes and Hofmann 1980a, Schultes and Hofmann 1980b.

## ADAM

Adam is an early name for MDMA, i.e. Ecstasy (see **Ecstasy**). The name was coined by American psychotherapists using it in their treatment of patients, the idea apparently being that it induced a state of innocence. It is also a near-anagram of MDMA.

## AFRICA, PSYCHOACTIVE PLANTS OF

A number of well-known African psychoactive plants are referred to elsewhere (see **Cannabis**, **Datura**, **Eboga**, **Qat**, **Yohimbe**), whilst lesser known ones that have only been reported sporadically are treated here. In addition to alcoholic drinks (especially beer which has a very long history in Africa), cannabis, tobacco and other substances of intercontinental importance, Africa has numerous psychoactive plants, many of which have been made use of by indigenous cultures. Unlike other areas of the world, such as Amazonia and Mexico, the use of hallucinogenic and narcotic plants in sub-Saharan Africa has received very little attention from researchers; some have even concluded that there is little to discover.

According to a 1658 entry in the diary of Jan van Riebeeck (who was the first governor of a Dutch settlement at the Cape of Good

Hope), cited by Brian Du Toit, the Hottentots of southern Africa make use of: 'a dry powder which ... [they] eat and which makes them drunk.' This powder was probably derived from *Leonotis leonorus*, the leaves of which were also smoked alone or in conjunction with tobacco. The Dobe Bushmen of Botswana use a local plant they call *kwashi* (a bulbous perennial, *Pancratium trianthum*) as a hallucinogen. By rubbing the bulb into cuts in the head visions are reported to be seen. The hallucinogenic bulb of *Boophane disticha* has been used traditionally by the Basuto people of South Africa in male initiation rites as it is believed to aid communication with the ancestors. The Basuto also use its bulb in their medicine, as an arrow poison and even as a way of committing suicide. Its use as a hallucinogen for contacting the spirits of ancestors is reported from Zimbabwe. In Zaire a plant named *niando* (*Alchornea floribunda*) is used for its aphrodisiac, stimulant and narcotic properties. It is also used as a hallucinogen by members of the Gabonese Byeri cult.

In 1966 a contributor to the academic botanical journal *Lloydia* surveyed a number of psychoactive plants used around the world, noting that:

perhaps the strangest of all the psychomimetic drugs employed by native peoples ... is the root of an obscure African plant which grows along the banks of the Ubangi River between the Congo and French Equatorial Africa. This reddish brown root, shaped like a foot, half human, half goatlike, is well-known to local medicine men who employ it as an ordeal poison ... because of the extreme secrecy in which the root is held by the West-African natives, practically no information concerning it is available in the pharmacognostical or toxicological literature. In fact, if *radix pedis diaboli* [devil's foot root] had not figured prominently in a murder case which occurred in the remote village of Tredannick Wartha, Cornwall, England in the spring of 1897, practically nothing about it would be known ... the records inform us that a quantity of the root was obtained in the Ubangi country by Dr Leon Sterndale, the well-known African explorer, [and] was stolen by Mr Mortimer Tregennis who employed it to dispose of his two brothers and a sister. A quantity of the drug was dropped on burning logs in a fireplace by Tregennis as he left the room, and the toxic vapour had a serious effect on his three relatives. The next day his sister was found dead, but his brothers, apparently of stronger constitution, were found in a demented state, laughing, shouting, and singing. Later, Tregennis died from the same poison, apparently by his own hand ... pharmacological studies have shown that the inhalation of the vapour given off by the burning root selectively stimulates the brain centres which control the emotions of fear.

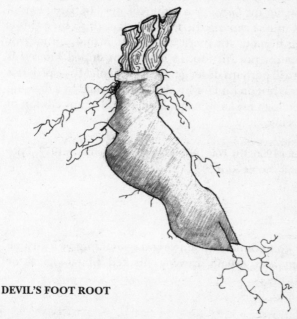

**DEVIL'S FOOT ROOT**

The author of this learned article then goes on to quote a daring psychonaut (the name sometimes given to scientific investigators of psychoactive substances who try them out on themselves) named J. Watson, who tried the dreaded root for himself:

at the very first whiff of it my brain and my imagination were beyond all control. A thick, black cloud swirled before my eyes ... in this cloud ... lurked all that was vaguely horrible, all that was monstrous and inconceivably wicked in the universe ... a freezing horror took possession of me ... the turmoil in my brain was such that something must surely snap ... my voice [was] distant and detached ... I dashed [into the open air] . . . the glorious sunshine [burst] through the hellish clouds of terror. Slowly it rose [and] peace and reason returned.

The bizarre murder performed with the help of the devil's foot root sounds like a case for Sherlock Holmes, which indeed it was, for the psychonaut was none other than the indomitable Dr Watson and the 'factual details' concerning the root are derived from Sir Arthur Conan Doyle's *The Adventure of the Devil's Foot*. Whether the writer for *Lloydia* was acting the devil by trying to fool his colleagues into accepting the fiction as fact (if so then this is truly dead pan humour for there is no levity in this journal!) or whether he simply put his foot in it and was duped himself is something we will perhaps never get to the root of. My suspicion is that the joke was not on him for his article is adorned by a drawing of the root which, to my knowledge, is not found in any edition of Conan Doyle's book.

**Sources:** De Smet 1996, Du Toit 1975, Rätsch 1992, Schultes 1977, Tyler 1966, Winkelman and de Rios 1989.

## ALKALOID

Basic organic compound of plant origin containing at least one nitrogen atom and usually causing marked physiological or psychological effects.

## AMANITA MUSCARIA see **Fly-Agaric**

## AMANITA PANTHERINA

Contrary to popular opinion, the panther fungus (*Amanita pantherina*) is not one of the deadly Amanitas (*A. verna, A. phalloides*) but a hallucinogenic species akin to *Amanita muscaria* (see **Fly-Agaric**). It has been a popular recreational drug in North America since the 1960s, especially in the Pacific Northwest. Psychoactive effects begin 2–3 hours after consumption and last 6–8 hours, depending on dosage. Jonathan Ott notes visual distortions, loss of equilibrium, mild muscle twitching and altered auditory and visual perceptions as the most significant effects. As is the case with *Amanita muscaria*, the psychoactive principle (ibotenic acid in its active form, muscimol) is voided unaltered in the consumer's urine. Whilst the experiences of intentional users have been, in the main, positive, many of those who have accidentally eaten *Amanita pantherina* reported adverse effects and required hospital treatment. The medical use of atropine in treating such cases has the opposite of the desired effect as it actually increases the effects of the drug it is supposed to neutralise. This demonstrates how poorly understood the properties of this mushroom are in medical circles. Although actual poisoning may occur in cases of excessive dosage, most negative experiences with this mushroom seem to be, at least in part, due to psychosomatic symptoms having their origin in the mycophobia (irrational and morbid fear of mushrooms and other fungi) of those who unwittingly consume them.

**Sources:** Ott 1993, Weil 1977.


## AMPHETAMINES

Amphetamines are a group of chemically related synthetic stimulant drugs. They have a structural resemblance to norepinephrine (NE), a chemical transmitter which is produced naturally by the body. Its chemical make-up is also similar to the psychoactive constituents of the plant *Ephedra* (see **Ephedra**), which has an extremely long history of use as a stimulant, perhaps going back 50,000 years to Neanderthal man. Amphetamines increase mental activity and physical energy as well as giving a euphoric feeling to the user.

As with the proverbial dinner there is no such thing as a free dose of amphetamines. Whilst the user may feel that they have twice as much energy as normal on the day or night that they take it, when its stimulating effects wear off they find themselves with half their normal energy. The 'comedown' effects sometimes include a general feeling of weakness and aching muscles and bones. If a user is not prepared to put up with these after-effects they have two chemical options – to take 'downers' to limit their body's awareness of the above effects or simply to keep going by taking more speed. Of course, neither of these options is problem free. The habitual use of 'uppers' and 'downers' interferes with the body's natural cycles and creates a 'see-saw' effect which can be very debilitating, as is the continual use of speed for extended periods of time; sooner or later the user has to face the 'come-down'. Habitual and chronic users may suffer much worse effects. Long-term use can cause general decline in health (e.g. damage to the blood vessels) and leave the user's body and face with the permanent imprint of premature ageing caused by unnatural weight loss. Paranoia and even psychosis may be the outcome for other users and there is evidence that speed may bring to the surface latent schizophrenia in particular individuals. The use of speed during pregnancy can be extremely harmful – embryo-toxicity, and physical malformation and brain damage of the foetus are all real dangers.

There are three basic types of amphetamine of different strengths. The weakest is laevo or d'l-amphetamine (trade name Benzedrine), twice as strong is dexamphetamine (trade name Dexedrine) and twice as strong again methylamphetamine (trade name Methadine). Amphetamines are taken in a number of ways. They can be swallowed in the form of pills (one common type being known as 'blues') or in powder form when wrapped in a cigarette paper (called a 'bomber'). Amphetamine sulphate has been the most widely available kind of speed on the street for at least twenty years and is a mixture of laevo-amphetamine and dexamphetamine. Often dubbed 'poor man's cocaine' this kind of speed is, like almost all street drugs, heavily cut. It is a dirty white or pink powder and has, according to Stephen Tyler, a leading expert on street drugs in Britain, become even more adulterated during the 1990s. Mildly psychoactive effects may be attributed to the inclusion of caffeine and Paracetamol, whereas other common additives are nothing more than a cheap 'filler' for the illicit manufacturers. These include baby milk, glucose, flour and talcum powder. The last two of these can be very dangerous if present in an injectable form of speed as they may clot in the veins. Amphetamines are known by a number of street names such as As, amp, speed, whizz (both on account of the drug's stimulant properties), sulph and sulphate.

German chemists first synthesised the drug in 1887 but little was done with it until the late 1920s when its medical potential began to be seriously investigated. It was first marketed by the pharmaceutical company Smith, Kline and French in 1932 as

Benzedrine in the form of a decongestant nasal inhaler suitable for asthmatics and those suffering from hay-fever and colds. Today amphetamines have a rather limited role in medicine, being used to treat narcolepsy (chronic sleepiness), hyperactivity and hyperkinetic children. In addition to these medical applications, speed, as it is commonly referred to, is used in two basic ways: First, it is used to increase short-term endurance and combat sleepiness when some physical or mental task needs to be accomplished; second, it is also a very popular recreational drug, used to stay awake and increase energy, not for the purpose of work but rather for play – to be able to party longer and drink more alcohol without 'crashing out'. There was widespread non-medical use of amphetamines in the mid-1930s and by the Second World War such use had already reached phenomenal proportions. Both Axis and Allied Troops were habitually fed amphetamine tablets; the actual amount consumed by military personnel during the conflict is estimated to run into hundreds of millions. It was not just the soldiers on the ground who took it, Adolf Hitler was apparently what would now be called a 'speed freak', taking both liberal amounts of tablets and daily shots of methylamphetamine. John F. Kennedy may not have had much in common with Hitler but there are reports that he did share the habit of injecting methylamphetamine. Even the more reserved British Prime Minister Anthony Eden said that he was constantly taking Benzedrine during the Suez Crisis of 1956.

Users from the world of music and entertainment included the American comedian Lenny Bruce and the greatest of all jazz saxophonists, Charlie Parker. Judy Garland, the film star most famous for her role as Dorothy in *The Wizard of Oz*, used amphetamines to try to keep her weight down, then picked up a barbiturate habit to help her sleep. The continual use of these two drugs with their opposite effects is seen as a major contributing factor to her severe depression which ended tragically in suicide. Because amphetamines suppress appetite, many models take them, as do many other women seeking a short cut to losing weight. The explosion in the use of amphetamines among civilian populations was due to soldiers returning from the war and by the 1950s speed was popular with students, housewives, truck drivers, American professional football players and other athletes, not to mention horse owners and trainers who fed their animals the drug to improve their performance in races. It was in Japan that overly enthusiastic (or greedy) pharmaceutical companies created a massive wave of amphetamine abuse which reached its social high in 1954 when it is estimated that over two million (of the then population of 88.5 million) people had become habitual users. The statistical stakes in the use of speed by the military were upped again when America was back at war. During the period 1966–69 the US Army used more amphetamines than *all* the combined Armed Forces of the USA and Britain in the Second World War put together.

Speed has been widely used by students taking exams in the belief that it allows them to write much more than they would otherwise be able to do. This is certainly true in many cases but whatever gains in quantity are made by this prop are counteracted by a corresponding loss of quality – the frenetic mental state induced by the amphetamines making it impossible to assess the value of what is rushing out of the pen. Methylamphetamine is the preferred form of speed used by injection. Injecting speed is a proliferating means of taking the drug and as with the similar use of heroin this has led to needle sharing with its attendant problems of HIV and Aids transmission. Ironically, intravenous injection of amphetamine was used in the 1960s as a treatment for heroin addiction. Since amphetamines do have certain medical applications they are legally classified as a Schedule II drug by both the UN and the US. Similarly, oral amphetamine is a Class B drug in the UK, but injectable amphetamine, having no recognised medical value, is Class A. In America, and more recently in the UK, a concentrated form of methylamphetamine in crystalline form has been manufactured and sold under the name of Ice. Ice is speed's answer to cocaine's freebase and crack (see **Cocaine**) and, although it can be injected, it is usually smoked in a glass pipe or with a more makeshift vessel such as a coke can or bottle.

**Sources:** Lukas 1985, Tyler 1995.

## AMYL NITRITE see Nitrites

## ANADENANTHERA

The two species of trees in the *Anadenanthera* genus (*A. peregrina* and *A. colubrina*) both have hallucinogenic properties and have been widely used to make powerful psychoactive snuffs in American Indian cultures. *A. peregrina* is found in Brazil, Guyana, Colombia, Venezuela, Paraguay and the West Indies. The more southerly species *A. colubrina* occurs in eastern Brazil, Bolivia, Paraguay, Peru, Chile and Argentina. In South America the snuff is known by a number of names, including *yopo*, *yupa*, *niopo*, *hisioma*, *angico*, *huilca* (*vilca*, *villca*), and *sebil*. The psychoactive effects of the resulting snuff include loss of muscular co-ordination, nausea, vivid waking hallucinations and macroscopia (the perception of objects as larger than they are normally), followed by deep sleep during which the hallucinogenic effects continue. The psychoactive principles found in the plant are tryptamine (DMT and bufotenine) and ß-carbolines.

The earliest written report concerning the use of this hallucinogenic snuff mixture dates from 1496 and concerns its use by the Taino Indians of the island of Hispaniola. This report states that it is: 'so strong that those who take it lose consciousness; when the stupefying action begins to wane, the arms and legs become loose and the head droops . . . and almost immediately they believe they see the room turn upside-down and men walking with their heads downwards.' Its use in the West Indies under the name *cohoba* has long since died out.

In South America there have been a number of secondary uses of *Anadenanthera*. In Bolivia its seeds are buried along with other items in the foundations of a newly constructed house in order to bring good fortune to the occupants. The seeds also have a number of medical applications and are used in treating urinary disorders and infertility as well as being made use of for their emetic, purgative and laxative qualities. Its ground seeds may have been taken by the Incas as a longevity drug, supposedly enabling them to reach ages of up to two hundred years. However, its primary role in native societies is as a hallucinogen, although sometimes adult males will take it in small stimulant doses on a daily basis (it is also given to hunting dogs to increase their alertness). The snuff is prepared by moistening the beans from the tree to make a paste. An alkaline additive is made using either the shells of snails or a plant source. The resulting mixture plays a key role in shamanic practices such as divination, trance, communication with the spirit world and the diagnosis of various illnesses. The Waiká Indians of Venezuela use huge amounts of the snuff, which is inhaled through foot-long tubes. The snuff is blown by a fellow shaman down the tube and into the nose of the user. Its effects are almost instantaneous. For a period of about half an hour the shaman is in a highly active state, dancing and shouting loudly; after this initial period he falls into a narcotic trance in which highly valued hallucinogenic dreams are experienced.

*Anadenanthera* is one of the four most widely used types of psychoactive substance in traditional South American Indian cultures, along with tobacco, *ayahuasca* and *Virola* species (see **Tobacco**, **Ayahuasca**, **Virola**). The antiquity of *Anadenanthera* use has been confirmed by important archaeological discoveries. At San Pedro de Atacama, a large oasis in the Atacama desert of northern Chile, a greater number of snuffing kits have been found than in any other location on the continent. Over the last forty years or so over 600 such kits have been found. At Solcor 3, one of the graveyard sites in the region, nearly 20 per cent of the individuals buried there had snuffing equipment with them. Almost all were found next to the bodies of men and only one with a small child and one other with an old woman. This indicates that the use of such snuffs was almost entirely a male prerogative (in many traditional societies post-menopausal women have a quasi-male status). Samples of the snuff were taken from a tomb at Solcor 3 (approximate date AD 780) and the resulting chemical analysis revealed the presence of the psychoactive substances DMT, 5-MeO-DMT and bufotenine. As the other major hallucinogenic snuff of South America (*Virola*) does not contain the alkaloid bufotenine, the snuff from the tomb was identified as deriving from *Anadenanthera*. Seeds found in nearby tombs were also definitively identified by Richard Schultes as belonging to the *Anadenanthera* genus. These discoveries have made the experts reconsider their former opinions that the use of such snuffs originated in the northern Amazon Basin and then diffused to the more southerly regions of the continent. It now seems that the reverse was the case, with its use originating in the Andes and then diffusing north.

**Sources:** De Smet 1985a, Reis 1979, Schultes and Hofmann 1980a, Schultes and Hofmann 1980b, Torres et al 1991.

**ANGEL DUST** see **PCP**

# ANIMALS

Although it is common knowledge that many plants contain psychoactive substances, the fact that certain animals also do is barely known. Modern research into the psychoactive fauna is still in its infancy. The seventeenth-century alchemist and physician J.B. van Helmont described alchemical research with animals as a quest for the 'Animal Stone' which is a 'mineral vertue' obtainable from the 'natural superfluities and excrements' of animals. Excrements should here be understood to mean all bodily secretions, not just faeces and urine. Early scientists and alchemists experimented with all kinds of animals. One such experimenter, Nicholas of Poland, is known to have made extensive use of toads, snake skins and scorpions. Christian Rätsch has noted that scorpion-bite victims report hallucinogenic symptoms and that their poisons still await scientific analysis to determine whether or not they have psychoactive properties.

There are a number of reports of the use of poisonous and other insects for their alleged psychoactive properties. Bees that have taken the nectar of the psychoactive plant *Atropa belladonna* (see **Belladonna**) thereby transfer the tropane alkaloids contained in it and these remain active in the resulting honey, which if eaten by humans has mind-altering effects. Multiple wasp stings are known to induce mildly hallucinogenic effects, such as increasing the intensity of colours and the perception of geometric forms. The use of ants for their apparent hallucinogen properties was once a common tradition among various Californian Indians (see **Ants**). A nineteenth-century French explorer named Augustin de Saint-Hilaire (1779–1853) has left behind descriptions of the use of *bicho de tacuara*, a 'bamboo grub' (which seems actually to be the larva of the moth *Myelobia smerintha*) by the Malalis, an indigenous people of eastern Brazil, and some Portuguese residents who had 'gone native'. He describes its use as follows:

When strong emotion makes them sleepless, they swallow, they say, one of these worms dried, without the head but with the intestinal tube; and then they fall into a kind of ecstatic sleep, which often lasts more than a day, and similar to that experienced by the Orientals when they take opium in excess. They tell, on awakening, of marvellous dreams; they saw splendid forests, they ate delicious fruits, they killed without difficulty the most choice game; but these Malalis add that they take care to indulge only rarely in this debilitating kind of pleasure.

As Saint-Hilaire did not actually witness the hallucinogenic effects he describes, this single anecdotal reference cannot be taken as definitive.

Mention should be made of the infamous aphrodisiac 'Spanish Fly' or cantharides. Cantharides is made from the wings of a beetle (*Cantharis vesicatoria*) and used to prolong erections, but in high doses it can be dangerous. The English physician William Salmon wrote in 1693 of the efficacy of distilled cantharides oil mixed together with other ingredients which if: 'annointed upon the soles of the Feet, Testicles, and *Perineum*, provokes and stirs up Lust, to a miracle, in both Sexes, and invigorates the feeble Instruments of Generation.' The scarab beetle, that was sacred to the ancient Egyptians, has been reported by the Egyptologist Wallis Budge to be ground up and drunk with water by Sudanese people. The Aztecs made a psychoactive salve or ointment which had among its ingredients poisonous insects, tobacco and the hallucinogenic morning glory *ololiuqui* (see **Ololiuqui**). Whether these insects contributed to the psychoactive effects of these Aztec mixtures is impossible to say as the species cannot be identified from the early, and unfortunately vague, accounts of these practices.

Toxic species of puffer fish have been identified as the key psychoactive ingredient in the making of the zombi drug (see **Zombi Drug**). A number of species of fish found as far afield as South Africa, Hawaii and Norfolk Island in the Pacific have been reported as 'dream fish' or 'nightmare fish' on account of the fact that they cause hallucinations. Eating the so-called 'dream fish' of Norfolk Island – a species of *Kyphosus* (it has been suggested that it may be *K. fuseus* or more likely *K. vaigiensis*) is reputed to cause dreadful nightmares. Christian Rätsch, the German anthropologist, states that the 'dream fish' contains large amounts of the hallucinogen DMT.

Reports by the local people of Hawaii of fish having psychoactive effects led researchers from the University of Hawaii to investigate this unusual phenomenon. They toyed with the idea of calling the syndrome ichthyosarcephialtilepsis but thankfully

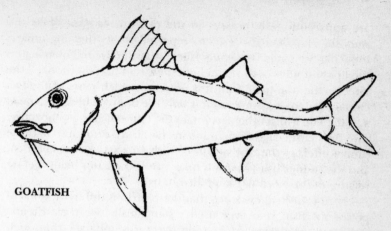

**GOATFISH**

decided on the more straightforward 'hallucinatory mullet poisoning'! In fact, four species of fish are known to cause such symptoms, two of the mullet family (Mugilidae), *Mugil cephalus* and *Neomyxus chaptalli*, and two belonging to the goatfish or surmullet family (Mullidae), *Mulloidichthys samoensis* and *Upeneus arge*. The last of these is known locally as *weke pahala* ('the nightmare weke') and a report from 1927 states that about thirty or forty Japanese labourers unwittingly ate the fish and suffered 'mental paralysis' and delirium. Not all those who eat it report having nightmares; some seemed to have enjoyed the hallucinatory effects. The symptoms vary from person to person. In the case of one family who shared the same fish, some members experienced intoxication whilst others were completely unaffected. That this could be due to some kind of allergic reaction has been rejected, as individuals who experience hallucinations and other effects when eating the toxic variety of fish happily consume the non-toxic variety regularly without any problems. Neither can the intoxication be explained away as psychosomatic; infants who have eaten it wake up screaming and try to get out of their cots, showing all the signs of having nightmares. What causes the psychoactive effects is something of a mystery; it is unlikely to be bacterial in origin since the fish is often eaten straight from the sea, allowing no time for decay to set in. Some local fishermen think that it may be due to the fish eating a certain kind of algae but researchers consider this unlikely. Hallucinogenic effects from these species of fish have been reported from two of the Hawaiian islands, Kauai and Molokai, and the toxins in question are apparently only present in the fish during June, July and August. Hawaiian fishermen reported that the nightmare-inducing fish could be distinguished by distinctive red blotches on the lips and sides of the head but others said that they looked the same as the non-toxic fish. It is not clear which parts of the fish contain the toxins; some say it is only the brain or head, the head and the tail, whilst others maintain the entire fish is psychoactive. Two further species of fish found in Hawaii are rumoured to cause similar effects – the tang or surgeonfish (*Acanthurus sandvicensis*), and the rudder fish (*Kyphosus cinerascens*), the latter being a close relative of the Norfolk Island 'dream fish'.

There is no real evidence that these various different kinds of poisonous fish were ever used systematically for their dream-inducing properties. Most reported cases indicate that such intoxication was, and still is, almost always accidental. Dr Bruce Halstead of the World Life Research Institute stated in 1959 that he had discovered the presence of a hallucinogenic substance in a fish, but did not name either the species in question or the location at which it was found for fear that the Russians would make use of it for developing nerve drugs. Rätsch has suggested that the yellow stingray (*Urolophus jamaicensis*) was used for its inebriating and aphrodisiac venom in pre-Columbian times by the Maya.

Amphibian toxins and venoms have also been attributed with psychoactive properties. Zoologists classify the *Amphibia* into *Anura*, the tailless amphibians (frogs and toads), and *Urodela*, the tailed amphibians, including newts and salamanders. Traditionally the venoms of a number of toxic species of frog have been used to provide hunting poisons which are applied to arrows and other projectiles. The reported uses of frog toxins for their purported psychoactive effects is still largely circumstantial and inconclusive. Nevertheless, the question of the use of frogs for their possible psychoactive effects is still open and as Richard Schultes, an expert on the hallucinogens of the Amazon, has said, the frog is a powerful and widespread symbol of intoxication in numerous native societies in South America. The Amahuaca people of the Peruvian Amazon are reported to use the poison from a frog (*Phyllomedusa bicolor*) to induce states of trance. The poison is rubbed into self-inflicted burns and believed to allow the hunters to communicate with animal spirits. Although this frog poison is dismissed as a 'pseudo-hallucinogen' by Andrew Weil and Wade Davis, these two researchers have, however, done more than anyone else to demonstrate beyond doubt that certain toads contain hallucinogenic drugs (see **Toads**). For a discussion of the possibility of psychoactive substances being found in salamanders, see **Salamanders.** Some newts have interesting toxic properties. Californian species belonging to the *Taricha* genus contain tarichatoxin, which is analogous to tetrodotoxin, found in octopuses and puffer fish (see **Zombi Drug**). European newts of the genus *Triturus* may also contain tarichatoxin.

Holy men in India are reported to smoke cobra venom for its psychoactive effects. Both the king cobra (*Ophiophagus hannah*) and common cobra (*Naja naja*) are used in this way; their dried venom glands or crystallised venom is often mixed with cannabis when smoked. There are possible indications that this practice may be of considerable antiquity. The *Sarngadhara Samhita*, an Indian text of the eighth century AD, likens the drug *bhanga* (i.e. *bang*; see **Mang**) to 'the saliva of a snake', perhaps a hint that snake venom was known not just as a poison but also as a psychoactive substance.

Stories of psychotropic birds are extremely rare. A sixteenth-century account of the Aztecs by Diego Múñoz Camargo describes how eating the flesh of the bird named *oconenetl* induces visions. It is not known to which kind of bird this refers, beyond the description of it as being red and black. It is possible that either the bird itself produced a psychoactive substance or it ingested the drug from a plant source. Batrachotoxins (i.e. amphibian poisons) have been recently discovered in the feathers and skin of South American birds of the genus *Pitohui*. Richard Schultes has reported that the bones of a certain bird that ate the fruits of a plant that was used as an additive to *ayahuasca* (see **Ayahuasca**) were known to be poisonous to dogs.

It is not only laboratory animals that experience drug states, some wild and domestic varieties seem to seek out such experiences. A Russian traveller in eastern Siberia in the late eighteenth century, whilst among the Chukchi people, reported a strange case of animal intoxication:

> In the last few days the Chukchi have had two dead reindeer and take the cause to be that they had given them too much human urine to drink. They give them some from time to time in order to make them strong and improve their

staying-power. The fluid has the same effect on the reindeer as intoxicating drink has on people who have fallen victim to the drinking habit. The reindeer become just as drunk and have just as great a thirst. At night they are noisy and keep running around the tents in the expectation of being given the longed-for fluid. And when some is spilled out into the snow, they start quarrelling, tearing away from each other the clumps of snow moistened with it. Every Chukchi saves his urine in a sealskin container which is especially made for the purpose and from which he gives his reindeer to drink. Whenever he wants to round up his animals, he only has to set this container on the ground and slowly call out 'Girach, Girach!', and they promptly come running towards him from afar.

The Chukchi are known to consume the fly-agaric mushroom (see **Fly-Agaric**) and sometimes they also drink their own or others' urine after eating this fungus, as its psychoactive properties are still effective in the urine. It seems that the above account must be referring to this urine as it is hard to believe that the reindeer would behave so irrationally if they had simply been drinking normal urine. Reindeer are also known to eat the fly-agaric of their own volition (as are Siberian bears in the rutting season who, according to native opinion, do so in order 'not to fear') and Siberians who find them in such a state bind them with ropes and quickly slaughter them to consume their flesh, which is psychoactive for a short time after death. Such reindeers are, of course, only psychoactive because of the mushrooms that they have eaten but there may be other mammals that are themselves psychoactive. In Russia it was apparently a custom that if a cat ate *mukhomor* (i.e. the fly-agaric mushroom) it was given the hemp or cannabis plant to sober it up!

To my knowledge there is no clearly proven case for the use of mammal parts for their own psychoactive properties. There are, however, some instances which would benefit from further investigation. The apparently hallucinogenic properties of the giraffe were first brought to my attention during a conversation with Professor Wendy James of the Institute of Social and Cultural Anthropology at the University of Oxford. The Humr tribe of Baggara Arabs who live in south-western Kordofan in the Sudan are keen hunters of the elephant and the giraffe. After killing a giraffe the hunters make camp and prepare a drink called *umm nyolokh* from its liver and bone marrow. The hunters say that the making of this drink is the main reason for hunting the giraffe. Ian Cunnison, an anthropologist who took part in one of their hunting expeditions, reported that among the Humr: 'it is said that a person, once he has drunk *umm nyolokh*, will return to giraffe again and again. Humr, being Mahdists, are strict abstainers and a Humrawi is never drunk (*sakran*) on liquor or beer. But he uses this word to describe the effects which *umm nyolokh* has upon him.' After drinking it, dreams of giraffes are commonly reported and Cunnison said that he actually heard a man wake up shortly after drinking it shouting 'giraffe on your left'. Waking hallucinations experienced under the influence of the drink also typically involve giraffes. The anthropologist did not really consider the possibility that this was a genuine hallucinogen (presumably because a psychoactive animal was too strange to even contemplate) and tried to explain it all away saying: 'I can only assume that there is no intoxicating substance in the drink and that the effect it produces is simply a matter of convention, although it may be brought about subconsciously.' Cunnison's explanation seems weak and we may well be dealing with a genuine case of a hallucinogenic mammal. DMT may be a psychoactive substance possibly present in the bone marrow of the giraffe.

The magic potions of numerous indigenous peoples of Africa, New Guinea and the Americas which are known to contain mind-altering plants also include diverse animal parts among their ingredients, few of which have ever been investigated for their possible psychoactive properties. Extant recipes that were used by the European witches often include faunal additives such as cats' brains and bats' blood, thus showing the famous witches' scene in *Macbeth* to be anything but purely poetic licence.

Human body parts and substances have long been used in medical practices, something which, of course, continues in our own times (such as organ transplants, skin grafts and blood transfusions). Yet because we tend to think of early medical practitioners as embroiled in superstition, many of the traditional uses of body parts seem to reek of witchcraft, which may often blind us to the practical and efficacious knowledge contained in the annals of ancient medicine. The corpses of young men who suffered a violent end were often sought out because they had not died due to illness, thus their flesh and organs were in a healthy state. The use of a dead young man's brain pounded in a mortar and mixed with the powder of a man's skull 'never buried' is a medicine mentioned by the seventeenth-century chemist John Hartman. Robert Boyle, one of the key figures in the foundation of modern chemistry, is often portrayed as releasing chemistry from the superstitious garb of alchemy, yet he also mentions the efficacy of remedies involving grated human skull (one of the constituents of the Haitian zombi poisons; see **Zombi Drug**). Oswald Crollius, one of the disciples of the great sixteenth-century physician and alchemist Paracelsus, describes what his master meant by the term 'mummy' in his writings on longevity:

> By mummy in this place our author means not that liquid matter which is found in the Egyptian sepulchers, in which Humane Bodies, embalmed with Aromaticks, have been kept for many years: But according to Paracelsus it is the flesh of a Man, that perishes by a violent death, and kept for some time in the Air.

Crollius goes on to tell us that Paracelsus also calls it *Mumia patibuli* (i.e. the flesh of a hanged man). The sixteenth-century physician William Bulleyn recommends that *mumia* (which to him meant 'dead bodies from Arabia') be beaten into the form of a powder, mixed into water and then squirted up the nose by means of a syringe in order to treat falling sickness and injuries!

The potent hallucinogens DMT and 5-MeO-DMT that are found in a number of psychoactive plants also occur in various mammals and in the cerebrospinal fluid of human beings. Scientific studies have found that the quantities of these psychoactive substances seem to be slightly higher in schizophrenic patients than in control groups of 'normal' subjects. However, these differences are marginal and no simple conclusions regarding a direct link between these substances and schizophrenic disorders can be made; 5-MeO-DMT has also been reported as being present in the blood of some schizophrenics. A story by the American writer Terry Southern called *The Blood of a Wig* is about a man who, in search of a new drug 'kick', consumes the blood of a schizophrenic. Whether Southern was aware of the scientific literature on this topic is unclear but the presence of DMT suggests that his bizarre story may not be pure fiction. That such hallucinogens can be made endogenously in the human organism suggests that the ancient alchemical quest for internal elixirs (see **Enchymoma**) may have involved the stimulation of such substances to achieve altered states of consciousness without introducing chemicals from outside the body. The *kundalini* serpent of the traditions of yoga and other similar descriptions of an 'energy' moving between the base of the spine and the head (e.g. among the Kung Bushmen of southern Africa) may also be references to the workings of such psychoactive substances.

**Sources:** Benet 1975, Britton 1984, Bulleyn 1562, Carmichael 1997, Corbett et al 1978, Crollius 1670, Cunnison 1958, Habermehl 1981, Helfrich and Banner 1960, Helmont 1688, James 1992, Love 1995, Ott 1993, Rätsch 1992, Saar 1991a, Salmon 1693, Schultes and Hofmann 1980b, Thorndike 1923–58, Wasson 1968, Weil and Davis 1994.

## ANTS

Native Americans of the southern part of California traditionally used a number of psychoactive plants, including tobacco and *Datura* (see **Datura**). Less well known is their use of certain species of ants for their apparently hallucinogenic properties. Whilst ants were sometimes swallowed as an emetic (i.e. as a medicinal means of causing vomiting) they were also employed in ritual ordeals in which the participants would have to endure the painful bites.

The ceremonial consumption of ants to obtain visions suggests that they may have had hallucinogenic effects. The anthropologist J.P. Harrington reported such a usage whilst doing fieldwork among the Kitanemuk Indians of the region in 1917. According to his account a Kitanemuk boy would undergo a three-day fast without even water and on the morning of the third day an elder would take him to a desolate place far away from home. The youth was then instructed to lie down whilst the elder dropped ants into his mouth, inhaling so that the insects were properly ingested. In the same region young Tubatulabal men in their late teens took ants to gain spiritual power. The decision to seek the aid of ants in the vision quest was the youth's own; there was no compunction to do so. If he so decided then he would have to wait until winter and then fast for three days. On the third day one of his grandfathers would lead him into the sweat lodge where he would swallow with water about seven balls of eagle down, each containing five yellow ants. When the youth's eyes were bloodshot it was considered by the elders that he had taken an adequate dose. He was then shaken violently to aggravate the ants into biting him. This caused him to fall into a stupor from which he would only awake that evening. The following morning he would be told to drink hot water to make him vomit. The balls of down would come up with the ants still alive. That night, having largely recovered from his ordeal, the young man would describe his visions of the previous day to his grandfather. The Kawaiisu people, neighbours of the Tubatulabal, also used eagle down as a wrapping for the ants. For them the ants provided a way to induce visions and obtain supernatural powers. Many other Indian peoples of south-central California used ants in their vision quests (including the Wukchamni, Miwok, Yokuts, Yauelmani, Yaudanchi, Mono, Paleuyami and Bankalachi).

The actual species or even genus of ants used by these native peoples is unknown. One myrmecologist, or specialist in the study of ants, has suggested that it may have been a species of the genus *Myrmacomecocystus*, possibly the yellow honey ant (*M. testaceus*). However, at the present state of biochemical research no compounds known to be hallucinogenic have been located in these type of ants. Certain other ants are known to contain three lactones related to nepetalactone, which is the psychoactive agent in catnip.

**Sources:** Blackburn 1976, Ott 1993.

## AYAHUASCA

*Ayahuasca* is the name given to both the central ingredient of a South American Indian psychoactive potion (a species of the *Banisteriopsis* genus) and the potion itself. Almost invariably other plants are mixed together with the jungle vine *Banisteriopsis*; about a hundred different species are known to have been added to the potion at different times and places. *Ayahuasca* has been used in a number of countries in South and Central America, including Panama, Brazil, Ecuador, Venezuela, Colombia, Peru and Bolivia, and by at least seventy different indigenous peoples of the Americas. In addition to *ayahuasca*, other native names include *yajé, caapi, natema, pindé, kahi, mihi, dápa* and *bejuco de oro,* the last meaning 'vine of gold'. *Ayahuasca* itself means 'vine of the soul'. *Ayahuasca* is made in the form of a drink or potion. The bark of the *Banisteriopsis* vine is either mashed to a pulp and then mixed with cold water or, in other regional methods of making the potion, it is boiled for a number of hours and then the resulting liquid is consumed. *Ayahuasca* gained a reputation for providing telepathic powers and a psychoactive alkaloid found to be present in it was named telepathine (now known to be the same as the alkaloid harmine found in Syrian rue; see **Peganum Harmala**). Harmaline is also present in both *ayahuasca* and Syrian rue. The reports of its telepathic powers have long since been rejected by experts, although the legend lives on in some quarters.

The presence of other plants alongside the *Banisteriopsis* species significantly increases the overall psychoactive effects of these native preparations. The psychoactive tryptamines contained in these additives are inactive when administered orally, unless substances called MAO inhibitors (monoamine oxidase inhibitors) are present. As both harmine and harmaline are MAO inhibitors they complement the tryptamines and the conjunction of the two kinds of alkaloid facilitates the powerful hallucinogenic effects of the *ayahuasca* mixtures.

Richard Schultes, during his many years of botanical research in the Amazon region, encountered a number of indigenous peoples who use *ayahuasca*. His overview of its effects and uses is highly illuminating:

Ingestion of Ayahuasca usually induces nausea, dizziness, vomiting, and leads to either an euphoric or an aggressive state. Frequently the Indian sees overpowering attacks of huge snakes or jaguars. These animals often humiliate him because he is a mere man. The repetitiveness with which snakes and jaguars occur in Ayahuasca visions has intrigued psychologists. It is understandable that these animals play such a role, since they are the only beings respected and feared by the Indians of the tropical forest; because of their power and stealth, they have assumed a place of primacy in aboriginal religious beliefs. In many tribes, the shaman becomes a feline during the intoxication, exercising his powers as a cat. Yekwana medicine men mimic the roars of jaguars. Tukano Ayahuasca-takers may experience nightmares of jaguar jaws swallowing them or huge snakes approaching and coiling around their bodies . . . shamans of the Conibo-Shipibo tribe acquire great snakes as personal possessions to defend themselves in supernatural battles against other powerful shamans. The drug may be the shaman's tool to diagnose illness or to ward off impending disaster, to guess the wiles of an enemy, to prophesy the future. But it is more than the shaman's tool. It enters into almost all aspects of the life of the people who use it, to an extent equalled by hardly any other hallucinogen. Partakers, shamans or not, see all the gods, the first human beings, and animals, and come to understand the establishment of their social order.

Schultes' understanding of the cultural significance of *ayahuasca* is in stark contrast to the derisory accounts of early travellers. The earliest Europeans to mention *ayahuasca* were Jesuits travelling in the Amazon. One of the earliest such reports of this 'diabolical potion' from 1737 describes it as: 'an intoxicating potion ingested for divinatory and other purposes and called *ayahuasca*, which deprives one of his senses and, at times, of his life.'

The serious scientific study of *ayahuasca* began with the field investigations of the English botanist Richard Spruce throughout the 1850s. In 1851 he collected samples of *Banisteriopsis* among the Tukanoan people of Brazil and sent them home for chemical analysis. *Ayahuasca*-type potions are still used by the Tukanoan peoples of the Colombian north-west Amazon, who call such preparations *yajé*. *Yajé*-induced geometric images play a highly significant role in shaping their cultural life. These hallucinatory signs are the raw visual data upon which is constructed a complex cultural code, each different sign representing a number of key social beliefs and institutions. These geometric forms and the states of visionary consciousness that they are perceived in are considered by the Tukano as pertaining to a higher reality than that experienced in ordinary states of consciousness. The powerful nature of these geometric forms is so pervasive in their cultural life that their decorative art is almost completely based on such designs. Their architecture, decorated pottery, sand drawings, masks, musical instruments, necklaces, stools, weapons, etc are all adorned in the same fashion. Even many of their songs and dances are said to be based on auditory and visual hallucinations resulting from their use of the potion.

The hallucinatory experiences of these peoples also have a marked sexual content. This applies not only to *yajé* but to hallucinogenic snuffs and other psychoactive substances used by them. Shamans in discussion with the anthropologist Reichel-Dolmatoff described hallucinogens as 'all semen' and the visions that they induce are states of sexual arousal and orgasm, often involving fantasies of incest. For the majority of native users of *yajé* the experience is a very positive one (although some find it literally nauseating or sometimes even terrifying) and in a few instances the erotic visions are transmuted into a mystical union with the mythical age and cosmic womb.

Among the Tukanoan peoples each of the tribes is the traditional 'owner' of one or more types of *yajé*. This indigenous form of classification is not based on botanical distinctions but on the different psychoactive effects of particular plants and their parts. Thus, the different altered states of consciousness, distinct fields of inner space, and the specific kinds of the drug are apportioned to the prevailing order and structure of Amazonian societies. Similar ways of classifying ayahuasca or *yajé* exist elsewhere in the Amazon. The Harakmbet Indians of the Peruvian south-west Amazon distinguish over twenty different types according to their meaning, effect and associated symbols. For example, one type, *boyanhe*, induces visions of hunting and fishing; *sisi*, known as the 'flesh of the ancestors,' gives visions of heaven; *benkuje*, or 'woodpecker', has leaves which contain a spirit that chops apart illness and so assists the healing process; *yari huangana* is a particularly potent type which causes delusions and should only be used with great caution: unconsciousness, even death await the reckless user. These selected examples can only give a glimpse of what is probably the most complex cluster of hallucinogen-using societies in the world today. The actual number of *ayahuasca* additives and preparations is impossible to calculate; many are the sole prerogative of single shamans. Whilst usage is by no means restricted to shamans, there is often a qualitative difference between the visions of shamans and others. The shaman's special knowledge of *ayahuasca* embraces the entire process of selecting, collecting, preparing and consuming the jungle vine and its additives in the potion. By supervising the doses administered to both themselves and others they are able to control, to an extent, both the content and intensity of the altered states of consciousness.

Ghillean Prance, now Director of the Botanic Gardens at Kew, has recorded an amusing anecdote he picked up in Amazonian Brazil: 'I met an air force captain who had once taken movies to show at Tarauacá to the Indians up river. He said that the Indians were distinctly disappointed by the movies (one a cowboy film, and the other a documentary about Brazil). They told him that they had seen all that and even more while under the influence of *cipó*, and they said that in the future they would use *cipó* instead.' Whilst the use of *ayahuasca* is culturally sanctioned in a great many Amazonian societies its use is shunned in others. In an ethnobotanical report on an isolated Indian group of eastern Ecuador, Wade Davis and James Yost note that:

> Amongst most Amazonian tribes, hallucinogenic intoxi-
> cation is considered to be a collective journey into the
> subconscious and, as such, is a quintessentially social event.
> The Waorani, however, consider the use of hallucinogens to
> be an aggressive anti-social act; so the shaman, or *ido*, who
> desires to project a curse takes the drug [*Banisteriopsis
> muricata*] alone or accompanied only by his wife at night in
> the secrecy of the forest or in an isolated house.

With the urbanisation of Amazonian peoples ayahuasca continues to be used for its magical and medicinal properties. The anthro-pologist Marlene Dobkin de Rios undertook a special study of its use among inhabitants of the city of Iquitos in the Peruvian Amazon. The slums of Iquitos are populated by people who have come in from the forest, and poverty, unemployment, malnutri-tion and crime dominate social life. Many of the slum dwellers seek out traditional ways of dealing with the myriad problems that they encounter; among these is the use of *ayahuasca* for its curative powers. Surgeries conducted by native healers take place at night in forest clearings on the outskirts of the city. These healers carefully screen their prospective patients and will not allow those suffering from extreme mental disorders to take part in the *ayahuasca* ceremonies for fear of disrupting the entire healing session. A communal cup is passed around and the amount consumed by each patient is monitored by the healer, who makes his or her assessment of the appropriate dosage according to each individual's body weight, physical condition and mental health. When all the patients have drunk from the cup

the healer will then also take *ayahuasca*. Throughout the ceremony the healer moves around the gathering shaking a rattle,
blowing cigarette smoke on some patients (tobacco smoke is
considered to have healing properties) and exorcising evil spirits
which are seen as the cause of various diseases and disorders.
Many of the problems which the native healers try to cure are what
we would call psychological traumas and depression. In the eyes of
the slum dwellers they are more often seen as caused by the evil
eye, witchcraft, and sorcery.

Rather like the Native American Church (see **Native American
Church**), whose members use the peyote cactus as a sacrament,
Neo-Christian churches have arisen in South America that use
*ayahuasca* in a similar way. These religious cults appear to have
begun at the beginning of this century and the most well-known of
them is called *Santo Daime*. Some of these cults have thousands of
members, many of whom do not come from societies where
*ayahuasca* was traditionally consumed. *Santo Daime* now has
branches in the United States and various European countries,
including Spain. Although these urban-based cults seem likely to
guarantee the continuing use of *ayahuasca* as an entheogen (see
**Entheogen**) there is also a growing interest in *ayahuasca* among
Western drug users. This has led to the growth of what Jonathan
Ott has called '*ayahuasca* tourism', i.e. groups of tourists visit the
rainforest to partake in the 'jungle drug', usually paying high
prices for the privilege. Since *ayahuasca* is not readily available in
the Western drug scene, its price is fairly prohibitive. Ott reports
that *ayahuasca* potions brewed in greenhouses in the United
States sell for as much as $800 a time. Bearing in mind that such
extortion is really pricing itself out of the market, Ott has noted
that:

> Americans, ever on the lookout for innovations, particularly
> in an open and unregulated field such as the underground
> drug market, have put considerable effort into the creation
> of temperate-zone analogues of *ayahuasca*, that is, combin-
> ations of temperate-zone plants which will supply a source
> of DMT and a source of ß-carbolines that, when combined,
> will yield an entheogenic potion similar to the decidely
> tropical *ayahuasca*. Dennis McKenna [the brother of Terence
> McKenna] has proposed the name *ayahuasca borealis* for
> temperate-zone *ayahuasca* analogues.

**Sources:** Davis and Yost 1983, Dobkin de Rios 1973, Ott 1993, Ott 1994, Prance 1970, Rätsch 1992, Reichel-Dolmatoff 1975, Reichel-Dolmatoff 1978, Reichel-Dolmatoff 1987, Reichel-Dolmatoff 1989, Schultes and Hofmann 1980a, Schultes and Hofmann 1980b.

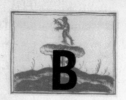

**BANG** see **Cannabis** and **Mang**

**BANISTERIOPSIS** see **Ayahuasca**

**BARBITURATES**

In 1863 Adolph von Baeyer, a research assistant in a Belgian laboratory, discovered barbituric acid. As the day of discovery was the feast day of Saint Barbara he named the acid in her honour. Barbiturates, which are derived from barbituric acid, thus get their name from her. Some forty years after von Baeyer's discovery the barbiturate named barbitone was synthesised. In 1912 another well-known barbiturate, phenobarbitone, was developed. Barbiturates were highly prized by the medical establishment as effective hypnotics and anti-convulsants and led the field as mass-market sedative drugs until the 1960s, when they lost much of their market share to Valium and Librium. They were available in many forms – elixirs, syrups, powders, capsules, tablets, suppositories and, in some cases, in injectable form. As was also to be the case with their successors, barbiturates were widely used outside the realm of medical practice. Such abuse reached its zenith in the 1950s and 1960s. With this shadowy social role that barbiturates took on came a whole host of slang terms for this group of drugs – barbs, goofballs and abbots among them. Their lethal properties are epitomised in the death of Jimi Hendrix, the greatest rock guitarist of them all. In the Notting Hill district of London at the age of twenty-eight Hendrix died when he choked on his own vomit after taking barbiturates. The drug slows the reflex action of the throat and depresses the respiratory system and so sealed his fate. Whilst barbiturates never really attained the glamorous

72|70

status of other drugs, they still feature in rock songs such as The Ramones' 'Go Mental'.

Sources: Henningfield 1986, Tyler 1995.

## BELLADONNA

Belladonna or deadly nightshade is a perennial plant that grows to a height of about three or four feet. It has ovate leaves, drooping bell-shaped purple flowers and its fruit is a shiny black berry. In England it flowers in July or August. The entire plant has psycho-active and poisonous properties. It grows in shady areas of woods and thickets and is often found near old buildings and hedges. It is native to Europe, but is also found in both North Africa and Asia and has escaped cultivation elsewhere in the world (including the United States). It contains the psychoactive tropane alkaloids hyoscyamine, atropine and scopolamine as well as traces of nicotine. The alkaloid content of the seeds is higher than that of the leaves and roots. There are conflicting accounts on what constitutes a fatal dose. Some state three or four berries may be eaten without any ill effects whatsoever, others say a single berry can kill. Charles Heiser, a distinguished botanist specialising in the nightshades, states that toxicity probably varies from plant to plant, also different individuals may be more or less tolerant to the effects. Children have been the commonest casualties in incidents of belladonna poisoning. The plant causes powerful hallucino-genic effects and ecstatic states which often involve frenzied activity and erotic fantasies.

The considerable number of names for belladonna indicate its cultural importance in Europe. The genus name Atropa is derived from Atropos, the name of one of the Fates in Greek mythology. Atropos, 'the inflexible one', cut the thread of human life with her shears. Both atropine and the generic term tropane alkaloids are named after Atropa. The nightshades were given three Latin names on account of their effects on the human organism – *Solanum somniferum* (sleeping nightshade), *S. manicum* ('raging' nightshade) and *S. læthale* (deadly nightshade). The name bella-donna comes from the Italian *bella donna*, meaning 'beautiful lady', and there are three accounts of how it came to get this name. The first and most popular of these states that Italian ladies,

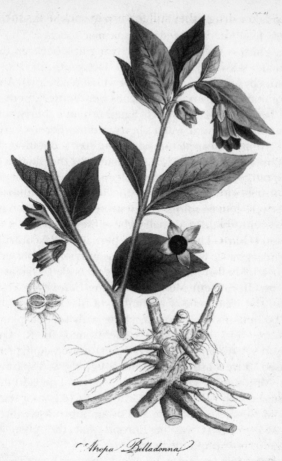

*Atropa Belladonna*

## BELLADONNA

especially those of Venice, used juice extracted from the plant to dilate the pupils of their eyes. This was said to make them more alluring and sexually attractive to the opposite sex. The second also involves belladonna's cosmetic use in Italy; the juice of the berries was applied to the face in order to make it appear paler. The other story attributes the naming of the plant to its use by an Italian poisoner named Leucota, who is supposed to have dispatched a number of beautiful female victims with its aid. Against the background of such conflicting tales, Linnaeus gave the plant this specific botanical name. In addition to referring to this botanical species, belladonna also refers to the medicinal drug prepared from it, as listed in pharmacopoeias. Throughout European history there has been a strong link between the plant and female sexuality that reached its zenith in the use of belladonna by European witches (for which see below). Among its other common and vernacular names were morrel, petty-morrel, hounds' berries, the Devil's herb, naughty man's cherry, sorcerer's cherry, apples of Sodom, witch's berry and murderer's berry. Such epithets give us a clear picture of the sinister reputation and uses of the plant. Dwale, another English name for the plant, is derived from the old Norse term meaning sleep, torpor or trance. To the Germanic tribes it was *Walkerbeere*, 'the berry of the Valkyries'. The Valkyries were female spirits who delivered warriors slain in battle to the heavenly castle of Valhalla where they would feast with the god Wotan (Odin). The berries may, perhaps, have contributed to the legendary battle frenzy of the Norse warriors or berserkers.

The use of belladonna can be traced back as far as written records go. In ancient Mesopotamia the Sumerians reportedly used it in the treatment of a number of illnesses thought to be caused by demons. Belladonna, along with related plants such as henbane and mandrake, is mentioned in R. Campbell Thompson's *Assyrian Herbal* as having many medicinal properties. It was used to treat asthma, chronic coughing and spasms of the bladder. Although there are sporadic reports of belladonna being used elsewhere in Asia and in North Africa (e.g. as a sedative in traditional Nepalese medicine and as an aphrodisiac in contemporary Morocco), it was in Europe that the plant became important in magic and medicine.

Belladonna juice is said to be one of the psychoactive additives to the wine drunk at the Bacchanalian orgies. Its intoxicating powers were seemingly a factor in inducing a state of frenzy in which the maenads (priestesses of Bacchus) tore apart animals, men and children. Aphrodisiac drinks containing belladonna were concocted in Greece and were a speciality of the witches of Thessaly. Roman priests are said to have drunk an infusion of belladonna before invoking Bellona, the goddess of war. According to legend the Scots, under the leadership of Duncan I, used the plant in a far more direct way to achieve their military ends in the war with King Sven Canute (*c.* AD 1035). They sent the enemy food supplies laced with lethal quantities of nightshade which effectively wiped out the Scandinavian army. Belladonna had a number of uses in the folk life of Europeans. In Eastern Europe its root was used in love magic. When it was removed from the ground, offerings to the spirit of the plant would be made. Elsewhere the root was used as an amulet (as was the root of its cousin the mandrake) for bringing good fortune in gaming and affairs of the heart. Central European hunters would eat several of its berries to increase their alertness on long hunting trips. But the central significance of belladonna in Europe was its role in the practices of the witches, especially as a ritual hallucinogen consumed at the sabbat. It was one of the key ingredients of the witches' hallucinogenic drugs (see **Witches' Ointments**) and as such naturally became demonised by the Church. According to one legend the plant is tended every night by the Devil, who only leaves it on Walpurgis night (the eve of 1 May) when he travels to the sabbat held on the Brocken peak of the Harz mountains in Germany. On this night one may see the plant transform into a beautiful, but deadly, enchantress.

Like so many other plants dealt with in this book, belladonna is at once a poison, a psychoactive substance and a medicine. John Gerard, the sixteenth-century herbalist, states that if the leaves (especially if moistened in wine vinegar) are laid on the temples of the patient severe headaches are relieved, allowing the patient to sleep. He also gives an account of the accidental poisoning of three boys of Wisbech (Cambridgeshire, England) who ate the attractive but poisonous berries. Two of the boys died within eight hours but the third was saved by being given a honey and water mixture which made him vomit up the berries. The English physician William Salmon wrote a more personal account of belladonna poisoning in the seventeenth century:

> The berries being eaten, bring present death in an hour or two at most; I speak by sad experience, for my part when very young, with some other Children, going into a Garden where this plant grew with ripe black Berries, we all gathered them, and eat them [sic]. I eat but 3 or 4 as I remember, being too luscious for me, and so escaped, but not without vehement Vomiting, sickness at Heart, and loss of my Hair, Nailes, and Skin; the other children who eat more of them, all died in an hour or two raving Mad, and extreamly swell'd, as if they would burst etc. But enough of this unpleasant and sad Subject, these lines being only written to give others warning.

Perhaps this tragic and no doubt traumatic incident may have affected Salmon's decision to become a doctor later in life.

In the eighteenth century belladonna was taken internally to treat cancer and in nineteenth-century homoeopathic treatments it was used as a preventative against scarlet fever. Even today it is an important source of medical drugs, including powerful and effective antispasmodic agents. Atropine, derived from belladonna, is used to dilate the pupils in contemporary opthalmic practice. It is also one of the two most important drugs used to treat cases of ergot poisoning (see **Ergot**), the other being papaverine, an alkaloid derived from opium. Its use in treating ergot poisoning – or St Anthony's Fire as it used to be known – has long been recognised; William Coles wrote in the seventeenth century that both the leaves and their juice were valued for this purpose.

Comte de Lautréamont, who was an obscure writer in his lifetime – he died age twenty-six – gained posthumous glory when André Breton, Salvador Dali and other surrealists recognised the frenzied and morally unrestrained writing of his *Maldoror* as a foreshadowing of their own artistic endeavours. In the book Lautréamont describes his anti-hero Maldoror as having a mouthful of belladonna leaves. The writing is so extraordinary and manic that it would not be surprising if the author himself wrote whilst in the throes of belladonna intoxication. Despite its considerable role in medicine, belladonna still retains an aura reeking of murder, baneful sorcery, frenzied imagination and dangerous but enchanting female sexuality.

**Sources:** Coles 1657, Emboden 1979, Gerard 1597, Heiser 1969, Ott 1993, Ratsch 1992, Salmon 1693, Salmon 1710, Schultes and Hofmann 1980b, Thorwald 1962, Turner 1568.

## BENZEDRINE see **Amphetamines**

## BETEL

The habit of chewing the betel nut mixture for its stimulating qualities is indulged in by between a quarter and a tenth of the world's population, which makes it one of the most popular of all psychoactive substances. It is used in an area stretching from east

Africa to Polynesia. Although it is commonly called betel chewing, this is not strictly correct since the 'nut' that is used is in fact the seed of the areca palm (*Areca catechu*) which is mixed with lime and then wrapped in a betel leaf (*Piper betel*). Nor is it really chewed, it is put between the cheek and tongue and left there, sometimes overnight! The main psychoactive constituent is arecaidine, which has stimulating effects akin to nicotine (sometimes it is 'chewed' with tobacco). The habit is thought to have originated in south-east Asia and there is archaeological evidence to support this view. The Spirit Cave site in Thailand yielded palaeobotanical remains of *Piper* and *Areca* which, since found at the same location, is circumstantial evidence for the practice of betel-chewing in prehistoric times. Since these remains are between 9,000 and 7,500 years old, this would make betel one of the earliest known psychoactive substances to be used in the world.

Betel chewing was – and still is – a custom that was integral to the social life of many south and south-east Asian societies. It played a major part in the etiquette of the royal courts and in the unwritten social grammar of Indian diplomacy. Unlike the more straightforward betel mixtures of Melanesia (which consist of only the three essential substances – areca nuts, *Piper betel* leaves and lime paste) and other regions, the Indians liked to add numerous flavourings and colourings to their betel preparations. It is the blending of these admixtures which constitutes the unique gustatory and aesthetic contribution of Indian culture to the world of betel chewing. The rich assortment of paraphernalia involved in making up betel mixtures included receptacles for each of the separate ingredients – mortars, dishes, spittoons, and cutters for the areca nuts. This last group of items are known as betel cutters and, of all the objects associated with the betel cult, these are the most ornate. A betel cutter is a hinged one-bladed instrument designed solely to cut the areca nut. Outside of the Indian sphere of influence the job was done simply with a knife. The importance of these distinctive forms of material culture is described by an expert and well-known collector Henry Brownrigg: 'cutters can . . . be seen as a sort of microcosm of Asian metalwork, with the craftsmen of a dozen different cultures producing items which are similar in function and general shape but utterly different in design and workmanship. It is this diversity which gives cutters their particular fascination.' Many of these regional designs make full use of the symbolic possibilities of the bipartite nature of the cutter to simulate erotic acts as the two parts come together in the cutting of the nut.

In New Guinea and other parts of Melanesia betel chewing is as avidly pursued as it is in India, mainland south-east Asia and Indonesia. Its Melanesian use is similar to our use of tea and coffee in the sense that it is an integral and informal part of the daily routine (although it is not without its ritualistic uses in the region). As in India and elsewhere, betel has been the inspiration for minor art forms and in Melanesia there are many finely decorated lime spatulas, lime containers and other objects incorporated into the betel-chewing kit. Betel was not always available and other plants were sometimes used in its place, as, for example, among the Kukukuku of south-east central New Guinea who substituted it with *Lactuta indica*.

**Sources:** Beran 1988, Blackwood 1940, Brownrigg 1991, Burton-Bradley 1972.

## BHANG see **Cannabis** and **Mang**

## BRUGMANSIA

Often called the 'tree *Daturas*', *Brugmansia* are now recognised by botanists as deserving of a distinct taxonomic status within the family Solanaceae. All species of the genus are native only to South America. The plant grows along the Andean and Pacific fringe of the continent from Colombia down to southern Peru and the middle of Chile. Various species (*B. arborea, B. sanguinea, B. aurea*) grow in abundance in the Andes above 2,000m. All these plants now only reproduce through being cultivated as there are no longer any truly wild species. The major alkaloid present in these species is scopolamine but hyoscyamine and atropine are also present. Scopolamine is the agent causing the powerful hallucinations. *Brugmansia* is also widely reputed to have aphrodisiac effects. *Brugmansia* species are known by a number of names, including angel's trumpet (a reference to the shape of the flowers) *yerba de huaca, campanilla, maicoa, tonga, toa, buyes, floripondio, chamico, huanco* and *huacacachu* and *borrachero*.

The anthropologist Weston La Barre maintained that the

Indians who entered and subsequently populated the New World were predisposed to the seeking out of psychoactive plants because of their archaic roots in Eurasian shamanism, which he believed built its religious life around the ritual use of hallucinogens. With this in mind he had the following to say about the Indian pioneers who pressed further south, already having sampled the *Datura* on their way: 'the morphological similarities between the flowers of *Datura* and *Brugmansia*, in addition to their similar chemical properties, would have made the latter readily accepted when encountered in the southern continent.' Whether one accepts the hypothesis of La Barre or not, we do know that most of the Indian peoples of western South America are aware of *Brugmansia* species and their hallucinogenic properties.

Native peoples drink hot and cold infusions of *Brugmansia* leaves and flowers, and also mix its ground seeds into their fermented maize beer (*chicha*). A traveller in nineteenth-century Peru gives the following description of the effects of such a psychoactive drink on an Indian man who was seen to be: 'falling into a heavy stupor, his eyes vacantly fixed on the ground, his mouth convulsively closed and his nostrils dilated. In the course of a quarter of an hour, his eyes began to roll, foam issued from his mouth, and his whole body was agitated by frightful convulsions. After these violent symptoms had passed, a profound sleep followed for several hours' duration and when the subject had recovered, he related the particulars of his visit with his forefathers. He appeared very weak and exhausted.' As well as using the plant as a way of communicating with the ancestors, native peoples have sought its aid in prophecy, divination, witchcraft and medicine and a number of less spiritually orientated pursuits such as finding gold and ancient graves, which, if found, could be plundered for treasure. So prevalent was this last activity in Peru that two of the local plant names cited above (*yerba de huaca* and *huacahaca*) actually mean 'plant of the tomb'.

Like all of its solanaceous relatives that possess psychoactive properties, *Brugmansia* species have their sinister applications. Among the pre-Conquest Chibcas of Colombia a concoction of *Brugmansia*, tobacco and maize beer was given to slaves and wives of dead kings in order to put them in a deep narcotic state so that they could be buried alive with their masters and husbands. An account from 1589 details just such an occurrence:

[a] dead chief was accompanied to the tomb by his women and slaves, who were buried in different layers of earth . . . of which none was without gold. And so that the women and poor slaves should not fear their death before they saw the awful tomb, the nobles gave them things to drink of inebriating Tobacco and other leaves of the tree we call Borrachero, all mixed in their usual drink, so that of their senses none is left to foresee the harm soon to befall them.

Schultes and Hofmann have identified the species in question to be *B. aurea* and *B. sanguinea*. It seems ironic that both those that lay dead in the tombs and those that plundered and looted such graves were there because of *Brugmansia* and its psychoactive effects. Yet perhaps it was also a kind of sympathetic magic on the part of the grave robbers. Other Colombian peoples are also known to have had similar practices; some graves belonging to the Quimbaya culture of Cauca Valley have been discovered to contain a large number of disc-shaped clay spindle whorls (items used in spinning thread) decorated with representations of what appear to be the intoxicating flowers of *Brugmansia* or *Datura*.

*Brugmansia* is also sometimes used in conjunction with tobacco. The present-day Tzeltal Indians of Mexico smoke the dried leaves of *B. suaveolens* with *Nicotiana rustica* in order to obtain visions that will indicate the cause of various diseases. According to Peter De Smet, the expert on the ritual use of enemas, the Jivaro Indians of eastern Ecuador and Peru (most famous for their unique contribution of headshrinking) used species of *Brugmansia* in a decoction which was taken as an enema by their warriors 'to gain power and foretell the future'. A Jivaro boy as young as six may take *Brugmansia* or another psychoactive preparation such as *ayahuasca* (see **Ayahuasca**) under the supervision of his father in order to create an 'external soul' which is a psychic 'organ' capable of communicating with the ancestors through visionary experiences. Among the Jivaro, children who suffer from what are currently described as 'behavioural problems' would sometimes be given a drink of *Brugmansia* and be admonished by the parents whilst the ancestors were present (due to the effects of the drink).

The plants are widely traded for both their psychoactive properties and ornamental value. The Kamsá and Ingano people of the Sibundoy Valley in the Columbian Andes distribute a number of species throughout the Amazon. The cultivation of the plant is supervised by shamans with special knowledge of their botany and pharmacology. In Sibundoy, as a rule, the use of *Brugmansia* for its psychoactive effects is restricted to shamans who drink it either in water or alcohol and see terrifying visions of jaguars (the most important shamanic animal in large parts of South America) and snakes. To withstand the assault of such powerful images one needs the psychological strength that is the prerogative of the shaman. Other psychoactive plants of the Solanaceae family are said to have a fragrance so strong that it can cause narcosis or sleep in those who inhale it (see for example **Mandrake**), and there is a similar belief concerning the *Brugmansia.* It is said that the scent of the flowers causes erotic dreams and for this reason it is incorporated into love magic.

**Sources:** De Smet 1983, Lockwood 1979, McMeekin 1992, Rätsch 1992, Schultes and Hofmann 1980b.

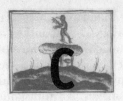

## CACTI

Although sometimes thought of as a kind of plant found only in hot deserts, cacti also grow in jungles and at high altitudes, as in the Andes. There are about fifty genera in the family Cactaceae and it is estimated that about 10 per cent of the species are hallucinogenic.

The most well-known hallucinogenic cacti are **Peyote** and the **San Pedro,** both of which contain mescaline. The Tarahumara people of Mexico are perhaps the most thorough investigators of the entheogenic (for an explanation of this term, see **Entheogens**) potentials of cacti. In addition to their peyote cult, they also know the following species as hallucinogens – *Ariocarpus fissuratus, Epithelantha micromeris, Mammillaria craigii, M. grahamii, Coryphantha compacta, Echinocereus triglochidiatus,* and *E. salm-dyckianus* and *Pachycereus pecten-aboriginum.*

**Sources:** Bye 1979, Richardson 1988.


## CAESALPINIA

*Caesalpinia sepiaria* is a shrubby vine found throughout southern China and Central Asia, the seeds, flowers and roots of which play a role in traditional Chinese medicine. Chinese sources say that the plant (known as *yun-shih*) has hallucinogenic properties. According to Li Shih-chen, the great sixteenth-century authority on medicinal plants, the flowers have the power to make one see spirits, to cause the sensation of levitation and impair motor function. In a Chinese work called the *Tao Hun-ching* it is said that the flowers, if put in water or burned, conjure up spirits. The burning of the seeds is said to have the same effect on those who inhale the resulting smoke. Schultes and Hofmann report that an alkaloid of unknown structure is contained in the plant. *Caesalpinia echinata* has been used as an *ayahuasca* admixture by Peruvian shamans (see **Ayahuasca**) and *C. bonduc* as a substitute for the mysterious *soma* plant of Asia (see **Soma**).

**Sources:** Li 1977, Ott 1993, Rätsch 1992, Schultes and Hofmann 1980b.

## CAFFEINE

Caffeine occurs naturally in well over 100 different plant species and as such is an active principle in numerous mildly psychoactive substances, including, of course, tea, coffee, cacao (the source of cocoa and chocolate)and numerous soft carbonated drinks such as Coca-Cola. It has rightly been called 'the world's most popular drug'. It is a stimulant but it functions in an indirect way, as Stephen Braun puts it: 'drinking caffeine is ... like putting a block of wood under one of the brain's primary brake pedals. Caffeine is an indirect stimulant: brain activity speeds up because it can't slow down. By itself, then, caffeine can't stimulate anything. It can only clear the way for the brain's own stimulants ... to do their job.' Up to four cups of coffee per day (or an equivalent intake of another source of caffeine) has a stimulating effect, anything more has no further effect or can even be counterproductive and make the user sluggish.

Although caffeine has a reputation as being an aid in weight-loss, the latest scientific findings tend to dismiss this. As a result of such research in 1991 the US Food and Drug Administration banned caffeine from all diet pills and allied products. However, the use of caffeine directly before an athletic competition undoubtedly has a positive effect, so much so that professional bicyclists are known to insert caffeine suppositories in order to enhance their performance. Braun, who, in his recent book *Buzz: The Science and Lore of Alcohol and Caffeine,* has applied the latest findings of neuroscience to study these two substances and their interaction, states that the: 'deep dichotomy between reason and irrationality can be seen in the world's tremendous appetite for alcohol and caffeine. Alcohol is the liberator of the irrational. Caffeine is the stimulator of the rational. It would appear that the human spirit craves both poles and turns to these most familiar of drugs to achieve those ends.' It is only in those rare moments of total drunkenness or complete sobriety that either of the poles is actually attained, the rhythm of daily life consisting largely of more subtle but perpetual mood swings between these distant poles. That the average adult usually has one or both of these psychoactive substances in his or her body at any given time means that our sense of the rational and irrational is permanently overlaid by the chemical dialogue of these culturally charged substances.

**Sources:** Braun 1996.

## CANNABIS

Although the cannabis plant is now ubiquitous, unlike other wide-spread types of hallucinogen (such as *Psilocybe* 'magic mushrooms' or *Datura*), it is not native to more than one continent. Cannabis is a plant native to Central Asia that has spread all over the world and is probably the most widely used recreational and usually illegal drug in the world, being smoked from the inner cities of America and Europe to the outlying atolls of Micronesia. The plant's natural homeland is most likely in the regions north of Afghanistan and the Altai mountains of southern Siberia. Its cosmopolitan distribution is no doubt due to a combination of cultural and natural factors. As Brian Du Toit, following Darwin, puts it: 'plant distribution can be brought about by winds, currents, and similar natural forces. It can also follow animal activity and migration by becoming attached to their feet or hooves, or by being eaten by birds.' In the case of cannabis, much still remains to be discovered about both these natural forces and the cultural contacts that were equally important.

Cannabis is a dioecious plant (i.e. an individual cannabis plant is either male or female). Whilst both produce good quality fibre it is the females that are the best producers of the cannabinoids, the psychoactive compounds present in the plant, the most significant of which is delta-1-tetrahydrocannabinol, most commonly referred to in its abbreviated form, THC. Of the three cannabis species, *C. sativa* has a number of strains sought out by smokers, such as Acapulco Gold and Durban Poison. *C. indica* is said to be the most potent psychoactive species whilst *C. ruderalis* comes in a poor third.

It is not yet clear where cannabis was first cultivated. Perhaps the peoples of Central Asia did so themselves – we must not be led to too readily assume that it must have been the more 'advanced' Chinese who would necessarily have preceded their more 'backward' Central Asian neighbours of the great steppes in using and subsequently cultivating hemp as either a fibre plant or a

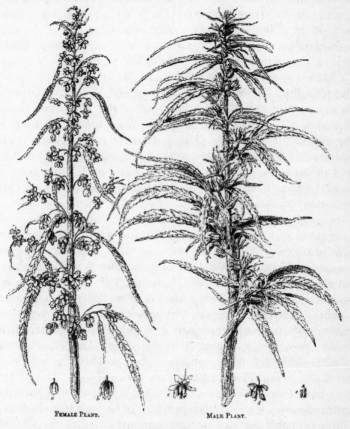

FEMALE PLANT.                    MALE PLANT.

### HEMP.

*Cannabis sativa.*

*a.* Unexpanded flower-bud.    *b.* Flower-bud beginning to expand.    *c.* and *d.* Expanded flower.
*e.* Female flower.

**CANNABIS**

drug. Central Asia, a vast land of deserts, steppes and oases is, despite its name, usually seen as of marginal historical influence, a kind of cultural vacuum between the great civilisations of China to the east, India to the south and the Middle East to its west. Yet, very early on, thriving trade routes passed through the region and these became known as the Silk Roads, on account of the importance of Chinese silk for both Muslim and Western merchants. It is known to archaeologists that Central Asia was an important centre for the transmission of new discoveries and religious ideas from prehistoric times onwards. The hemp plant, being of major technological importance as a fibre and being one of the most influential psychoactive plants in human culture, was most likely a key trade item from a very early date. The anthropologist Weston La Barre was of the opinion that cannabis use goes as far back as the Mesolithic (Middle Stone Age) period as part of a religio-shamanic complex. Certainly the use of the plant had already spread across an area stretching from Romania to China before the end of the Stone Age. There are three main cultural routes which cannabis took. Firstly east to China, secondly south to India and on to south-east Asia, and last, and certainly not least, to western Asia, from where it diffused to Africa, Europe and eventually the Americas.

It seems most likely that the cultivation of hemp may have originated in north-east Asia (north and north-east China and south-eastern Siberia). It is the only fibre plant of any great importance in the region and, as such, must have been eagerly sought out for its numerous technological uses. The earliest indirect evidence of hemp use is from decorated Chinese Neolithic pottery having cord impressions on it (see below for similar pottery from prehistoric Europe). Painted pottery from Honan province belonging to the Neolithic Yang-shao culture (C.4200–3200 BC) also indicates the probable presence of cultivated hemp. Pieces of what are thought to be hemp cloth have been found on the inside of a jar belonging to a Neolithic culture at a site in the western province of Gansu (2150–1780 BC). Other probable finds of hemp fragments dated to the Chinese Neolithic period have been discovered at a site in Chekiang province. The earliest uncontroversial find of fibre cloth is from the Western Chou era. The indications are that in early China hemp seeds were also a significant foodstuff. North-east Asia is still associated with shamanism today and it was surely important throughout North, Central and East Asia during prehistoric times. If the cannabis plant was practically important as a fibre plant to these early societies then it was probably equally important in their spiritual life. Direct and incontrovertible evidence for this comes from a later prehistoric period of southern Siberia (see below).

In Chinese hemp is known as *ta-ma,* meaning 'great fibre' (*ma* being 'fibre'). In the ancient Chinese script *ma* is supposed to represent fibres placed on a rack inside a roofed shelter. Yet this technological use for hemp does not appear to have been the only one, as Hui-Lin Li says:

> that the stupefying effect of the hemp plant was commonly known from extremely early times is also indicated linguistically. The character *ma* very early assumed two connotations. One meaning was, 'numerous or chaotic,' derived from the nature of the plant's fibers. The second connotation was one of numbness or senselessness, apparently derived from the properties of the fruits and leaves which were used as infusions for medicinal purposes ... as a character it [*ma*] combines with other characters to form such bisyllabic words as *ma-tsui,* narcotic (*ma* and 'drunkenness'); *ma-mu,* numb (*ma* and 'wood'); and *ma-p'i,* paralysis (*ma* and 'rheumatism').

The earliest of the Chinese pharmacopoeias, the *Pên Ching,* dating from the first century BC but containing much material undoubtedly of older date, makes it clear that the Chinese knew the psychoactive properties of cannabis: 'To take too much makes people see demons and throw themselves about like maniacs. But if one takes it over a long period of time one can communicate with the spirits and one's own body becomes light.' The Taoists used cannabis as a hallucinogen by adding it to other ingredients in incense burners (something also done by the Assyrians). In the sixth-century AD work *Wu Tsang Ching,* or 'Manual of the Five Viscera', there is the following instruction for magicians: 'If you wish to command demonic apparitions to present themselves you should constantly eat the inflorescences of the hemp plant.' It was also believed that using cannabis and ginseng together gave one visionary powers to see into the future.

Despite the numerous Chinese references to cannabis it has

never played a comparable role in Chinese social life to that it achieved in the Middle East and India. Hui-lin Li has suggested that the austere and somewhat puritanical system of ethics and social behaviour founded by Confucius put a stop to the widespread use of cannabis as a psychoactive substance. The often unpredictable effects of cannabis could easily result in a very un-Confucian way of behaving. Opium, says Li, with its narcotic effects, was far more socially acceptable. Whilst a superficially persuasive explanation for the marginal role of cannabis use in China, it fails to explain why alcohol – surely *the* most un-Confucian of all inebriants! – should have played such an important role in Chinese history. The real explanation may lie elsewhere. That cannabis may have been one of the main psychoactive substances used by the shamans of archaic China may have resulted in the decline of the habit along with the shamanism that gave its use its meaning. The other reason for its marginal place is that traditionally China has seen itself as the unmoving centre and the surrounding barbarians of its northern and western borders as a volatile threat. Cannabis, as the chosen drug of many of these neighbouring peoples, would have been an unsavoury choice for many Han Chinese, who didn't wish to indulge in 'barbarian habits'. This still holds true today. In Chinese Turkestan (Xinjiang) the local Muslim peoples, mainly Uighurs, are still associated with cannabis by the Han Chinese, According to Owen Lattimore, a great traveller and expert on Central Asia, in 1937–38, 42 per cent of exports from Chinese Turkestan to India down one of the old silk routes were in the form of cannabis resin. That cannabis may have been one of the main psychoactive substances used by the shamans of archaic China may have resulted in the decline of its use as the cult of shamanism gave way to religion organised on a larger scale. Hemp does not seem to have been used to any significant degree for its psychoactive properties by the Japanese people, although hemp strands were an important symbol in betrothal and marriage (as were hemp seeds in Europe, see below). The *gohei*, a sacred rod used by Shinto priests to banish impure spirits, has traditionally been made of hemp.

In contrast to the history of hemp in China, cannabis (*bhang*, *ganja*) has been widely used in India throughout its history and down to the present day. In the ancient text the *Artharvaveda*, cannabis is described as one of a number of herbs that 'release us from anxiety'. Various psychoactive preparations containing cannabis were sacred to the gods, particularly Shiva and Indra. One of Shiva's epithets was 'Lord of *Bhang*'. (For details of the sacred role in India of cannabis when smoked with the powerful hallucinogen *Datura*, see **Datura**) Cannabis has been widely used in the Tantric tradition as an aphrodisiac incorporated into cere-monial sexual practices. Cannabis seems to have been introduced into south-east Asia around the sixteenth century. Since almost all the common terms for the plant have their etymological root in the Sanskrit word *ganja* (in Laos hemp is *kan xa*, in Vietnam *can xa*, in Thailand *kancha* or *kanhcha*, and in Cambodia *kanhcha*), it is clear that it was under Indian influence that cannabis spread into the region.

The method of use of the plant for its psychoactive effects in south-east Asia has been in the form of 'grass', i.e. the leaves, flowering tops and stalks were smoked, usually with tobacco. In Cambodia the plant is sometimes boiled and some of the resulting liquid is sprinkled on tobacco and then it is smoked. The smoking of cannabis resin in the region seems to be due to recent foreign influence. Although Cambodians are reported to be light smokers of the plant, in Thailand the problems that sometimes occur with chronic habitual smoking are traditionally treated by native medicine men who employ a certain root to wean the inveterate smoker off the drug. At least until the current 'drug problem' (introduced and caused by Western foreigners) it was common-place in Thailand to employ cannabis for its analgesic and other medical uses. An infusion of the tops was given in small quantities (to avoid intoxication) at meal times to women who had just given birth. Similar practices are reported from Cambodia (although there the hemp is an ingredient in an alcoholic decoction). Fewer medical applications for cannabis are reported from Laos which, according to the researcher Marie Alexandrine Martin, is most likely due to the ready availability of opium derivatives which are used instead. For both their psychoactive effects and flavour, hemp leaves are popular in the local cuisines of the region, being variously used in soups, curries, fish fritters and other dishes.

Hemp moved westward out of its Central Asian home at a very early date. Evidence for its use in eastern Europe as a psychoactive substance can be traced to the later part of the third millennium BC. Two archaeological finds are of particular interest. The first was found in a pit-grave burial in Romania and is an artefact known as a 'pipe cup'. This particular pipe cup and another one, roughly contemporaneous, from a north Caucasian early Bronze Age site, both contained the charred remnants of cannabis seeds. This evidence, in conjunction with other finds across Europe (such as the great number of hemp seeds found in Neolithic contexts in central Europe) has been interpreted by the Oxford archaeologist Andrew Sherratt as foreshadowing the later ritual use of cannabis. There is further prehistoric evidence that cannabis was widely used as a psychoactive substance on the steppes. Russian archaeologists have discovered large-scale Iranian fire temples in the Kara Kum desert region of western Central Asia which contain the remains of cannabis, opium and *Ephedra* (see **Ephedra**, **Soma**) in ritual vessels. These ancient temples are dated to the first millennium BC.

In the fifth century BC the Greek historian Herodotus wrote of the use of cannabis by the Scythian people of the Black Sea region:

> On a framework of tree sticks, meeting at the top, they stretch pieces of woollen cloth. Inside this tent they put a dish with hot stones on it. Then they take some hemp seed, creep into the tent, and throw the seed on the hot stones. At once it begins to smoke, giving off a vapour unsurpassed by any vapour bath one could find in Greece. The Scythians enjoy it so much they howl with pleasure.

Amazingly, almost identical hemp-smoking equipment was found by the Russian archaeologist Rudenko at the Pazyryk site in southern Siberia at the other end of the vast steppes of Asia. Not only was the equipment the same but the dating of the site makes it contemporary with the report of Herodotus from the Black Sea area thousands of miles from Pazyryk. No clearer proof could be found to indicate that the ritual use of cannabis was widespread in prehistoric Asia and Europe.

Cannabis was also widely used in the ancient Near East. It was used by the Assyrians as a fumigation to relieve sorrow and grief, which is surely an indication of psychoactive use. Hemp was widely used in Ancient Egypt as a rope fibre. Remains of hemp have been discovered in the eighteenth-dynasty tomb of Akhenaten (Amenophis IV) at el-Amarna and cannabis pollen was found on the mummy of Rameses II (nineteenth dynasty). The suggestion that cannabis was *kaneh bosm* (one of the ingredients of the Holy

Oil which God instructed Moses to prepare; see Exodus 30:23) has been rejected by most authorities.

Its use among the Islamic mystical orders of Sufis and Dervishes has been equally controversial. Many contemporary Sufis have wanted to distance themselves from what has now become a disreputable substance to many governments. Nevertheless, bearing in mind the long tradition of cannabis use in Central Asian and Middle Eastern religious life, that the Sufis made no use of it is something difficult to believe. Sufis have been called 'the hippies of the Arab world' by Ernest Abel in an otherwise accurate book on cannabis, but this is a trite and unfounded comparison. Sufism has been a continuous mystical tradition for over a thousand years and is a spiritual path that has been followed by many of the greatest poets, thinkers and scientists of the Islamic world. The hippy movement (if indeed it is such) has been around for just over thirty years and the literary and philosophical output (let alone the scientific!) scarcely bears comparison. Certainly cannabis was, and still is, widely used for recreational purposes in Muslim countries and this was certainly the case in Arabic Egypt. The diffusion of the plant into sub-Saharan Africa seems to have been partly due to migrant communities of Muslims from the north and to Arab merchants trading along the east African coast. Although it seems difficult to believe cannabis was not, at least according to some experts, present in West Africa before the Second World War.

In a source cited by Brian Du Toit, the famous explorer David Livingstone describes the use of *matokwane* (cannabis) by the Makololo people:

we had ample opportunity for observing the effects of this matokwane smoking on our men. It makes them feel very strong in body, but it produces exactly the opposite effect upon the mind. Two of our finest young men became inveterate smokers, and partially idiotic. The performances of a group of matokwane smokers are somewhat grotesque; they are provided with a calabash of pure water, a split bamboo, five feet long, the great pipe, which has a large calabash of kudu's horn chamber to contain the water, through which the smoke is drawn Narghille fashion, on its way to the mouth. Each smoker takes a few whiffs, the last being an extra long one, and hands the pipe to his neighbour. He seems to swallow the fumes; for, striving against the convulsive action of the muscles of the chest and throat, he takes a mouthful of water from the calabash, waits a few seconds, and then pours water and smoke from his mouth down the groove of the bamboo. The smoke causes violent coughing in all, and in some a species of frenzy which passes away in a rapid stream of unmeaning words, or short sentences, as, 'the green grass grows', 'the fat cattle thrive', 'the fish swim'.

Potted histories of cannabis often imply that hemp's intoxicating properties were virtually unknown in Europe until the eighteenth and nineteenth centuries when travellers to Egypt and other parts of the East 'discovered the drug'. Such versions of events are built on the false premise that alcohol is and always has been the inebriant *par excellence* of European culture and that other substances like cannabis and opium are recent arrivals. The evidence for the use of hemp in prehistoric Europe has already been mentioned and there is no shortage of early historical references to its use throughout European history. Palaeobotanical studies have shown that hemp was cultivated (presumably as a fibre first and foremost) in eastern England by the Anglo-Saxons from AD 400 onwards. A cloth made of hemp was found in the late sixth-century tomb of the Merovingian queen Arnegunde in Paris. Its use among the Vikings is known from the discovery of plant remains at a castle in Denmark, fishing line and cloth made of hemp from Norwegian graves and cannabis seeds found in one of their ships.

Antoine Rabelais, who was the father of François Rabelais (*c.*1494–1553), the famous doctor and writer of the immortal *Gargantua and Pantagruel*, is known to have cultivated hemp on a large scale at his property at Cinais, south-west of Chinon in France. It was perhaps in helping out on his father's property that the young Rabelais first gained knowledge of cannabis. In the aforementioned work he dedicates three chapters to hemp, which he calls 'the herb Pantagruelion'. Under King Henry VIII of England a law was passed that instructed all subjects having arable land to put aside some of it for the cultivation of hemp or flax to provide sufficient fibre for the making of rigging for ships. In England, as elsewhere in Europe, hemp was indispensable as a fibre plant; its use permeated all spheres of life. William Bulleyn

(1500–76), who was related to Anne Boleyn, Henry's second wife, extolls it thus: 'no Shippe can sayle without hempe . . . no Plowe, or Carte, can be without ropes . . . the fisher and fouler muste have hempe, to make their nettes. And no archer can wante his bowe string: and the Malt man for his sackes, with it the belle is rong, to service in the Church.' The word canvas is derived from cannabis on account of its use as a fibre.

Cannabis was known by numerous names – neck weed, gallows grass (this because of its being the fibre from which the hangman's noose was made) and Welsh parsley among them. In certain parts of Britain (such as the Welsh border, Herefordshire and Oxfordshire) the seeds of the hemp plant were used in a very specific form of folk divination. In order to see a vision of her future husband a girl would have to retire alone at the witching hour to a churchyard, and whilst throwing the seeds over her left shoulder, enchant the following short rhyme:

Hempseed I sow, Hempseed, grow.
He that is to marry me,
Come after me and mow.

If she was lucky a spectral form of her husband-to-be mowing with his scythe would be there when she looked behind her. If she were not so fortunate she would see a coffin behind her, signifying that she would die whilst still young and unmarried. Such a use of hemp seed is known from the seventeenth century and certainly continued into the nineteenth and, perhaps, even the twentieth century. What is remarkable is the fact that very similar folk practices are also known from the Ukraine. Ukrainian girls with hemp seeds in their belts jump on a pile of hemp, crying out:

Andrei, Andrei,
I plant the hemp seed on you.
Will God let me know
With whom I will sleep?

Then they take off their blouses, fill their mouths with water to spit on the hemp seeds and run around their houses a magical three times. Dances involving hemp were also common in eastern Europe, sometimes in connection with magically aiding the hemp crop to grow and sometimes as part of marriage feasts and other wedding celebrations. Sula Benet sees another cultural role of hemp as having archaic roots:

> [a] custom connected with the dead in parts of eastern Europe is the throwing of a handful of seeds into the fire as an offering to the dead during the harvesting of hemp – similar to the custom of the Scythians and of the Pazyryk tribes, two-and-a-half-thousand years ago. There is no doubt that some of the practices, such as funeral customs, were introduced by the Scythians during their victorious advance into southeast Russia, including the Caucasus, where they remained for centuries ... hemp never lost its connection with the cult of the dead. Even today in Poland and Lithuania, and in former times also in Russia, on Christmas Eve when it is believed that the dead visit their families, a soup made of hemp seeds, called *semieniatka*, is served for the dead souls to savour.

As the use of hemp goes back far further into European prehistory than even the Scythian period (see above) such customs may have their ultimate origins even further back than Benet supposes.

Hemp also had a number of uses in early medicine, being used to treat gout, worms, tumours and inflammation. Nor were its psychoactive properties forgotten. Bulleyn warns that it can bring madness and it was a seventeenth-century belief that apothecaries and others that traded in cannabis often became epileptics, an effect attributed to the seeds. Although the seeds of cannabis are the last part of the plant that we would associate with psychoactive effects, this was a widespread idea in past centuries. William Turner (*c*.1508–*c*.1568) quotes an earlier author called Simeon Sethy (or Sethi) who wrote that: 'hemp sede if it be taken out of mesure taketh mens wittes from them.' Turner himself says it is the powder of the dried leaves that makes men 'drunk'. William Salmon, writing in 1693, says that cannabis seeds, leaves, juice, essence and decoctions were readily available in druggists' shops at the time, thus showing that cannabis was a widely used medicine.

Despite precursors such as Rabelais, sustained interest in cannabis among the literati may be said to have begun with *Le Club des Haschischins*. This informal club met in the privately owned baroque palace known in the 1840s as the Hôtel Pimodan at 17 quai d'Anjou on the Isle St Louis in Paris. Whilst many of its members were prominent in the artistic community (Honoré de Balzac, Alexandre Dumas, Théophile Gautier, Gérard de Nerval and Charles Baudelaire) its driving force – and supplier of the hashish in the form of a green paste (an echo of the witches' drugs which were greenish ointments; see **Witches' Ointments**) – was a psychiatrist named Jean-Jacques Moreau de Tours (1804–84). Moreau, who also experimented with the possible medical applications of *Datura stramonium* (see **Datura**), is often described as the first psychiatrist interested in the use of psychoactive substances as a means of treating mental illness. In fact, even though Anthony Störck was too early to be called a psychiatrist (he published the results of his work in 1762) he conducted systematic experiments – very much in the modern style – with henbane and thorn-apple specifically to ascertain their potential in treating mental disorders (see **Datura** and **Henbane**).

The first cultivation of hemp in the Americas seems to have been in Nova Scotia in 1606 and it subsequently became widely grown across North America for its use as a fibre. It seems, however, that there was no awareness of its psychoactive properties until the middle of the nineteenth century. In two books published in the 1850s the popular writer Bayard Taylor wrote of his hashish experiences in Egypt in a manner not unlike that of some members of the Parisian Hashish Club. Although rarely read today, his books were, for many of his numerous readers at the time, the first they had heard about the psychoactive effects of the hemp plant. The author of *The Hasheesh Eater: Being Passages from the Life of a Pythagorean* (1857), Fitz Hugh Ludlow, who is often considered to be one of the best writers on the subjective effects of hashish, never reached the contemporary audience that Taylor did, despite his posthumous fame.

It was not, of course, only writers that began to spread the word. Dubious figures in the unofficial world of medicine (better known as quackery) seized upon the 'new' drug and peddled it as an aphrodisiac. Ernest Abel has unearthed what must be one of the earliest and certainly one of the best lurid headlines concerning drugs. It is from the *Illustrated Police News* of 2 December 1876, and next to a drawing of elegant young women lounging in a swish apartment in a state of intoxication are written the immortal words: 'SECRET DISSIPATION OF NEW YORK BELLES: INTERIOR OF A HASHEESH HELL ON FIFTH AVENUE.'

It was not just the media but also the medical profession that were becoming increasingly aware of cannabis. Although doctors used it in treating many disorders (ranging from epilepsy and hysteria to alcoholism and asthma) the demonisation of drugs that began with opium was soon to spread to other psychoactive substances, including cannabis. As the anti-opium movement was intertwined with bigotry against the Chinese so with marijuana it was to be the turn of the Mexicans and then the Blacks. In 1915 California became the first state to make it illegal to possess cannabis. By the 1920s marijuana (called muggles or moota and later mezz, sassfras or tea; marijuana cigarettes or joints were known, as they still sometimes are, as reefers) had become a major 'underground drug'.

It was the first psychoactive substance (apart from alcohol) that became a common subject in modern popular music, with jazz classics from the 1930s such as Louis Armstrong's *Muggles* and Cab Calloway's *That Funny Reefer Man* topping the bill of marijuana-inspired fare. In opposition to the positive portrayal of cannabis in the jazz scene were wildly sensational accounts – supposedly based on fact – of the intimate connection of the drug with violence (drawing on the tradition of the Assassins, an Islamic sect who were supposed to take cannabis before committing murders) and sexual promiscuity. Finally, in 1937, through the considerable persuasive powers of Harry J. Anslinger, the first commissioner of the Federal Bureau of Narcotics, the Marihuana (Marijuana) Tax Act became federal law and in 1956 the drug was incorporated into the more comprehensive Narcotics Act.

Although the most well-known anti-marijuana film, *Reefer Madness*, was designed to shock young people with its vivid portrayal of the drug menace, it seems to have had little effect. Today it is something of a cult movie (mainly among cannabis smokers!) since its plot of moral and social decline is so utterly unconvincing and ludicrous. A less well-known film about hemp was made by the US Department of Agriculture and was entitled *Hemp for Victory* (1942). It was made as a propaganda film to encourage the growing of the plant for its fibre by American farmers during the Second World War as, due to the conflict, sufficient overseas supplies were unavailable. Due to the controversy surrounding the psychoactive use of cannabis the very existence of the film was later officially denied; having seen it myself I can attest to its existence.

*Grifos* was a name given to cannabis in the Caribbean and derives from the Spanish *grifos,* meaning 'crinkly', which some have seen as a description of the female plant's flower heads. The word found its way into America by its use among Puerto Ricans. In 1920s Harlem it became anglicised as 'reefers' but also continued to be known as 'griffs' or 'griff'. There are innumerable vernacular and slang names for cannabis. Among the most common are weed, blow, gear, grass, draw, smoke, shit and herb. Other terms have a more restricted use, as is the case with the name 'lamb's bread' used by Rastafarians, for whom it is a sacred psychoactive plant or entheogen. A number of medical uses for cannabis have made the whole debate about its legalisation a major issue. Cannabis is known to have real value not only in pain relief but also as a preventative medicine.

**Sources:** Abel 1980, Benet 1975, Bulleyn 1562, Coles 1657, Du Toit 1975, Emboden 1997, Godwin 1967, Herodotus 1880, La Barre 1980, Li 1974a, Li 1974b, Manniche 1989, Martin 1975, Merlin 1972, Moreau de Tours 1973, Needham SCC 5/2, 5/4, 5/9, 6/1, Opie and Tatem 1992, Radford and Radford 1980, Richardson 1988, Salmon 1693, Salmon 1710, Sarianidi 1994, Sherratt 1991, Sherratt 1996a, Stearn 1975, Thorndike 1923–1958, Turner 1568.

## CHOCOLATE

Chocolate is made from the beans of the cacao tree (*Theobroma cacao*) which is thought to be a native of the Amazon although it had already been transplanted to Mexico before the arrival of the Spanish. The name chocolate is derived from the Aztec word *chocolatl* meaning 'food of the gods'. The Aztec nobility indulged themselves by drinking it from gold vessels and its luxurious aura soon captured the attention of the conquistadors. Once known as the 'manna from Caracas', chocolate was imported to Europe along with its reputation as an aphrodisiac. William Coles (1626–62), an Oxford-educated herbalist, wrote affectionately of it as: 'of wonderful efficacy for the procreation of children; for it not only vehemently incites to *Venus,* but causeth Conception in Women.' The Jesuits were highly instrumental in the popularising of chocolate. Piero Camporesi describes them as its emissaries, eulogists, pioneers and importers. Despite, or perhaps because of, its link with the Society of Jesus, chocolate never caught on in the same way in other spheres of Catholic society. The Dominicans, as old rivals of the Jesuits, felt obliged to condemn the use of this exotic stimulant.

The erotic reputation that has surrounded chocolate since the time of the Aztecs continues unabated; one has only to watch chocolate commercials. Although it is a mild stimulant (containing caffeine and theobromine) and 'chocaholics' are not exactly hard-core drug addicts, chocolate is, at least in the Western world, the first drug that most individuals experience; the toddler's desire for more chocolate foreshadows the use of other, more potent, psychoactive substances later in life.

(See also **Caffeine**).

**Sources:** Camporesi 1994, Coles 1657, Emboden 1979.

# COCA

The coca plant (*Erythroxylum coca*) is a bush or shrub that grows to a typical height of about 1m. The chewing of its leaves is a traditional practice in a wide area from Central America and throughout the Andes and into the Amazon region. There are fourteen different alkaloids that are contained in the leaves of the coca plant, the most famous, of course, being cocaine (nicotine is also present in smaller quantities). The 'chewing' of the coca leaf is something of a misnomer but since the use of the term is so widespread, I have retained it. Whilst the leaves of the coca plant may be chewed when first put in the mouth (in order to make them form a quid), after that it is placed between the cheek and gums and not really chewed as such. Invariably an alkaline substance is added to the quid in order to facilitate the release of the psychoactive properties of the leaves. A wide variety of sources of these alkalis are known and they include a woody cactus, the bark of trees, shells and plant stalks. The alkaline mixture is carefully put in the quid so that it does not burn the inside of the mouth. What is remarkable is that the various stimulating plants that are chewed in various disparate parts of the world almost all contain alkaline additives. This is true of the traditional chewing of tobacco on the Pacific north-west coast of North America, the tobacco and *pituri* chewing in Aboriginal Australia, and the chewing of betel in India, south-east Asia and Melanesia (see **Tobacco**, **Pituri**, **Betel**).

According to archaic indigenous beliefs, coca 'chewing' is essentially harmless. This was given a modern scientific vindication by the Peruvian pharmacologist, Fernando Cabieses Molina, who wrote just after the end of the Second World War that traditional coca consumption has certain features that distinguish it markedly from cocaine abuse. The amount of the cocaine alkaloid is, of course, far lower than in chemically pure extracts from the plant. By introducing the coca leaf orally its psychoactive properties are absorbed slowly and without ill-effects by the digestive system. It is a stimulant and used to suppress hunger, to increase physical endurance and, in the Andes, to help cope with high altitudes. Distinguished visitors to Bolivia, including Pope John Paul II and Princess Anne have drunk coca tea (*mate de coca*) as it is the traditional way of avoiding altitude sickness. Impartial and scientific investigations have shown that regular use of coca is not harmful and no major social problems are known to have resulted from its traditional, and millennia-long, use in the Andes. This contradicts the claims of its ill-effects contained in reports by the United Nations and other official bodies, which seem to be based more on prejudice, ethnocentric bias, and the desire to portray the natural source of cocaine as negatively as possible in order to justify plans for eradicating coca in its homeland.

The ethnobotanist Richard Martin has eloquently highlighted the plight of the coca-using Indians when confronted by the irrational forces of Western civilisation:

confusion about the effects of crude coca leaves and those of cocaine has caused many people to regard the chewing of coca leaves as practised by the Indians of South America as merely an addictive vice, with the result that coca is now being suppressed even in the areas where the Indians have relied on its stimulating and medicinal properties for thousands of years, and where it has formed a significant part of their religious and cultural heritage . . . to deny the use of coca to the Indians is as serious a disregard for human rights as would be an attempt to outlaw beer in Germany, coffee in the near east or betel chewing in India. The recent attempts to suppress and control the use of coca can be interpreted only as the latest step in the white man's attempt to exterminate the Indian way of life and make him completely dependent on the alien society and economy which has gradually surrounded him.

There is archaeological evidence for the ancient use of coca. At a burial site in the Chilean Andes a frozen mummy of an Inca boy was discovered, accompanied by a number of articles including a feathered pouch containing coca leaves. Peruvian Mochican ceramics from around AD 500 are often decorated with motifs clearly indicating the use of coca. Many such vessels show people with their cheeks bulging in the place where the coca quid is held inside the mouth. To the Incas, coca was the entheogen *par excellence* and the places where it grew were considered to be holy places. In the heyday of their empire coca use was largely restricted to priests and nobles. Court orators also used it to stimulate their powers of memory whilst reciting incredibly long oral histories. The sacrifice of coca accompanied almost all of their rites and ceremonies. Coca leaves were placed on fires and the way that they burned was interpreted by diviners. Scrying (divination by the visual appearance of things) is a custom reported throughout the world and can be considered to be one of the foundations of magic. The Inca reading of the coca leaves is analogous to the reading of tea leaves so widely practised in Europe, although the latter practice is debased. When the Spanish invaders brought the Inca empire and its hierarchy to its knees, coca use was no longer restricted to the elite and it became widely used throughout Andean society. Its entheogenic status nevertheless remained intact and it is still venerated as such today. The Quechua Indians make offerings of it to Mother Earth and the dead are not only believed to rest better with a coca quid in their mouths but also to attain paradise by this means.

The Colombian anthropologist Gerardo Reichel-Dolmatoff dedicated most of his professional life to the study of the use of psychoactive substances in native South American cultures. In addition to his highly influential work on the use of *ayahuasca* in the Amazon, he also conducted fieldwork among the coca-using Kogi Indians of the Sierra Nevada de Santa Marta, Colombia, who were later to reach an international audience when a BBC film crew came to hear their dire warnings concerning the destruction of Mother Earth by the world powers, whom the Kogi condescendingly called 'younger brothers', on account of their own superior wisdom. Reichel-Dolmatoff gives the following account of the Kogi views concerning their chosen entheogen:

> Upon the effect of the coca, the Kogi emphasises in the first place that its consumption brings a certain mental clarity which one ought to take advantage of for ceremonial gatherings and any religious act in general, being conversations, personal rites, or group rites. Evidently the coca causes a euphoric state which lasts for a long period and is prolonged by the gradual consumption of larger and larger quantities. The individual turns into an animated speaker, and says that he feels an agreeable sensation of tingling over all the body and that his memory is considerably refreshed which permits him to speak, sing, and recite during the following hours. In the second place the Kogi say that coca appeases hunger. According to them, however, this never is the object of consuming coca but only an agreeable consequence, seeing that during the ceremonies or ceremonial conversations the consumption of food is prohibited and the assistants ought to fast. Another effect which is attributed to coca is insomnia. Here again the Kogi see an advantage since the ceremonial conversations should be carried on at night and individuals who can speak and sing for one or several nights without sleep, merit high prestige. The Kogi ideal would be to never eat anything beside coca, to abstain totally from sex, to never sleep, and to speak all of his life of the 'Ancients', that is to say, to sing, to dance and to recite.

According to tests carried out by Svetla Balabanova on ancient Egyptian mummies, some of them show traces of cocaine. Although her tests have been widely criticised (many critics suggesting contamination of the samples in question) others have seen this as strengthening the possibility of transatlantic links between Egyptian voyagers and the inhabitants of the New World, as no plants native to the Old World are known to contain cocaine.

In those Indian societies where coca has been regularly used its beneficial effects in various aspects of life are taken for granted as manifestly obvious. There are abundant accounts of the powerful stimulating effects of coca. So intimately is it connected with the indigenous lifestyle of the Indians of the Peruvian Sierra that long journeys are calculated in units called *cocada*. Each *cocada* represents the distance that can be covered whilst chewing a single quid of coca. Since the distance that can be traversed depends on the terrain the *cocada* is as much a unit of time as of space. One visitor to the Andes has recorded the powerful effects of coca on a sixty-two-year-old man he hired to undertake some very strenuous digging work. The labourer worked almost continually for five days and nights, averaging two hours of sleep per night. Throughout this period he ate no food but simply chewed a coca quid every three hours. As if this wasn't enough he then proceeded, having finished digging, to accompany his employer on a two-day-long journey, all the time keeping up on foot whilst his employer rode a mule!

Coca's reception in the modern urban-based world has been a mixed one. In Bolivia and Peru, where coca is legal, it is used in toothpaste, chewing gum, wine and, most widely in the form of a tea (*mate de coca*). The cultural story of coca was radically different from that of the crass glitzy beginnings and subsequently sordid short life of its extract cocaine. Increasing demand for cocaine in North America and Europe has caused an inevitable increase in supply from the Andes. Since 1989 the US has sought to take the War on Drugs to the source and attempt to cut down the cultivation of coca; this has failed because, as an anonymous writer for the Catholic Institute for International Relations put it:

> The Andean strategy has failed because the premises upon which it is based are flawed. Most critically it assumes that it is possible significantly to reduce cocaine supply from the Andes while demand in the US remains high. Indeed it relies on supply reduction as the chief method of reducing demand. The Bush administration hoped that by curtailing supply they could force up the price of cocaine on the streets, making it prohibitively expensive for users and thus forcing a drop in actual demand. In doing so the Bush administration overestimated its capacity to impede traffickers and underestimated the power of the first law of the free market: demand elicits supply.

The long and seemingly golden age of traditional coca use has been rudely interrupted by the prostituting of *mama coca* (as the plant is known to the Indians) to the rich hedonists of the West and the pimps of crack.

In 1992 the Bolivian President Jaime Paz Zamora began his campaign to have coca use (but not cocaine use) made legal throughout the world. Not only would this preserve the rights of Andean people to pursue their ancient traditions of coca use unimpeded by foreign powers but would provide a legitimate world market for products containing coca and thus divert at least some coca cultivation away from the production of cocaine. Unless there are radical changes in the West away from the cultural shadow-boxing of the War on Drugs then such practical and economically sound ideas will continue to fall on deaf ears.

**Sources:** Andrews and Solomon 1975, Anon 1993, Antonil 1978, Grinspoon and Bakalar 1985, Martin 1970, Mortimer 1974.

## COCAINE

In 1860 Albert Niemann of the University of Göttingen discovered the way to isolate a psychoactive alkaloid from the leaf of the coca plant and he named it cocaine. Carl Koller discovered its use as a local anaesthetic and from then on cocaine became an important medicinal drug. From the 1860s onwards the stimulating and pleasurable qualities of both coca and cocaine resulted in a number of diverse preparations being launched on the inter-national market. These included cocaine cigarettes, ointments, nasal sprays, and most popular of all, alcoholic drinks laced with coca and cocaine. The most famous of these was Vin Mariani, developed by the Corsican Angelo Mariani. Mariani was enrap-tured with coca and its lore. He wrote a book in its honour, tended it in his garden and avidly collected Inca artefacts and other paraphernalia relating to the plant. Vin Mariani was launched in 1863, and made by steeping selected coca leaves in wine. Despite many imitators Mariani's wine reigned supreme. In the British Library there are thirteen *de luxe* volumes of comments made by the rich and famous extolling the virtues of his drink. Vin Mariani was enthusiastically quaffed by a great many eminent individuals, including among royalty Queen Victoria, King Alphonse XIII of Spain, Albert I Prince of Monaco, George I King of Greece and the Shah of Persia. Leading religious figures also admired it very

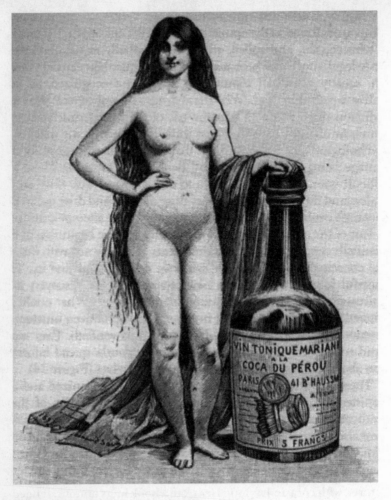

**ADVERTISEMENT FOR VIN MARIANI**

much, as their comments written in the various volumes of the book make abundantly clear. The Grand Rabbi of France Zadoc Kahn wrote: 'My conversion is complete. Praise be to Mariani's wine!' Pope Pius X was also an enthusiast and Leo XIII gave Mariani a gold medal in thanks. Cardinal Lavigerie wrote the somewhat perverse compliment: 'your coca from America gave my European priests the strength to civilise Asia and Africa.' Its stimulating properties made it a favourite of Louis Blériot, the first man to fly across the English Channel, who took a flask of Mariani wine with him on the flight. Dr Jean Charcot, who led the French Antarctic Expedition of 1903, expressed his plan to take a supply of it with him on the arduous journey. Vin Mariani had many advocates in the world of letters, Alexandre Dumas, Anatole France, Edmond Rostand, Jules Verne, H.G. Wells and Henrik Ibsen among them. There is even a communication from the secretary of William McKinley, the President of the United States, which reads:

Executive Mansion, June 14, 1898.

My dear Sir,

Please accept thanks on the President's behalf and on my own for your courtesy in sending a case of the celebrated Vin Mariani, with whose tonic virtues I am already acquainted, and will be happy to avail myself of in the future as occasion may require.

Very truly yours,

John Addison Porter,
Secretary to the President.

This missive displays a rather different attitude to coca than that of either Reagan or Bush! Even inventors such as Thomas Edison (the inventor of the gramophone) and the Lumière brothers (who invented the cinema) were regular drinkers of Vin Mariani. Both Vin Mariani and cocaine were used by opera singers to relieve sore throats, an occupational hazard.

Coca-Cola was originally developed by a pharmacist from Georgia named Styth Pemberton in 1886. The most famous carbonated soft drink in the world, Coca-Cola contained cocaine until 1906. Sigmund Freud, in his 1884 paper 'On Coca', eulogised the drug as a harmless panacea. The celebrated fictional detective, Sir Arthur Conan Doyle's Sherlock Holmes, was portrayed by his creator as resorting to injecting himself with cocaine when his mind was not working on a case. Legend has it that Robert Louis Stevenson wrote the famous story Dr Jekyll and Mr Hyde under the influence of cocaine. Stevenson is known to have written this 60,000-word book in six days and nights in

October 1885. This achievement is doubly impressive since after three days he destroyed the manuscript and started again from scratch! It has even been suggested that the story is an allusion to the cocaine abuse that by this time had begun to appear among members of the medical profession. Although it had been widely used in the treatment of alcoholism and opiate addiction (as suggested by Freud and other leading figures of the time) this effectively ceased when its own habit-forming properties became known. One of the early critics of the use of cocaine in this way was Louis Lewin, one of the founders of ethnopharmacology, whose book Phantastica: Narcotic and Stimulating Drugs is still a very useful work today. In his final publication on the drug in 1887 (Craving for and Fear of Cocaine) Freud retracted his support for the use of cocaine in treating opiate addiction but denied that cocaine itself was addictive. Freud himself used cocaine sporadically but does not seem to have had any problems with it; his chosen drug seems to have been nicotine administered in the form of cigars.

It is in the 1880s that the historian of cocaine, David Courtwright, sees the rise of the first cocaine 'epidemic' in the United States that continued until the 1920s. The press had, by the 1890s, begun to associate the drug with the fringes of society – with criminals, prostitutes, pimps, gamblers and racial minorities. The use of the word 'coke' as an abbreviation for cocaine goes back at least to the turn of the century. A well-known prostitute working in Fort Worth, Texas at this time was called 'Queen Coke Fiend'. Legal restrictions in the US around the turn of the century meant that doctors and druggists could no longer supply many of those who were reselling it. Not surprisingly, this led to an expansion of the black market which would ultimately lead to the development of the Colombian drug cartels. Cocaine's popularity waned in the 1930s, in part because of the readily available amphetamines which provided users with an alternative and similarly potent stimulant drug. Nevertheless there were still many users in Europe, particularly in Germany. Among the most notable consumers of the drug was Hermann Goering, who was also a morphine addict.

The revival of cocaine as a leading recreational drug took place in the 1970s. The image of cocaine at this time was one of glamour, sophistication and class. It was portrayed as a rich man's drug and was popular in media and modern musical circles. Songs such as J.J. Cale's 'Cocaine' (later covered by Eric Clapton) demonstrate the easy-going attitude towards the drug at this time. The solid silver cocaine-sniffing spoons of the era epitomise the acceptance of the drug in certain chic circles of society; they are a type of artefact akin to the snuff-boxes and paraphernalia of a more genteel time. Whilst cocaine was reborn with a silver spoon in its nose its image was soon to be shattered by the powerful media images of the crack baby. Cocaine prices dropped dramatically from 1980 onwards as the drug cartels successfully expanded their client base, bringing in many people who previously could not afford to use the 'champagne drug'.

The changing face of cocaine and its economic anatomy is epitomised in the career of the most famous of the South American drug barons – Pablo Escobar. Pablo Emilio Escobar Gaviria was born in 1949, his father was a peasant farmer and his mother a primary school teacher. He was raised in Medellín which was to become, in the words of Escobar's biographer Simon Strong, 'the epicentre of the world's cocaine industry'. As a teenager Pablo was already involved in petty crime, serving his apprenticeship in car theft and protection. Escobar was fond of marijuana and the occasional drink but apparently did not use the cocaine which was to make him his fortune. Despite his ascending the ranks of the criminal classes to the high status of kidnapper, smuggler and murderer, Escobar nevertheless managed to convince himself that he was a Robin Hood figure. More particularly he identified himself with the famous Mexican bandit Pancho Villa and collected rare paraphernalia and bibliographic items relating to his chosen exemplar.

Escobar began a business partnership with Carlos Lehder, the son of a beauty queen and a German immigrant, who hero-worshipped Hitler. Lehder was able to bring to the negotiating table an established network that led directly, among other places, into the heart of Hollywood. According to Escobar's brother-in-law, the partners in crime were fully aware not only of the economic power that could be gained through the cocaine industry but also its political potential. The political effects were to be diverting billions of dollars out of America and into the coffers of the cartel, the reduction of US influence on the internal affairs of Latin American states and the enfeebling of the American youth by their craving for cocaine. Escobar's personal fortune became vast, it is estimated that by 1983 he was worth $5 billion dollars. By this time he had already established business links with the Mafia and in deference to them he named his 3,000-hectare ranch *Nápoles*. Besides Pancho Villa artefacts, he also collected vintage cars made in the 1920s and 1930s with an unsurprising penchant for those models most closely identified with the infamous Chicago gangsters. In order to complete the effect he is said to have shot through a vintage Chevrolet with bullet holes and left it beside the driveway at *Nápoles*. Getting his livestock on the black market he set up a zoo, open to the public and boasting elephants, zebras and hippopotamuses.

In 1984 there was the first real crackdown by the Colombian authorities against the drug lords; Escobar was forced to flee the country and the Medellín cartel had to switch its headquarters to Panama. This new arrangement soon ran into problems when the US forced the Panamanian authorities to send the army in to destroy the cartel's illegal laboratory in the jungle close to the Colombian border. It was not only the Colombian, Panamanian and American authorities that were bearing down on Escobar's empire; relations with the rival Cali cartel had degenerated to the point of no return and Escobar's own home was bombed by them in 1987. Meanwhile the Colombian government were in pursuit but, apparently due to a tip off, Escobar narrowly escaped a pre-dawn raid which involved 1,000 soldiers backed up with tanks and helicopters. This was only the first of several embarrassing incidents for the authorities and Escobar escaped two similar attempts to catch him in 1989. Escobar fought back by paying hitmen $4,000 for every policeman killed in Medellín. The situation was now escalating on all fronts with the Cali cartel upping the stakes by offering a $1.5 million bounty for his head.

By 1992 Escobar was running out of options and turned himself in. He was placed in a special jail along with fourteen of his accomplices. Accounts of life in the jail suggest that it was hardly the punishment it was supposed to be – 64″ TVs adorned every room and jacuzzis were installed especially for the prisoners' comfort. This farcical state of affairs had its more sinister side and there were reports of Escobar and his entourage torturing *their* prisoners within the confines of this most open of prisons. The outrage against this lenient treatment of Escobar meant that his being moved to a top-security location was on the cards. He decided to escape, which, considering his criminal status, was achieved in a ludicrously simple fashion. He bribed a guard and went through a hole in the perimeter fence, taking his brother with him. This final humiliation for the Colombian authorities impelled them to track him down and finish the job. The financial stakes reached a new height with an official jackpot of nearly $7 million (much of it being put up by Interpol, the CIA, the FBI and the DEA) offered for his capture, closely followed by the 'black market' Cali bid of $5 million. The final act took place on 2 December 1993 when Escobar phoned his family from a hideaway, was tracked down by scanners and shot dead by order of the authorities.

Needless to say the death of Escobar did little to alter the cocaine trade; others eager for riches and power took his place. Although it was an operation somewhat overshadowed by cocaine production, during the 1980s the drug barons were investing heavily in the cultivation of the opium poppy in Colombia. Chemists who had been working in the heroin business on the Indian subcontinent were hired to oversee production. So successful was the operation that official sources estimate that by 1992 Colombia had replaced Mexico as the world's third largest producer of heroin. The profits that can be gained from heroin production far exceed those derived from cocaine.

The widespread use of freebase and crack also radically alter the image of cocaine. Freebasing seems to have begun in California in 1974. It is a process by which adulterated powder cocaine is converted into cocaine freebase. By heating cocaine hydrochloride in a water solution with ether and ammonia a pure crystalline form of cocaine can be made. This can then be smoked in a pipe and gives the user a stronger 'hit' than powder cocaine. In 1980 the comedian Richard Pryor had a near fatal accident, catching on fire in the process of making freebase. In practical terms most of the freebase (also called 'base' or 'rock') made in the 1970s was not made by any sophisticated means that produced a 'pure' product, it was made using baking soda and was crack in everything but name. The simple technique used in the preparation of crack consists of heating cocaine hydrochloride in a baking soda and water solution and smoking the resultant cocaine residue. Crack gets its name from the crackling sounds made by the 'rocks' (i.e. lumps of the drug) when they are smoked in a pipe. Thus, crack appeared much earlier than its discovery by the media would suggest. The word crack seems to have been first used in the media in the *New York Times* on 17 November 1985. In its post-glamour phase the image of cocaine has been projected as intimately connected with social deviance, the polar extremes being the tycoons of the cocaine trade on the one hand and the crack fiend of the streets on the other. The media has had a field day with stories relating to crack cocaine and despite the inaccuracies and scare-mongering in such tales there are, unfortunately, many stories from real life to show the human degradation and suffering that is caused by the drug.

In the tradition of earlier ethnographic reports of urban drug use (such as those on PCP; see **PCP**), a series of anthropological field studies was conducted on crack use and the subordination of women who sell themselves for crack. In these studies, which were undertaken in major American cities, including New York, Chicago, Los Angeles, Miami and San Francisco, a common theme emerged in which an underground economy exists in which (mainly) female habitual crack users prostituted themselves not for money in order to buy the drug but for the drug itself. In this way crack acts as a currency, a sinister but economically ideal product akin to William Burroughs' descriptions of heroin (see **Heroin**). Dr James Inciardi, Director of the Centre for Drug and Alcohol Studies at the University of Delaware, who has been studying crack use in Miami since 1986, describes an all too typical scene:

My first direct exposure to the sex-for-crack market came in 1988, during an initial visit to a North Miami crack house. I had gained entry through a local drug dealer, who had been a key informant of mine for almost a decade. He introduced me to the crack house door man as someone 'straight but OK'. After the door man checked us for weapons, my guide proceeded to show me around. Upon entering a room in the rear of the crack house (what I later learned was called a freak room), I observed what appeared to be the gang-rape of an unconscious child. Emaciated, seemingly comatose, and likely no older than fourteen years of age, she was lying spread-eagled on a filthy mattress while four men in succession had vaginal intercourse with her. After they had finished and left the room, however, it became readily clear that it had not been forcible rape at all. She opened her eyes and looked about to see if anyone was waiting. When she realised that our purpose there was not for sex, she wiped her groin with a ragged beach towel, covered herself with half of a tattered sheet affecting a somewhat peculiar sense of modesty, and rolled over in an attempt to sleep . . . upon leaving the crack house a few minutes later, the dealer/informant explained that she was a house girl, a person in the employ of the crack house owner. He gave her food, a place to sleep, and all the crack she wanted in return for her providing sex – any type and amount of sex – to his crack house customers.

Many similar horror stories from crack culture are told by the other ethnographers involved in the study. Crack use affects those of all ages, even foetuses in the womb. Foetuses, newly born babies and children can be directly affected by powder cocaine or crack (putting aside all the family problems that will arise in a cocaine-using household) if the mother has used either during pregnancy or if the father has in the week before conception. The extent of the problem in the United States is difficult to assess. Government figures from 1989 state that some 375,000 children were affected as a result of alcohol or other drug use by their mothers during pregnancy. This figure may be far too low; some estimates suggest that 400,000 babies per year are born affected by cocaine abuse. Among the catalogue of problems that occur as a consequence of cocaine and crack use are damage to neurotransmitters which effects the workings of their nervous system, strokes, brain damage, genital deformities, cerebral palsy, addiction withdrawal symptoms and a number of disorders which interfere with the process of bonding such as 'gaze aversion' (when the baby avoids eye contact) and 'touch aversion'. A whole new series of problems may confront the crack-affected child as he or she grows – hyper-activity, incontinence, eating and sleeping disorders, learning problems and alienation.

With such a horrific social scenario it is hardly surprising that many people approve of the War on Drugs and believe that it can achieve its goal of reducing drug-related harm. But, whether or not one approves of the War on Drugs, it does not appear to be working and there is a growing movement that seeks to seriously explore other options, including the legalisation of hard drugs. The rationale behind this is basically to distinguish between the medical and social problems caused by the drug itself and the problems resulting from its illegal status. Criminal activity may be divided into two types – the drug trade itself and criminal acts committed by users seeking to sustain their habits. Obviously the two are not entirely distinct, but those who call for the legalisation of the hard drugs argue that the extreme violence associated with the black market trade in these substances would be eliminated if the drugs were available legally, and if they were legal and affordable there would be no need for habitual users to resort to theft and prostitution to guarantee a continual supply of the drug. Since the illegality of various drugs dissuades their users from seeking medical or social help to deal with their problems (fearing arrest) the rise in addiction and habituation continues unabated. Another point often stressed by those who wish to see an end to the War on Drugs is that the police and other law enforcement agencies would save a great deal of time and money and could therefore pursue other aspects of their work more effectively. Furthermore it is argued that taxes derived from the sale of such drugs could provide funds to deal with the enormous health problems arising from their use. Finally it is argued that legalisation would result in quality control of the drugs in question and eliminate dangerous adulterants that are so common in street drugs. Clearly there are objections to such plans for a 'cease fire'. The counter-arguments to this suggest that to legalise is to condone or even encourage (clearly if such drugs were legally manufactured and marketed by pharmaceutical companies there would be advertising, even if it were of the restricted kind, as in the case of tobacco products). Such a drastic change in legislation could result in an explosion of drug abuse on a scale hitherto unknown and at present contained only by legal sanctions. There is, of course, no simple answer but present policies do not seem to be working, no victory against the 'evil' of drugs seems imminent.

The American academic David Lenson has made a strong case for a radical review of current drug policy in the United States. He argues that the War on Drugs with its battle cries 'Just Say No' and 'Zero Tolerance' put all presently illegal substances into a single group without differentiating them in regard to their potency, addictive or non-addictive properties or psychoactive effects. He sees the War on Drugs having come into its own in the 1980s as a monolithic enemy needed to replace a waning Communism. The strategies and tactics that were used in the anti-Communist propaganda of the Cold War period were recycled in order to vilify the new enemy that was 'infecting' the body politic. As Lenson puts it the new: 'scapegoat could . . . be totally Other (Colombian, Peruvian, Panamanian, Bolivian) and at the same time as close as one's own bloodstream' and 'as close and distant as Bolshevism, with a needle and pipe instead of a hammer and sickle'. With a large percentage of the American population using illicit substances, Lenson also questions the wisdom of criminalising citizens purely on the basis of their use of drugs. He sees important civil liberties threatened in an uncomfortably intimate way: 'What crosses the blood-brain barrier is now open to the same surveillance as what crosses international borders. There is a customs in the cranium, a Checkpoint Consciousness.'

Recent research conducted by the Scottish Cocaine Research Group has shown how inaccurate a picture of the typical cocaine user is painted when the polar images of the cocaine yuppie and the crack ghetto child are taken as the starting point. The Group make the very obvious, but highly important, point that the users of cocaine (and, by implication, other illicit drugs) who are usually made the subjects of the social studies that generate meaningful statistics are, almost invariably, made up of individuals who have either been caught by the police or sought out medical assistance. But what about all the other users who do not appear in these statistics, the invisible majority? That is whom the Group sought out through confidential interviews. At least as far as Scotland goes they found these users were not: 'particularly young, particularly delinquent, particularly poor or deprived, nor particularly wealthy.' In fact, the typical cocaine-using Scottish man is in his mid-twenties, has a university degree and a job at which he earns £10,000–£15,000 a year. He takes cocaine occasionally as one of a number of drugs of choice that he uses. He takes it because it makes him relaxed and self-assured but complains that it is expensive and causes insomnia. Despite these rather minor reservations about the drug, he doesn't worry about getting hooked to cocaine.

The research team that undertook this survey of cocaine users felt that the 'psycho-pharmacological witch-hunting' of present drugs policies are rather inappropriate, particularly as so many of those users interviewed were clearly rather 'normal' citizens. The message of this study is that the silent majority of users of illicit substances are integrated in mainstream society and cannot be pigeonholed simply as medical patients or anti-social criminals.

(See also: **Coca**.)

**Sources:** Andrews and Solomon 1975, Courtwright 1995, Ditton and Hammersley 1996, Grinspoon and Bakalar 1985, Lenson 1995, Lewin 1964, Mortimer 1974, Ratner 1993, Strong 1995, Waller 1993.

## COFFEE

*Coffea arabica* is the tree that yields the coffee bean that has become probably the most widely used stimulant in the world, along with its caffeine-bearing rival the tea plant. It is thought that *C. arabica* originated in the Ethiopian Highlands and from there it was taken to Arabia around the time of Muhammad. Long before its use caught on in Christian societies it was the stimulating social and intellectual fuel of the Muslim world. In the seventeenth century news of the novel beverage hit Western Europe. It was introduced into England in 1601 and soon gained a following among the intelligentsia. By the 1630s it was drunk at Balliol College, Oxford and in 1650 Oxford boasted its first coffee house, The Angel. A café on the same site still serves coffee today.

The spread of coffee drinking during the Enlightenment was partly due to the fact that it fitted so well with the prevailing notions of the era, as Wolfgang Schivelbusch put it: 'Coffee functioned as a historically significant drug . . . it spread through the body and achieved chemically and pharmacologically what rationalism and the Protestant ethic sought to fulfil spiritually and ideologically. With coffee the principle of rationality entered human physiology.' This view is vindicated by the fact that a number of key intellectual figures of the time, such as Kant, Voltaire and Rousseau, were enthusiastic coffee drinkers.

The reading of tea-leaves is still widely practised but a similar kind of divination involving coffee grounds seems to have fallen by the wayside. In an Irish newspaper dated 4 June 1726 there is an advertisement which reads: 'Advice is hereby given, That there is lately arrived in this City, the Famous Mrs Cherry, the only Gentlewoman truly Learned in that Occult Science of Tossing of Coffee Grounds; who has . . . for some time past, practised, to the

General Satisfaction of her Female Visitants ... Her Hours are after prayers are done at St. Peter's Church, till Dinner.' It may be that coffee and tea divination may be a continuation of earlier European practices of 'reading' the leaves of herbal beverages that would have been drunk before coffee or tea were available.

(See also **Caffeine.**)

**Sources:** Braun 1996, Camporesi 1994, Opie and Tatem 1992, Sherratt 1987, Tyler 1995.

# CRACK see Cocaine

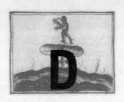

## DATURA

The traditional use of species of *Datura* is known from various parts of North and South America, Africa, Europe and Asia, making it one of the most widely dispersed hallucinogenic plants of all. There are approximately fifteen to twenty species, the most well-known of which is *Datura stramonium*. This species is an annual plant which usually grows between 1 and 3 feet tall. It has coarse leaves and the entire plant gives off an evil odour. The flowers are white or purplish and its capsular fruit is typically covered with spines. The various species have often been given different names, which can create a certain amount of confusion. The *Datura* plant is an extremely tenacious weed and an experiment with forty-year-old seeds gave the result that 90 per cent of them germinated. Although the 'tree *Daturas*' (*Brugmansia* spp.) were once classed by botanists as belonging to the *Datura*, they are now universally accepted as being a distinct genus (see **Brugmansia**).

The tropane alkaloids typically found in other psychoactive plants of the Solanaceae family – atropine, hyoscyamine and scopolamine – are also present in the various species of *Datura*. The highest concentration of the alkaloids is in the roots. There are many accounts of the extremely powerful and often dangerous effects produced by these plants. A high dose can result in a state of intoxication that can last for days; there are even reports of its effects continuing for up to twenty days! As with belladonna (see **Belladonna**), *Datura* species can be dangerous, particularly to children; many such poisonings have occurred in South Africa.

The generic name *Datura* is from the Indian word *dhatura* or *dhattura*. In India *Dhat* is the name of a poison prepared from the

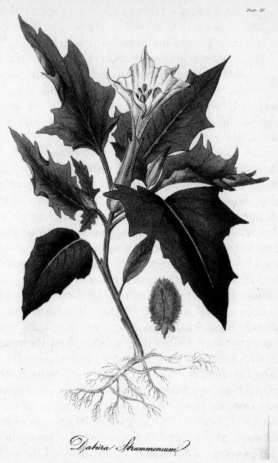

**DATURA**     *Datura Strammonium*

plant and *Dhatureas* the name of a criminal gang who used the poison to stupefy their victims. However, according to Charles Heiser, a botanist specialising in solanaceous plants, Linnaeus, who accepted the name, wanted to find a Latin root for it, however tortuous, and so decided on *dare* ('to give'), the reason being that the plant is given to those whose sexual powers are weak. *Dutroa* was a seventeenth-century variant of the word *Datura*. Other names for the plant include thorn-apple (because of its spiky fruit), sorcerers' herb, Jimson weed (a contraction of Jamestown; see below for the story of how this name came about), stinkweed (on account of its unpleasant smell), stramonium,

Devil's apple, and angel's trumpet (referring to the shape of its flowers). Other early names mention the New World, such as apple of Peru and *Hyoscyamus Peruvianus,* which means 'henbane of Peru'. This latter name shows how herbalists and early botanists sought to classify the new plant in terms of those they already knew. Henbane has similar medical and psychoactive properties to *Datura* (see **Henbane**) and tobacco when it became first known in Europe was also seen as a kind of henbane and was called 'yellow henbane' (see **Tobacco**).

The plant was also known to the Greeks and Romans. Dioscorides records the widespread knowledge of this plant and its psychoactive properties nearly two thousand years ago. The root being drunk in a dragm (from which comes our unit of measurement the dram) of wine causes 'not unpleasant phantasies'. Larger amounts induce temporary insanity or even death. *Datura* was known by a number of names at this time, including Anydron, Thryon and Persion. Robert Beverley suggested that it was *Datura* that Mark Antony's army met on their way back from the Parthian War. Having run out of food they accidentally consumed a plant of which it was said that: 'whoever ate of it forgot all that he had hitherto done and recognised nothing.' If this plant was indeed *Datura* then this incident foreshadows the Jamestown incident detailed below.

In India the *Datura* plant has, since time immemorial, been considered a holy psychoactive plant or entheogen. According to the *Vamana Purana, Datura metel* sprang forth from the chest of the great god Shiva. One of the many secondary names of this god is *unmatta,* 'the crazy one', and *Datura* is called *unmata,* 'divine madness'. The followers of Shiva smoke cannabis and *Datura* together for reasons explained by Claudia Müller-Ebeling and Christian Rätsch:

> both plants are sacred to Shiva ... the smoking mixture of *ganja* [cannabis] and dhatura corresponds to one of the cosmological principles of the god, namely his androgyny. *Ganja* is the female aspect and dhatura the male; the mixture of the two is the perfect primordial unity and cosmic creative energy of Shiva, the androgynous ... the smoking blend must be ignited with two small pieces of wood. These represent his feminine and his masculine aspects and, when transformed by Shiva's aspect as the god of fire, awaken the

aphrodisiac creative power and activate the kundalini snake (*Lakshama*) which is rolled up and resting in the pelvis. When the kundalini has been unleashed, it snakes along the spinal cord through the seven chakras, the non-material energy centres, and causes them to blossom like the flowers of the lotus. The universal consciousness of the unity of the cosmos pervades the being. In this way, the plant of the god becomes the sacred aphrodisiac of man.

It has also been reported that enraged Indonesian women have taken revenge on unfaithful lovers by feeding beetles with *Datura* leaves and using the insects' toxic excrement to poison them. In the Philippines *Datura* is smoked to relieve the symptoms of asthma. In present-day Nepal the smoke given off by frying *D. stramonium* seeds in oil is inhaled to alleviate toothache. To my knowledge there is only one report of the use of a *Datura* in traditional Australia. Two Aboriginal boys got accidentally 'drunk' when they unknowingly ingested *D. leichhardtii*.

Leaves of *D. inoxia* have been used as a psychoactive drug in East Africa. In Tanzania *Datura* is added to beer to give it a real kick; a similar use of plants containing the tropane alkaloids is known from native America and Europe. There are also reports that *Datura* has been used in Tanzania to drug victims who are then robbed. Wade Davis' study of the zombi lore of Haiti led him to suggest that *Datura stramonium* was given to the zombified victim as a kind of antidote to the drug that had first made him or her a zombi (see **Zombi Drug**).

The archaeological evidence for the prehistoric use of *Datura* in the Americas is rather indirect but is, nevertheless, persuasive, particularly in the light of the rich ethnographic record of *Datura* use as an adjunct to Amerindian shamanistic practices. Excavations of rock shelters in the Lower Pecos River region that spans the border between Texas and Mexico have shown that they have been occupied by humans on and off for thousands of years and right into the historical period. In addition to large quantities of botanical remains, an impressive body of rock art has also been discovered. Researchers divide the art into four distinct and consecutive stylistic periods, the earliest of which is called the Pecos River style; the various examples of which are between 4,200 and 2,950 years old. Over half the depictions of human-like figures (identified as shamans) portray them in conjunction with a motif which has been convincingly identified as the fruit of the *Datura* plant. Whilst finds of *Datura* seeds in these rock shelters have been rather sparse elsewhere, at a site in New Mexico about 900 seeds were found on a floor on which ceremonial equipment was also discovered. In addition to these archaic rock paintings and botanical remains there is a later but equally persuasive body of archaeological evidence to indicate that *Datura* was as important in the remote past as it has been in more recent times. There are a number of kinds of prehistoric pottery vessels that have been found in the south-western part of the USA, Mexico, Guatemala and El Salvador that have forms that have long puzzled archaeologists. These ceramic artefacts are usually called 'spiked' or 'hobnailed' on account of their spiky surfaces. No satisfactory explanation for this curious type of decoration was put forward until William Litzinger from the University of Colorado identified them as representations of the spiny fruit of species of *Datura*. Many kinds of prehistoric and ancient pottery have skeuomorphic designs. That is to say that their shape and decoration imitate natural objects or artefacts made of other materials. Whilst many pots were made in imitation of baskets and leather or metal vessels and containers, some also represented plants. Although Litzinger seems to be unaware of the fact, another researcher had shown some years earlier that pottery found in ancient Egypt mimicked the shape of another psychoactive plant, in this case the opium poppy. The

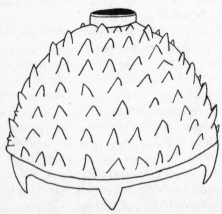

**PREHISTORIC INCENSE BURNER FROM NORTH AMERICA IN SHAPE OF DATURA FRUIT**

spiked ceramic forms that Litzinger has identified as *Datura* skeuomorphs include lidded jars, bowls, small containers and incense burners. Most of these artefacts date from the period AD 850–1200.

*Datura* use in historical times has been recorded from a number of native North American societies, including the Navajo, Zuñi, Tewa, Costanoan, Yokut and Hopi. Among the Costanoan Indians of California the leaves of *Datura meteloides* were dried and then smoked. The ensuing hallucinations were believed to reveal one's future. They also smoked a mixture of *Datura* seeds and tobacco for its aphrodisiac effects. The Navajo, whilst revering the plant and its prepared forms with the epithets 'Great Flower of the Sun 'and 'Decoction of the Beautiful Path', were also fully aware of its potential for abuse and also named it 'Imbecile-Producer'. Matilda Stevenson, an anthropologist with an intimate knowledge of the culture of the Zuñi Indians of New Mexico, wrote an account of how the powerful anaesthetic properties of *Datura* were made use of in native medicine at the beginning of the century:

> The late Nai'uchi, the most renowned medicine man of his time among the Zuñi, gave this medicine before operating on a woman's breast. As soon as the patient became unconscious, he cut deep into the breast with an agate lance, and, inserting his finger, removed all the pus; an antiseptic was then sprinkled over the wound, which was bandaged with a soiled cloth . . . when the woman regained consciousness she declared that she had had a peaceful sleep and beautiful dreams. There was no evidence of any ill effect from the use of the drug.

Stevenson also reports that the Zuñi use the plant for 'seership'. Bye, an ethnobotanist who was collecting plants in Mexico, was warned by the local Tarahumara people not to pick *Daturas* as this was only to be done by people of authority. Unsuprisingly, he ignored his hosts' advice in the name of science and went ahead and picked them. The locals were very angry as he had failed to treat the plants with the reverence they expected and he was accused of mistreating the *Datura*. For days afterwards they refused to talk to him.

One of the main centres for the religious use of *Datura* was native California. *Datura inoxia* (often called *D. meteloides* in the literature) was widely used in the region and the Luiseños Indians made use of its powerful effects in initiation ceremonies. According to one account of such a usage:

The plant itself is called by the Luiseños *Naktamush*, or *Naktomush*; the ceremony is known as the *mani* or *manish-mani*. When it grows dark the masters of the ceremony, called *paha*, go from house to house to collect the candidates for initiation, sometimes carrying in their arms little boys who have already fallen to sleep to the place of assembly. The strictest silence is observed, and it is necessary that the *paha* be a shaman, or wizard skilled in magic. A large *tamyush*, or stone bowl, is placed before the chief, who, sitting in the darkness, pounds with a stone *mano*, or pestle, the dry scraped root of the plant, to the accompaniment of a weird chant, while the boys stand waiting. The powdered root is then passed through a basket-sieve back into the stone bowl and water is poured on it. The boys are enjoined to keep silence. As each boy kneels in turn before the big bowl to drink the infusion, his head is supported by the hand of the master of ceremonies, who raises it when enough has been taken. It is a solemn occasion, a spiritual rebirth, suggesting the rites of baptism or confirmation. During the entire ceremony both the men and the boys are quite nude. When the drink has been administered to all the candidates, dances are performed in the darkness, accompanied by cries in imitation of birds and beasts; and when these are finished the candidates are marched around a fire, chanting a ceremonial song. As the effects of the narcotic plant overcome them, one by one they fall to the ground and are carried to another place and left until they regain consciousness. After this the dancing is resumed and kept up through the entire night. At daylight they return to the place where the drink was administered, and after a day of fasting they witness feats of magic performed by the shamans, from whom, after having been dressed in feathers and painted, they receive wonder-working sticks. The boys are also instructed by their elders in certain mysteries and rules of conduct, somewhat corresponding to one's duties towards God and to one's neighbour, as taught in the catechism. The initiatory ceremony is followed by two or three weeks of abstinence from salt and meat, after which a ceremony with a rope, called *wanawut*, is performed. When this is finished the candidates are free.

The Algonquin Indians of Virginia seem to have used another species (*D. stramonium*) in their male initiation rites and an early report concerning such ceremonies suggests that the effects of the *Datura* lasted from eighteen to twenty days as the initiates were intermittently given more of the infusion to drink. As William Emboden has suggested, the administering of *Datura* by way of an enema is the most likely means of extending its psychoactive effects over such an extended period.

Although it has often been suggested that *Datura* was a novel import to Europe brought in from the New World, the discovery of it in an Early Bronze Age context in western Hungary shows that the use of *Datura* species is of great antiquity in the Old World. It has been suggested by Sherratt that 'grape-cups', a type of Early Bronze Age pottery found in Britain, may be an Old World equivalent of the New World pottery identified by Litzinger as vessels imitating the fruit of *Datura* (see above).

According to the account of Robert Beverley, writing at the turn of the eighteenth century, unsuspecting soldiers sent to Jamestown to crush the uprising known as Bacon's Rebellion (1676) ate *Datura*, whence the name Jimson weed sometimes given to the plant. His account is worth quoting in full:

The JamesTown weed (which resembles the Thorny Apple of Peru, and I take to be the plant so call'd) ... was gathered very young for a boiled salad, by some of the Soldiers ... and some of them eat plentifully of it, the Effect of which was a very pleasant Comedy; for they turn'd natural Fools upon it for several Days: One would blow up a Feather in the Air; another would dart Straws at it with much Fury; and another stark naked was sitting up in a Corner, like a Monkey, grinning and making Mows at them; a Fourth would fondly kiss, and paw his Companions, and snear in their Faces, with a Countenance more antick, than any in a Dutch droll. In this frantick Condition they were confined, lest they should in their folly destroy themselves; though it was observed, that

all their Actions were full of Innocence and good Nature.
Indeed, they were not very cleanly, for they would have
wallow'd in their own Excrements, if they had not been
prevented. A Thousand such simple tricks they play'd, and
after Eleven Days, return'd to themselves again, not remem-
bering anything that had pass'd.

*Datura stramonium* was first introduced to England by the herbalist
John Gerard with seeds from Constantinople given to him by Lord
Edward Zouch. *Datura stramonium* is known to have been used in
European witchcraft (see **Witches' Ointments**) and its reputation
prompted one nineteenth-century historian to falsely attribute
the entire witch mania to the introduction of this plant into
Europe. This is clearly wrong as not only do the witches' hallucinogenic preparations precede the re-introduction of *Datura*, but
also there are a number of recipes for these ointments that
include other psychoactive plants that were far more commonly
used, particularly belladonna (deadly nightshade), henbane and
mandrake, all of which, however, are closely related to *Datura* and
have similar effects when taken. Gypsies are purported to have
drugged their victims with *Datura* during the Middle Ages,
although there is no clear evidence for this and it may be just a
typically anti-Romany story.

The modern era of the study of the psychological effects caused
by *Datura* may be said to start with the work of Anthony Störck. In
1760 Störck heard that even to smell the thorn-apple could cause
intoxication. Despite the fact that he was a very sober individual
(he states in the introductory passages to his book that 'loss of
judgement appears a more grevious calamity to me than death
itself'), he decided to see for himself. Having smelled the plant
and suffered no ill effect he proceeded to express its juice in a
marble mortar and this too had no effect. Finally he evaporated
the juice to the consistency of an extract by heating it in an
earthenware vessel over a low heat, stirring it regularly to prevent
it burning. The extract was then allowed to cool and the resulting
product was then given to mentally disturbed patients. He
concluded from these experiments that thorn-apple was
successful in treating temporary mental disorders, convulsions
and fits. During both the World Wars the United States was unable
to import sufficient quantities of belladonna (the main source of
the alkaloid atropine) and thus initiated the widespread

cultivation of *Datura* as an alternative source of this important medicinal drug.

**Sources:** Beverley 1705, Bocek 1984, Boyd and Dering 1996, Bye 1979, Camporesi 1989, Davis 1983, Ellis 1946, Gerard 1597, Gunther 1959, Heiser 1969, Litzinger 1981, Manandhar 1995, Mehra 1979, Peterson 1979, Rätsch 1992, Richardson 1988, Safford 1922, Schenk 1956, Sherratt 1996a, Stevenson 1915, Störck 1763, Thorwald 1962, Watt and Breyer-Brandwijk 1962, Withington 1917.

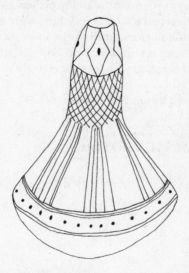

**PRE-COLUMBIAN SPINDLE WHORL IN FORM OF DATURA FLOWER, QUIMBAYA CULTURE, COLOMBIA**

## DEADLY NIGHTSHADE see Belladonna

## DIGITALIS

The drug digitalis is derived from the common purple foxglove *Digitalis purpurea*. The medicinal use of this plant is very old, it is mentioned in the Anglo-Saxon herbals and in preparations used by the Welsh 'Physicians of Myddrai', an ancient lineage of physicians who can be traced back to the eleventh century and who continued their herbal traditions into the nineteenth century. According to folk beliefs in Scotland the foxglove is considered an inauspicious plant. The foxglove has a number of names in folk botany such as Witches' Thimble, Fairy Weed, Dead Man's Bellows and Bloody Man's Fingers.

It has long been used for the treatment of a number of heart complaints and even before Dr Withering pioneered its use in modern medicine it was taken in the form of a herbal tea to treat dropsy. Digitalis was at the centre of a large-scale insurance scam that hit America in the 1930s depression years. Individuals in collusion with their lawyers and crooked doctors were given digitalis to interfere with their natural heartbeat in order to create the illusion of a heart attack. This was done with sufficient skill to dupe the examining doctors hired by the insurance companies. It is estimated that several hundred thousand dollars was paid out – a huge amount at this time – before the whistle was blown.

**Sources:** Radford and Radford 1980, Williams 1947.

## DUBOISIA HOPWOODII see **Pituri**

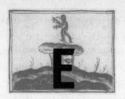

## EBOGA

The West African shrub (*Tabernanthe iboga*) from which the hallucinogen *eboga* (sometimes spelt *eboka* or *iboga*) is prepared is found both in the wild and around native villages. The root (particularly the root bark) is most widely used for its aphrodisiac qualities but in small doses it acts as a stimulant by increasing endurance and muscular strength. Its use as a hallucinogen is restricted to ritual use, as in the case of the West African Bwiti cult, for whom it is an entheogen, or sacred psychoactive plant. The formation of this cult by the Fang people of Gabon was one of many revitalisation movements that arose in reaction to the encroachment of foreign, particularly European, values. The activities of the cult take place at night and are dedicated to *Nyingwan Mebege*, the feminine principle of the universe. The cult fuses traditional and Christian (especially Catholic) symbolism and its ceremonies are conducted in chapels where its members hope to achieve *nlem mvore*, the state of 'oneheartedness'. The cult is committed to giving its followers an experience of the beyond in order for them to come to terms personally with death. It also seeks to re-establish contact with the ancestors, something which had become severely disrupted under the forceful influence of missionary evangelism. *Eboga* use is considered central to fulfilling both these needs. Cult members are called *ndzi eboga*, or '*eboga* eater'.

The consumption of large doses of *eboga* can be dangerous, even fatal. In a period of forty years about a dozen cases of manslaughter or murder were brought against leaders of the Bwiti cult after initiates who had used the plant died. Initiates are made aware of these dangers and, except in the very clearly defined and delineated context of the initiation itself, the cult leaders do not condone the taking of strong doses. Initiation is a six-stage process. Firstly, on the night before the initiation is to take place, the candidate is assessed by the cult leaders who then decide whether or not he or she will be accepted. Sometimes at this juncture a little *eboga* may be given to the candidate. The second stage involves the day-long consumption of large quantities of *eboga* in the chapel. When the candidate has reached the appropriate state of consciousness they are taken out to the forest and ritually prepared (third stage) to re-enter the chapel and join in with the general ceremonial activity taking place there whilst continuing to consume *eboga*. Around midnight the initiate usually collapses in a state of extreme intoxication (known as '*eboga* death') which marks the fourth stage, which represents entry into the land of the dead. There is no further use of *eboga* and the initiate is taken out of the chapel to finish his or her visionary state in a tranquil environment (fifth stage). The final stage takes place the next morning when the initiate has fully recovered and is able to recount the details of the whole experience, and subsequently is integrated into the Bwiti community. The visions seen under the influence of *eboga* by an initiate are usually of a similar nature to those experienced by other members. This is due to the conscious orchestration of the experience by the cult leaders who not only control administration of the drug and supervise the ceremonial environment of the chapel, but also tell candidates what they are likely to experience with *eboga*. The entheogenic experience with *eboga* involves two sacred journeys – one a return to the womb and the primal collective (via the individual's ancestors) and the other a travelling forward to the land of the dead. There is no contradiction between the journeys; even though, from a rational point of view, they seem total opposites, mystically they represent the theme of eternal return in which beginning and end merge in mythical time.

**Sources:** Fernandez 1972, Fernandez 1982, Pope 1969, Schultes and Hofmann 1980b.

## ECSTASY

MDMA, or Ecstasy as it is commonly known, is often defined as a psychedelic amphetamine. It is usually taken orally (in the form of a pill, capsule or sometimes in powder form) and when digested in the stomach then enters the bloodstream. It releases serotonin and dopamine, two of the neurotransmitters. The MDMA is then metabolised by the liver and then the kidneys and expelled in the urine. Like the psychoactive principles of the fly-agaric mushroom, the drug still retains its mind-altering properties in the urine; some two thirds of the ingested MDMA is voided in the urine. MDMA is an analogue of MDA (3,4-methylenedioxyamphetamine) which first surfaced as a recreational drug in the mid-1960s.

There are a number of different street names given to Ecstasy pills, many varieties of which contain additives which may be harmful. White Dove, which may be white, cream, yellow or light green in colour and is impressed with the symbol of a bird, when analysed generally showed MDMA (or in some cases MDEA, a closely related substance) to be present. MDEA or Eve is the psychoactive substance of other varieties, including some batches of Buffalo (also known as Matador or White Bull), and pills with the 'PT' impress, known as Pete Tong or Party Time. The aptly named Sitting Duck, also white with a bird design, was found to contain a group of potentially hazardous substitutes for genuine MDMA: ketamine, selegiline and ephedrine. Another type known as Strawberry, red and pink in colour, and sometimes made with a strawberry fragrance, often contains the same substitutes as Sitting Duck. The type known as Shamrock (or Green Clover) may also be well-named as being a sham form of Ecstasy samples which contain not only no MDMA or MDMA analogues but apparently no other psychoactive substances. However, some users of this type report hallucinogenic effects. Other varieties are known to contain caffeine and/or amphetamine; placebo drugs are also sometimes sold as Ecstasy.

The two basic effects of the drug are as a stimulant and a relaxant. Some users report that Ecstasy is an aphrodisiac but many of them said that whilst sexual desire intensified the actual physical ability to perform was impaired. More commonly sex seems to take a back seat. As Nicholas Saunders, Britain's leading advocate for, and writer on, Ecstasy, puts it:

One reason why women are not into sex at raves is that men on Ecstasy have less interest in sex and do not expect sex. Most men have the opposite to an erection: a shrinking penis. 'Sex is not one of the foremost pleasures offered by Ecstasy. The motivation for raving is more likely to be sensations of the mind, body and soul. The pleasure of dancing with expression and empathy pushes sex into the background.' The attraction of raves for women derives from being in a pleasurable group setting, from which the pressure towards and emphasis on sex from men has been removed, in contrast to alcohol-based night life. Interviews indicated that sex is the last thing women have in mind when going to a rave. The sexual safety of raves is an attraction for girls, compared to alcohol-based clubs, which are seen as cattle markets. Girls sometimes enjoy kissing at raves because it feels good but is 'safe', not going to involve sex. One girl reported being with other girls walking through a dangerous part of the city when they were approached by a gang of men. They were scared until they realised the men were on E, 'then heaved a sigh of relief'.

Ecstasy is not, generally speaking, used by people alone but almost always with others. It produces a feeling of empathy and easy sociability and breaks down inhibitions. On the down side certain regular users complain of 'paranoia' which may be due to latent psychological problems brought to the surface by use of MDMA (or indeed any other drug), fear of persecution or arrest because the drug they are consuming is illegal or the actual chemical effect of the drug on certain users. A typical example is that of a user who said that: 'after nearly four years of using E every weekend, I got paranoid walking down the street, thinking that everyone was looking at me. I work as a bank clerk, and sometimes felt that all the customers I served were planted to test me, like I was under investigation.'

Although some research suggests that Ecstasy causes brain damage in laboratory animals it is not yet clear whether or not human brain cells are adversely affected by it, and there is also some research that indicates that it may have some positive effects on the functioning of the brain. Almost all deaths caused by taking Ecstasy are from heat stroke. This may occur when a user exerts themselves by dancing for hours without sufficient fluid intake in a hot environment. The use of Ecstasy in conjunction with other psychoactive substances is likely to exacerbate the danger. The dangers of heat stroke are widely known now and most clubs provide 'chill-out' areas and often a free supply of water. Intervals in the playing of the music also help by breaking the trance of the dancers and giving them the opportunity to 'chill out'.

MDMA was first known as Adam (see **Adam**) and only later received the name by which it has now become universally known – Ecstasy. The distributor of MDMA apparently preferred to call it Empathy but, thinking that many of his customers would not know what the word meant, decided on his second choice of name. MDMA was first made by the Merck pharmaceutical company in Germany in 1912 and apparently sold as a slimming pill. It was just one of many drugs tested on animals by the US army during the early 1950s for its possible applications in chemical warfare. It was given the title Experimental Agent 1475. Despite these early uses, the real story begins with the investigations of the chemist Alexander Shulgin, who not only made the drug in his laboratory in the mid-1960s but also tried it out on himself. Over the years Shulgin and his entourage have personally experimented with numerous substances, including a great many synthesised by Shulgin himself. Many of these belong to that group of psychoactive substances known as the phenethylamines.

In the late 1970s a number of professional psychotherapists, having tried it themselves, began to give it to their patients. In 1983 MDMA began to be distributed vigorously by what has become known as the 'Texas Group'. It was brazenly sold in bars in Dallas and Austin and soon became a highly sought after recreational drug, now in the open and outgrowing its rather elitist status within a psychotherapeutic coterie. By 1984 its use in the USA was widespread and the inevitable soon occurred when in the following year the Drug Enforcement Agency put a ban on various 'new' drugs, including Ecstasy. It is a Schedule 1 drug in America. The initial spread of Ecstasy in Europe during the mid to late 1980s is reportedly due to followers of Bhagwan Rajneesh bringing it over from the US and ravers using the drug in Ibiza (then known as 'XTC island') bringing it back to Britain for use in the warehouse parties that took place all over the country, replacing LSD as the drug of choice in the Acid House music scene. Due to concerted efforts by the police to end these raves (no doubt spurred on by a hysterical media campaign against these modern versions of the witches' sabbats) and a consolidation of the impromptu beginnings of dance culture into a more business-like approach, there was a shift of the movement into a club scene and the smaller scale Acid House scene expanded into the nation-wide Rave culture.

Ecstasy is seen by some of its users as having the status of an entheogen, i.e. a sacred drug that brings spiritual awareness. As such it is embraced by many people in the New Age movement who see its effects as entirely harmonious with an ecologically correct ideology. Among such 'techno-hippies' the tribal spiritualities of the Australian Aborigines or the Native Americans (with their emphasis on both ecological living and music and dance as key elements in the spiritual life) have, to some extent, taken the place of practices that were drawn from the oriental spiritual traditions (such as yoga, meditation and Zen) by their LSD-using forebears of the sixties. The New Agers, however, represent a hardcore, whereas most regular users of Ecstasy have no ideology fuelling or articulating their use – it is, for most, simply a recreational drug of choice. Ecstasy has become so popular in Britain that it has become a serious threat to the alcohol industry. Its reputation for inducing peacefulness and empathy has been reported to have, on occasions, dissolved the barriers between users in Northern Ireland. As one raver put it: 'At the warehouse doors, no one asks your religion . . . the raves are the last meeting ground for the children of Catholic and Protestant violence . . . we've never known anything but hatred . . . it's always the same: them over on one side, you on the other, except at raves.' Studies of rival football fans also indicate that Ecstasy may dissipate an interest in violent confrontation.

Although the typical user is the young raver, many others have also found Ecstasy a valuable experience, including a Benedictine monk interviewed by Nicholas Saunders. This monk stated in a letter to Saunders that:

> MDMA always propels me into an intimate space in conversation. There is a special quality to this conversation. One feels a heaviness, a sense of the weight of the moment, of something profound, of the seriousness of life itself. It is a space that is inner, without masks, without pretence, utterly open and honest. It is not an erotic intimacy, but a philosophical and mystical intimacy . . . one has the consciousness that this is an inner communication rarely achieved in ordinary discourse. There really are no adequate words to

express this state of awareness, only to say, that it is essential in my experience.

**Sources:** Beck and Rosenbaum 1994, Saunders 1995, Tyler 1995.


## ENCHYMOMA

A term coined by the distinguished historian of science, Joseph Needham, meaning 'an elixir created within the body by physiological means rather than by chemical means'. He derived it from the Greek *en* 'within' and *chumos* 'juice'.


## ENTHEOGEN

Since they found the existing terminology misleading that refers to the properties and uses to which psychoactive substances have been put, R. Gordon Wasson and his collaborators Carl Ruck, Jeremy Bigwood, Danny Staples and Jonathan Ott proposed that a new word should be used to clarify the rather hazy nomenclature that has plagued the study of such substances. In a seminal article published in *The Journal of Psychedelic Drugs* in 1979 they set out their aim of replacing the terms 'psychedelic' and 'hallucinogen' with the word entheogen. They wrote:

We ... propose a new term that would be appropriate for describing states of shamanic and ecstatic possession induced by ingestion of mind-altering drugs. In Greek the word *entheos* means literally 'god (*theos*) within', and was used to describe the condition that follows when one is inspired and possessed by the god that has entered one's body. It was applied to prophetic seizures, erotic passion and artistic creation, as well as to those religious rites in which mystical states were experienced through the ingestion of substances that were transubstantial with the deity. In combination with the Greek root *gen*–, which denotes the action of 'becoming', this word results in the term that we are proposing: *entheogen*. Our word sits easily on the tongue and seems quite natural in English. We could speak of *entheogens* or, in an adjectival form, of entheogenic plants or substances. In a strict sense, only those vision-producing drugs that can be shown to have figured in shamanic or religious rites would be designated entheogens, but in a looser sense, the term could also be applied to other drugs, both natural and artificial, that induce alteration of consciousness similar to those documented for ritual ingestion of traditional entheogens.

The term entheogen has, as a result of this article been used by a number of writers on the chemistry, botany and history of psychoactive substances and it seems that such usage will become more common as its value is appreciated. The derivative term entheobotany, meaning the study of entheogens, has also been proposed and is also gaining converts.

**Sources:** Ott 1996, Ruck et al 1979.

## EPHEDRA

*Ephedra* is a plant that contains alkaloids with stimulant properties similar to amphetamines (see **Amphetamines**). Among these are ephedrine and norpseudoephedrine. Norpseudoephedrine, which is also present in **Qat**, is a far more powerful stimulant than ephedrine but occurs in *Ephedra* only in low concentrations. *Ephedra* is perhaps the earliest known psychoactive plant in human history. Pollen remains of six plants (including *Ephedra altissima*) were found in a 50,000-year-old Neanderthal grave at Shanidar cave in Iraq. This unusual archaeological discovery seems to show that these six plants were intentionally placed in the grave, perhaps as part of a funerary rite. The excavator Solecki and the paleobotanist Leroi-Gourhan originally thought that the flowers were put there for their aesthetic value, as flowers are placed on the graves of lost ones today. However, a few years later Solecki came to believe that the plants may have been of medicinal rather than ornamental value to the Neanderthals. Five of the plant types found at the site are known to have medical properties, mostly in the treatment of wounds. *Ephedra* may have been used by the Neanderthals as a stimulant whilst hunting, although this is pure speculation.

*Ephedra* has been put forward as a candidate for the sacred *Soma* plant used by the ancient Indian and Iranian peoples (see **Soma**) but since it does not have hallucinogenic properties – unlike *Soma* – this identification has been rejected. However, recent archaeological finds of the plant in prehistoric temples in Central Asia (in contexts relating it to both cannabis and opium) indicate that it could have been an important additive in psychoactive preparations. Species of *ephedra* (*ma huang*) have been used since ancient times by the Chinese to combat coughs and lung complaints. In North America species of the plant have also been used medicinally. *Ephedra nevadensis*, when made into a hot water infusion is also known as Teamster's tea and Mormon tea. Such a beverage was used by the Zuñi Indians of New Mexico for treating first stage syphilis. In 1887 a Japanese chemist named Nagai first extracted ephedrine from the *Ephedra* plant, although its importance as a central nervous system stimulant was not realised in Europe until the 1920s. It was first used in the treatment of asthma during the 1930s.

**Sources:** Kalix 1991, Lietava 1992, Stevenson 1915, Thorwald 1962.

## ERGOT

Ergot (*Claviceps purpurea*) is the name given to a parasitic fungus that is found in diseased grasses and sedges, most markedly in rye crops. In early Europe and elsewhere rye infected with this fungus was sometimes eaten, causing mass outbreaks of ergotism, the effects of which are detailed below. The psychoactive alkaloids of ergot are mostly derivatives of lysergic acid and have hallucinogenic effects. LSD (see **LSD**) was synthetically derived from ergot by Albert Hofmann.

Archaeologist Jeremy Dronfield has suggested that some of the art that adorns the dramatic passage-tombs of Neolithic Ireland may have been inspired either by ergot or other hallucinogenic fungi. There are references to grain contaminants in Assyrian and Zoroastrian sources which may indicate that ergot poisoning was a problem in antiquity. A distinguished trio of scholars (the chemist Albert Hofmann, whose knowledge of the pharmacology of ergot is second to none, R. Gordon Wasson, the ranking ethnomycologist of his generation and specialist on the hallucinogenic fungi, and the classicist Carl Ruck, whose particular expertise is in the botany of the Greeks) put forward the argument in their *The*

*Road to Eleusis: Unveiling the Secrets of the Mysteries* (1978) that ergot was the entheogen used in the Eleusinian Mysteries of ancient Greece. As the authors say:

> the ancient testimony about Eleusis is unanimous and unambiguous. Eleusis was the supreme moment in an initiate's life. It was both physical and mystical: trembling, vertigo, cold sweat, and then a sight that made all previous seeing seem like blindness, a sense of awe and wonder at a brilliance that caused a profound silence, since what had just been seen and felt could never be communicated; words were unequal to the task. These symptoms are unmistakably the experience induced by a hallucinogen. Greeks, and indeed some of the most famous and intelligent among them, could experience and enter fully into such irrationality.

Whilst ergot may well have been instrumental in the spiritual lives of the Greeks, its role in later European history was anything but exalted. Ergotism was the cause of terrible suffering in Europe, particularly during the Middle Ages, when it was called St Anthony's Fire, the Divine Wrath and *sacer ignis* or Holy Fire. England was largely unaffected as rye was only a minor constituent of the human diet. There are records of ergotic outbreaks as early as AD 857, and to give some idea of the scale of this affliction 40,000 people are said to have died in Aquitaine in the year 994. Ergotism had extreme effects on both the body and the mind. It caused convulsions, severe mental disturbance and precipitated epileptic fits. Even worse was the gangrenous infection that it caused. The limbs went black and swelled up and the loss of hands, feet and even whole limbs was commonplace. One grisly anecdote will suffice to demonstrate the appalling suffering caused by ergotism. A woman who was suffering with the disease was riding to hospital on an ass when her leg knocked against a shrub; the force of this contact was enough to make her leg fall off. She is then said to have carried it in her arms to the hospital.

Ironically ergot also had a role in Medieval medicine. Among the archaeological discoveries made at the site of a hospital run by Augustinian monks from about 1190 to 1460 were sixteen ergots (*Claviceps purpurea*) mixed with juniper berries. The excavation reports suggest they may have been used as a means of inducing

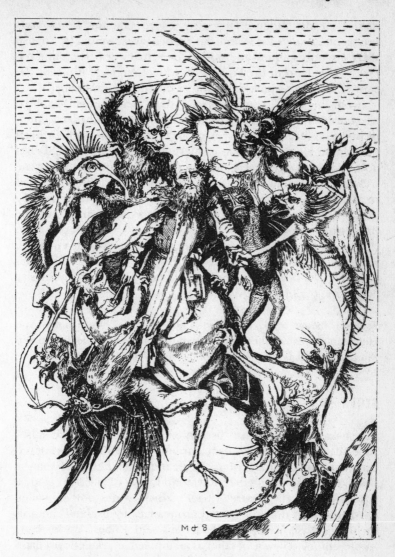

**SAINT ANTHONY BESIEGED BY DEMONIC APPARITIONS**

abortions. It is known to have been used by midwives throughout
Europe to induce labour. The great importance of ergot in
Europe is demonstrated by the fact that in the German tongue
alone Schultes and Hofmann have found sixty-two vernacular

names for the fungus. They also record that the Dutch have twenty-one names for it and the French over twenty. In English there are only seven in addition to the actual word ergot, which is taken directly from the French (in which language it means the spur of a cock to which the shape of the fungus was likened).

According to Christian Rätsch, some 'acid heads' (habitual users of LSD) consider St Anthony their patron saint on account of his close links with ergot. Various ergot derivatives have been used for their psychoactive properties, most famously **LSD** but also, and more rarely, pergolide mesylate. The latter is used in the treatment of Parkinson's disease, and in 1995 a case was reported in which an experienced drug user who had read up on the psychoactive potentials of ergot alkaloids experimented with the drug, which he obtained from a relative who was suffering from the disease. About half an hour after taking the drug he entered a state of dissociation that lasted forty-five minutes. This was followed by a two-hour period of hallucinations in which the size and shape of objects were altered.

**Sources:** Barger 1931, Dronfield 1995, Rätsch 1992, Schultes and Hofmann 1980a, Schultes and Hofmann 1980b, Wasson, Hofmann and Ruck 1978, Watt and Breyer-Brandwijk 1962, Wilcox 1995, Williams 1947.

## ETHER

Ether was perhaps first discovered by the Arab alchemists. Albertus Magnus made an 'aqua ardens' by the distillation of red wine, quicklime, tartar, common salt and green figs which may be described as a kind of ether. Raymond Lully (1234–1315) made a substance he called 'sweet vitriol', which would now be called ethyl ether. A number of other European alchemists and chemists including Basil Valentine, Paracelsus and Robert Boyle made 'proto-ethers'. The use of ether as an inhaled anaesthetic predates that of nitrous oxide, better known as laughing gas (see **Inhalants**).

Ether was often abused for its psychoactive effects even though its primary use was as an anaesthetic agent. The hypocrisy of those who abused ether whilst espousing temperance was ridiculed in the satirical 'Ether Song', the lyrics being written by Douglas MacLaren to the tune of 'Yankie Doodle':

Intoxication's a disgrace,
Teetotalism growls, Sir;
But ladies, with unblushing face,
Get now as drunk as owls, Sir.

Ether was a popular inebriant at student parties in the first half of the nineteenth century. Such 'frolicking' became so notorious that a contemporary French writer cited such behaviour as proof of the growth of decadence in Anglo-Saxon cultures. Ether drinking was also rife among the Irish in the mid-nineteenth century. In Draperstown and Cookstown on market days the air was redolent with the smell of ether. Irish peasants of the time used to drink up to about 400g a day, washed down with water to reduce the rate of

## WONDERFUL EFFECTS OF ETHER IN A CASE OF SCOLDING WIFE.

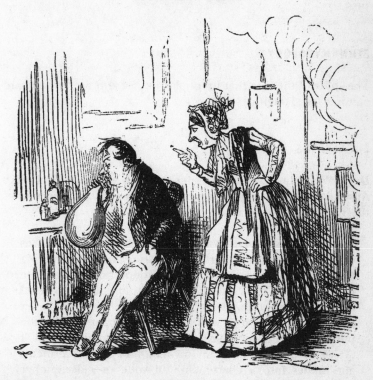

*Patient.*—" THIS IS REALLY QUITE DELIGHTFUL—A MOST BEAUTIFUL DREAM."

evaporation of the ether, thus getting the full effects. Ether abuse was also reported to be endemic at one time in Norway, Russia and Lithuania. Echoing the beserker frenzies of the Vikings were reports that German troops in the First World War were given ether to drive them into a state of bloodlust. Ether has also been used by occultists in their attempts to tap into hidden powers of the psyche. Kenneth Grant, a disciple of Aleister Crowley, records how he was introduced to ether by his master in 1946, a year before the death of the 'Great Beast', as Crowley liked to call himself. In a magical experiment devised by Crowley ether was inhaled in order to test the visionary aptitude of his would-be initiates. Grant reports that the occult symbols he was shown by Crowley under the influence of ether appeared intensely bright.

**Sources:** Ellis 1946, Grant 1972, Kohn 1992, MacLaren 1873, Schenk 1956.

## ETHNOMYCOLOGY

The study of the role that fungi play in past and present human cultures (see **Fungi**).

## EUCALYPTUS

David Bunce, a traveller who spent over twenty years exploring Australia in the first half of the nineteenth century, described how the Tasmanians made an alcoholic drink:

> the natives obtained from the cider-trees of the Lakes (*Eucalyptus resinifera*) a slightly saccharine liquor, resembling treacle. At the proper season they ground holes in the tree from which the sweet juice flowed plentifully. It was collected in a hole at the bottom near the root of the tree. These holes were kept covered over with a flat stone, apparently for the purpose of preventing birds and animals coming to drink it . . . when allowed to remain any length of time, it ferments and settles into a coarse kind of wine or cider, rather intoxicating if drunk to excess.

The aboriginal Tasmanians have been described as one of the most 'primitive' societies to be encountered in recent history, and partly because of this reputation the idea that they could have discovered by themselves a means to make alcoholic drinks has been treated with some scepticism. Bunce's account seems to be unique and this has led to it being dismissed as hearsay. Whether or not one believes that the Tasmanians made such a fermented drink depends entirely on the weight one puts on the report of Bunce.

**Sources:** Roth 1899.


## EVE

Street name given to the MDMA-related drug MDEA and clearly inspired by the early epithet, Adam, given to MDMA (see **Ecstasy**). Also called simply MDE.

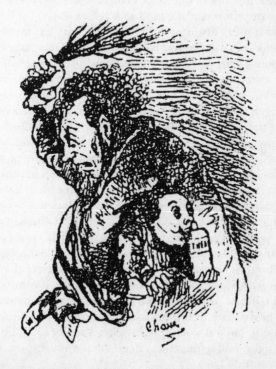

**ETHER**

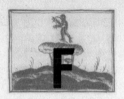

## FLY-AGARIC

The fly-agaric mushroom (*Amanita muscaria*) is found in both the Old World and the New World and typically grows at the base of the birch, larch and fir trees. The Old World variety has a bright red cap covered with white warts and is easily recognised as it is the prototype for the toadstool depicted in fairy stories. In North America this variety is found in the north-western part of the continent whilst the fly-agaric of central and eastern regions has an orange or yellow cap adorned with yellow warts.

In Siberia users distinguish between the smaller, more potent mushrooms (i.e. with young fruit bodies) and the larger, flatter topped ones (mature). They recommend the former should be used for a stimulant effect as required for work tasks involving considerable physical labour, and the latter for experiencing hallucinogenic effects. Yet, in eastern Siberia, the native people warn that the: 'big fungi are not so obedient as small ones, they may deceive; small fungi are stronger than the big ones but more submissive.' They also say that it is important to tell the mushroom (either out loud or to oneself) what you want from it, otherwise it may lead you astray. Its stimulating properties have been confirmed by reliable witnesses who have seen such users perform remarkable physical tasks. Vladimir Bogoraz, a Russian anthropologist, said that a Siberian man with whom he was travelling would happily take off his snowshoes and stride through deep snow for hours without fatigue under the influence of the fungus. Similar stories from Siberia detail how eating the mushrooms helped in other arduous tasks, such as hauling heavy boats, carrying heavy loads and long-distance running. As one Chukchi person put it: 'an old woman runs 30km and does not die.'

Among the hallucinogenic effects of the mushroom are the

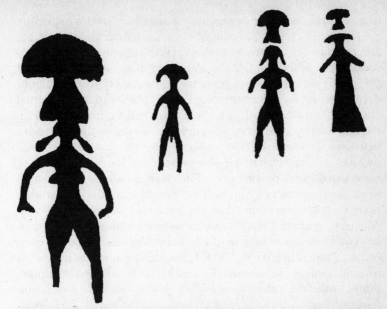

**PREHISTORIC SIBERIAN ROCK ART DEPICTING FLY-AGARIC PEOPLE**

perception of objects as either larger than they are (macroscopia) or smaller than they are (microscopia), as well as auditory and visual hallucinations. Among some Siberians the hallucinogenic effects of the fungus are best experienced during sleep and so they eat them just before going to bed. There are a number of ways in which the fly-agaric may be taken. It has usually been eaten raw and fresh, raw and dried, cooked, or taken in the form of an extract or decoction. The fungi can be soaked in water or fruit juice and the resulting liquid drunk. The use of the juice of the bog bilberry (*Vacinium uliginosum*) is said to increase the potency of the fly-agaric's psychoactive effects. *Epilobium angustifolium*, or fireweed, was also used as an additive. Another fairly common practice – at least in Siberia – was to drink one's urine after consuming the mushroom as the psychoactive properties were still active in the urine. People would also drink the urine of another person who had taken the mushroom. Not surprisingly the Russian and other European witnesses to such events were disgusted by this practice. Smoking the fungus has been reported from Mexico (see below) and been described in a story recounted by the renowned Ojibwa Indian artist Norval Morrisseau, but not from Siberia. As to the dosage that is required for the hallucinogenic effects to take place, the Siberian sources vary widely. There are a number of reports of such effects using only a single mushroom. At the other end of the scale there is an isolated report of the taking of twenty-one, but this is most likely to be a figure derived from sacred numerology (3x7) rather than an actual amount. The Khanty of western Siberia believe it is unlucky to consume an even number of fungi and therefore always ensure that they consume an odd amount. The Siberians made three provisos to ensure that the altered states of consciousness they experienced were positive ones. First, if an individual was deemed weak then they were given only an extract from the mushroom. Second, they made sure that the user was not interfered with during such altered states in order to avoid both a 'bad trip' and any chance that the user might accidentally injure themselves or come to any other harm. Finally, the mushroom was not taken with alcohol as the two were seen to be highly incompatible. Whilst under the influence of his beloved mushroom a user would perceive a man who was drunk on vodka, in the words of a Russian investigator: 'as being a filthy force, black even in colour, detrimental to men, and he passes him by from afar.'

The custom of eating the fly-agaric exists in both western and eastern Siberia and it is probable that it was used right across the far north of Asia in early times; the northerly migration of Altaic tribes (who had no tradition of *Amanita muscaria* use) from the south seems to have created a 'wedge' between the two present areas of fly-agaric consumption. Among the western peoples who have used the mushroom were the Khanty (once called the Ostyak), the Mansi, the Forest Nenets, the Nganasan and the Ket. In the east it was taken by the Koryak, Chuckchi, Kamchadal (Itelmen) and some of their neighbours, perhaps including the Siberian Eskimos. Although the mushroom was used freely in most of these societies, some, such as the Kets and the Forest Nenets, restricted its use to shamans. In certain areas only some shamans or magicians took the fly-agaric, and those who could perform their work without its aid were considered the stronger. The spiritual and magical activities with which fly-agaric use has been associated include communicating with the dead and with other spirits, the interpretation of dreams, divination undertaken to locate stolen or lost property, clairvoyance, visions of and visits to the upper and lower worlds (which, to the Koryak and Chukchi are the future and the past respectively) and learning the special language of the spirits.

There are numerous Russian and other European travellers to Siberia who have recorded the use of the psychoactive mushroom *Amanita muscaria* among the native peoples of this vast region; the earliest, by a Polish prisoner of war, was written in 1658. Stepan Krasheninnikov, an explorer of the Kamchatka peninsula in eastern Siberia, wrote in 1755 the following description of fly-agaric (or *mukhomor* as it is known to the Russians) use by the native Kamchadals:

> The first and usual sign by which one can recognise a man under the influence of the *mukhomor* is the shaking of the extremities, which will follow after an hour or less, after which the persons thus intoxicated have hallucinations, as if in a fever; they are subject to various visions, terrifying or felicitous, depending on differences in temperament; owing to which some jump, some dance, others cry and suffer great terrors, while some might deem a small crack to be as wide as a door, and a tub of water as deep as the sea. But this applies only to those who overindulge, while those who use a small quantity experience a feeling of extraordinary lightness, joy, courage, and a sense of energetic well-being.

The same writer also relates an incident in which a Cossack who had been posted to this far-flung outpost of Russian influence took the mushroom and experienced a religious vision in which he:

> had a vision of Hell and a terrifying fiery chasm into which he was to be cast; for which reason, following the orders of the *mukhomor*, he was forced to get down on his knees and confess all the sins that he could remember committing. His friends, of whom there were a great many in the common room where the intoxicated man was confessing, heard this with great amusement, while he seemed to believe that he was confessing his sins in the privacy of the sacrament to God alone. Because of this he was made the butt of much deliberate ridicule, since, among other things, he related some things which should have best remained unknown to others.

The antiquity of the eastern Siberian use of the fly-agaric was demonstrated by finds made from 1965–68 by N.N. Dikov of the Magadan Institute of Archaeology, who discovered a series of petroglyphs (rock carvings) at Pegtymel in Chukotka near to the arctic seas, an area where the mushroom is still used today. These carvings clearly show both men and women with mushrooms on their heads. Among the eastern Siberians (Chukchi, Koryak and Kamchadal) the fact that small beings known as 'fly-agaric men' and also as 'amanita girls' are seen under the influence of the mushroom shows that in this region of the world – as in so many others – there are strong links between a belief in 'the little people' and the use of psychoactive substances. *Czelkutq and the Amanita Girls*, a Kamchadal folk tale collected by the Russian anthropologist Jochelson, recounts the story of a man who was literally 'away with the fairies', abandoning his family for the love of the mushroom. I reproduce the translation in full below. As Siberian singers and storytellers used fly-agaric themselves before performing perhaps this tale was once told under the influence of the mushroom!

There lived Czelkutq. He wooed Kutq's daughter Sinanewt and worked for her. He brought in much wood. Czelkutq married Sinanewt. They began to live. They amused themselves well. Sinanewt gave birth; a son was born. Czelkutq set off into the woods, where he met the beautiful amanita girls. Czelkutq stayed with the girls and forgot his wife. Sinanewt thought of her husband and waited for him. She thought: 'Where is he, long ago he was killed!'

With them there lived an old aunt of hers, Kutq's sister, who said: 'Well, Sinanewt, stop waiting for your husband; long ago he stayed with the amanita; send your son to his father.'

The little boy set off to his father. He began to sing: 'My father is Czelkutq, my mother is Sinanewt, father has forgotten us.'

Czelkutq heard his son singing and said to the girls: 'Go and burn him with burning brands, and tell him that I am no father to him.'

The girls took the burning brands and burned the boy all over, they burned his little hands all over. 'It is hot! Mother they burn me!' he cried, and back he went to his mother. She asked: 'Well, what did your father say?'

'He said: "I am no father to you;" he ordered the amanita girls to burn me with hot brands; he burned my hands all over; it is hot and hurts me. I will not go to my father again, or they will burn me with hot firebrands.'

The next day his grandmother sent him to his father again, saying: 'Go once more, sing again, say "Father, tomorrow all of us will leave, you will stay in the forest here with the amanita; afterwards you will surely starve".'

The little boy set off to his father and began to sing: 'Father, tomorrow all of us will leave together. You will remain in the forest with the amanita; afterwards you will surely starve.'

Czelkutq, hearing his son singing, became angry and said: 'Go, girls, and beat him thoroughly with a leather strap and burn him with fire; tell him to stop coming here.'

Thus the girls took firebrands and leather strap and began to beat him and burn him; thus they drove him away. The boy cried, and started back to his mother. He was burned all over when he arrived, but his grandmother blew at him and made him well. The old woman said: 'Well, Sinanewt, let us get ready to go, we shall go into the woods.'

They began to get ready; they tied up all the animals and took them all, leaving nothing. They started into the woods. When they arrived, they picked out a high mountain, climbed up to the top, and poured water all over the mountain, making a sheet of ice.

Czelkutq began to go into the woods. He did not kill any animals at all; all the traces had gotten lost. He and the girls began to starve. What could they eat? Then Czelkutq remembered his wife and son and went home. He came to his house, but did not find his wife and son. He began to weep: 'Where did all my people get lost? I am starving, Sinanewt, I am hungry. Where did you and our son go away?'

He followed his wife by their traces, and reached that high mountain. 'How to get up? The ice is very slippery.' From below he called up: 'Sinanewt, pull me up!'

Sinanewt threw down a leather cord and called out: 'Well, Czelkutq, catch the cord!'

He caught the cord. She began to pull him up to the top of the mountain, but when he was ready to step onto the top, she cut the cord with a knife. Czelkutq flew downwards, he fell, he died, he revived, and again he called out: 'Sinanewt, pull me up, I am starving!'

'Why don't you live with the amanita? Why don't you live with the amanita? Why do you come to us? You tortured your son, and now you are being paid back; it's you yourself who began that sort of life.'

'Sinanewt, stop being angry, pull me up, I am hungry!'

She threw down the cord again, saying: 'Well, catch, I shall pull you up now.'

Czelkutq caught the cord and she pulled him up. When he got near the top, she again cut the cord with a knife; he flew down, he fell, he died, he lay there, he came to life again, and cried out: 'Sinanewt, stop being angry!'

'If I pull you up, will you go on living like that afterwards?'

'No, I won't, Sinanewt, I shall stop living like that.'

She threw down the cord, he was pulled up, dried out, and became happy: he ate, he became satiated. Again they began to live as before, amusing themselves. The amanita dried up and died.

Clearly the fly-agaric was seen as potentially harmful to the family and social life in general as well as being, at the same time, a socially sanctioned psychoactive substance. This dual social nature of the fly-agaric in Siberia has, in this respect, certain parallels with the role of alcohol in Western societies in which drinking is seen as a cultural norm but alcoholism socially debilitating. As with alcohol in our society, mushrooms were often used in a recreational way at major social events such as weddings, house parties and hunting feasts. Yet, very much in contrast to the case of alcohol, violent behaviour is almost completely unheard of in relation to fly-agaric use. In areas of Siberia where the mushroom did not grow in abundance a single fly-agaric could change hands for considerable sums. In the nineteenth century Russian traders could get $20 worth of furs per fungus and in the internal exchanges of the Siberians one could fetch three or four reindeer.

The fly-agaric was known in China as *ha ma chün* (meaning 'toad-mushroom') and by the later name *tu ying hsin* ('fly-killing mushroom') both of which display remarkable parallels to the connotations of the European names. Joseph Needham, author of the monumental *Science and Civilisation in China*, is of the opinion that not only were the psychoactive effects of this mushroom known to the shamans of ancient times but also to the Taoist adepts. This is supported by the many reports, dating from the Han dynasty onwards, that state that the Taoists drank urine, which may indicate the use of the fly-agaric. In line with his central idea that the ancient hallucinogen *soma* was the fly-agaric, Wasson believed that the Chinese interest in this mushroom was largely due to the influence of India (see **Soma**). It seems more likely that the Taoist use of the fly-agaric was either a continuation of an indigenous shamanic tradition or inspired by shamans further north, namely eastern Siberia, an area in which the use of *Amanita muscaria* is both well-documented and ancient. It would be false to think that a so-called 'higher culture' (such as that of China) would only import ideas and practices from other 'advanced' cultures (such as India) and not from the 'lowly' Siberian peoples. One need only think of the European adoption of tobacco and chocolate from the native American peoples as a case in point. An isolated case of the traditional use of the fly-agaric in the Hindu Kush mountains of Central Asia is reported, which could be seen as corroborative evidence for Wasson's thesis that the mushroom was the *soma* of the Indo-Iranian peoples who originated from this part of the world. However, the fact that the mushroom is called 'raven's bread' in the Hindu Kush seems to point more towards a link with the folklore of eastern Siberia, where the peoples who use the fly-agaric have a mythology in which the raven is a fundamentally important figure.

In response to Wasson's *soma* theory (published in 1968), the leading French anthropologist Claude Lévi-Strauss wrote a wide-ranging survey of the use of fungi by native North Americans, in which he gives an early sixteenth-century reference in the *Jesuit Relations* to the native use of a sacred mushroom. This passing reference is found in a letter from Pére Charles l'Allemant in Quebec to his brother in France. It is dated 1 August 1626. In it he discusses the local Algonkian Indians who: 'assure you that after death they go to heaven where they eat mushrooms and hold inter-course with each other.' Lévi-Strauss had informed Wasson of this letter and its contents in the early sixties, many years before he published an extract of it, and it had stayed in the back of Wasson's mind, nagging him over the years. Finally, in 1975, through a series of fortuitous meetings, he encountered Keewaydinoquay, a female herbalist of the Ahnishinaubeg (Ojibwa) people who was still using the fly-agaric as a sacred substance or entheogen. The Ahnishinaubeg are one of the Algonkian peoples of the Great Lakes region, and Wasson had no hesitation in now viewing the early Jesuit letter (which preceded the earliest reference to the fly-agaric in Siberia by a century) as referring to none other than the fly-agaric. He also suggested that this mushroom cult must have extended into Quebec and was perhaps part of the culture of the Abenaki and Montagnais Indians.

Keewaydinoquay, who at this time was in her sixties, lived a hermit-like existence on a tiny island in Lake Michigan. When Wasson visited her there she presented him with a birchbark scroll which described the legend of the origin of the fly-agaric (*miskwedo* or 'red top' in her native tongue) in the form of pictures. His colleague Reid Kaplan was initiated by her into the ceremony of the mushroom in August 1977. According to the accounts of Keewaydinoquay herself, she was taught herbalism at an early age by an older woman named Nodjimahkwe, for whom she had great respect. Nevertheless this first teacher was fiercely opposed to the use of fly-agaric. Keewaydinoquay was, however, eager to learn about the forbidden mushroom and was initiated into the use of it by another herbalist when she was about fourteen. From that time on she used it sparingly and always with reverence. Although Keewaydinoquay has had a book published under the auspices of the Botanical Museum of Harvard University, a number of manuscripts relating to her collaborations with Wasson and Kaplan are kept under lock and key in a library at Harvard University which are not available to researchers until some years into the twenty-first century, presumably to protect the Ahnishinaubeg people from the unwanted attention of thrill-seeking intruders (particularly in the light of what had happened to the Mexican healer María Sabina after she had introduced Wasson to the mushroom cult of her people, for which see **Psilocybe**).

Another case of fly-agaric use in recent times comes from the account of Joel, a Brooklynite who, during the 1960s, went to work in a fishing camp near the Mackenzie mountains in northern Canada. Whilst there he met a Dogrib Indian shaman named Adamie, who took on his visitor as an apprentice. After a tough series of preliminary ordeals Adamie gave Joel the fly-agaric mushroom to eat. Joel described it thus: 'I ate the mushrooms . . . and there was drumming and a seance. It was a very frightening experience. The drug felt toxic and I didn't know how to deal with it . . . it was like eating belladonna . . . like there's no way out now because those things with big teeth are coming . . . it was hell, an endless chaotic battle with no real point.' Although his experiences later made more sense to him he felt he had to leave the barren landscape of the region and the strange psychic world he had been initiated into and return to the urban white world.

Both Lévi-Strauss and Wasson appear to have missed an account which seems to hint that the fly-agaric may also have been used on the Pacific north-west. Captain Bourke of the US cavalry was a keen student of the more unusual aspects of culture, particularly the variety of uses to which urine and excrement have been put. His book on this subject, published a century ago, includes the following report concerning the Makah Indians of Cape Flattery on the Olympia peninsula in Washington state:

> As was learned from Mr Kennard, US Coast Survey, whom the writer had the pleasure of meeting in Washington DC, in 1886, the medicine men distil, from potatoes and other ingredients, a vile liquor, which has an irritating and exciting effect upon the kidneys and bladder. Each one who has partaken of this dish immediately urinates and passes the result to his next neighbour, who drinks. The effect is as above, and likewise a temporary insanity or delirium during which all sorts of mad capers are carried on. The last man who quaffs the poison, distilled through the persons of five or six comrades, is so completely overcome that he falls in a dead stupor.

This inebriation is so close to descriptions of the Siberians' use of fly-agaric that this appears to be another genuine example of the use of the mushroom in native North America. This conclusion is further supported by the fact that fly-agaric is the only known naturally occurring hallucinogen that retains its psychoactive properties in the urine (the synthetic drug MDMA also has this unusual property; see **Ecstasy**). The Nez Perce Indians have a word *petuqes*, which means both 'toadstool' and 'silly' or 'berserk'; this may also be a reference to a hallucinogenic mushroom known to the native Americans.

There are also reports of the fly-agaric being used in Mexico and in the Philippines. In order to assist them in identifying the causes of illnesses, native healers, or *curanderos*, in the Puebla Valley in Mexico are said to consume the fly-agaric in a rather unusual fashion, namely dried and smoked with tobacco. A reliable experimenter with the fly-agaric has confirmed to me that smoking the fungus can cause hallucinogenic effects. An unpublished ethnographic manuscript by Dennis Alegre, cited by the German anthropologist Christian Rätsch, reports that the Sagada Igorots of the mountainous regions of the island of Luzon in the Philippines maintain a cult of the fly-agaric for use in their traditional rites of passage. They are said to make a hallucinogenic beverage out of six fresh mushrooms.

Reid Kaplan has suggested that motifs depicted in the prehistoric art of Scandinavia represent the sacred mushroom but this remains controversial. There is no evidence for the traditional use of the fly-agaric in Britain but it does turn up as an influence on Charles Lutwidge Dodgson, a don at Christ Church, Oxford, better known to the world at large as Lewis Carroll, author of the classic children's story *Alice's Adventures in Wonderland*. Dodgson appears to have read about the psychoactive effects of the mushroom in the writings of Mordecai Cooke, a mycologist with a particular interest in narcotic substances. Cooke mentions the fly-agaric in two books: *The Seven Sisters of Sleep: Popular History of the Seven Prevailing Narcotics of the World* (1860), a title which would have had a peculiar resonance for Dodgson, who had seven sisters himself, and *A Plain and Easy Account of British Fungi* (1862). Cooke describes the macroscopia and microscopia induced by the mushroom, which is seen as the inspiration for some of the transformations undergone by Dodgson's young heroine. In a recent article Michael Carmichael has suggested that this was not just a literary influence but one that encouraged Dodgson to experiment with the mushroom itself. In a meticulous study of the various medical books in Dodgson's personal library Carmichael shows that he would have been aware of the effects and properties of numerous psychoactive substances. There are also numerous veiled references to drug-induced altered states of consciousness in Dodgson's writings. The fly-agaric was supposed to be taken by members of a witches' coven that was based in the New Forest in southern England during the 1930s and 1940s and into which the founder of the modern witchcraft movement, Gerald Gardner, was initiated; there is no real evidence of this and it may be mere hearsay.

**Sources:** Bourke 1891, Carmichael 1996, Cooke 1860, De Smet 1985, Dunn 1973, Hajicek-Dobberstein 1995, Halifax 1979, Kaplan 1975, Keewaydinoquay 1978, Needham 5/2 6/1, Rätsch 1992, Saar 1991a, Wasson 1968, Wasson 1979, Worth 1961, Yefimenko 1995.

**FLYING OINTMENTS** see **Witches' Ointments**

**FOXGLOVE** see **Digitalis**

**FUNGI**

Most of the main hallucinogenic species of fungi belong to the class Basidiomycetes, which includes *Amanita muscaria* (see **Fly-Agaric**), *A. pantherina* (see **Amanita Pantherina**) and the numerous *Psilocybe* species (see **Psilocybe**) as well as the puffballs (see **Puffballs**).

The academic discipline called ethnomycology (the systematic study of the role of fungi in culture) was pioneered by R.Gordon Wasson(1898–1986). At first glance one could not conceive of a

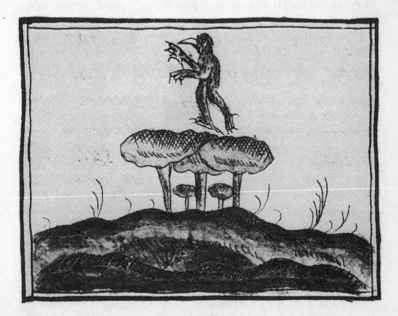

**DEMON OF THE MUSHROOM FROM THE FLORENTINE CODEX**

more unlikely figure to uncover to the world at large the profound role that hallucinogenic mushrooms and other fungi have played in the development of religion. Although starting his professional career as an academic, Wasson soon shifted his attention to journalism, contributing a daily financial column for the *Herald Tribune*. He entered the world of banking in 1928 and joined J.P. Morgan & Co. in 1934. He became vice-president in 1943 and remained with the company until his retirement in 1963. His interest in mushrooms was first stimulated by his wife Valentina who, as a White Russian, was, in the tradition of her people, a mycophile, or mushroom lover. The story of Wasson's enrapturement with mushrooms is something of a legend and is best told by the man himself:

My wife and I embarked on this our intellectual foray late in August 1927. A little episode started us on our way. Valentina Pavlovna was Russian, a Muscovite by birth. I was of Anglo-Saxon ancestry. We had been married less than a year and we were now off on our first holiday, at Big Indian in the Catskills. On that first day, as the sun was declining in the West, we set out for a stroll, the forest on our left, a clearing on our right. Though we had known each other for years, it happened that we had never discussed mushrooms together. All of a sudden she darted from my side. With cries of ecstasy she flew to the forest glade, where she had discovered mushrooms of various kinds carpeting the ground. Since Russia she had seen nothing like it. Left planted on the mountain trail, I called to her to take care, to come back. They were toadstools she was gathering, poisonous, putrid, disgusting. She only laughed the more: I can hear her now. She knelt in poses of adoration. She spoke to them with endearing Russian diminutives. She gathered the toadstools in a kind of pinafore that she was wearing, and brought them to our lodge. Some she strung on threads to hang up and dry for winter use. Others she served that night, either with the soup or the meat, according to their kind. I refused to touch them . . . This episode, a small thing in itself affecting only a peripheral aspect of our busy lives, led us to make inquiries, and we found that the northern Slavs know their mushrooms, having learned them at their mother's knee; theirs is no book knowledge. They love these fungal growths with a passion that, viewed with detachment, seemed to me a little exaggerated. But we Anglo-Saxons reject them viscerally, with revulsion, without deigning to make their acquaintance, and our attitude is even more exaggerated than the Slavs'. Little by little my wife and I built up extensive files concerning this modest corner of human behaviour.

In 1952 Robert Graves informed Wasson of the discovery by the ethnobotanist Richard Evans Schultes (who was later to become both the Director of the Botanical Museum at Harvard and a lifelong friend of Wasson) of the continuing use of hallucinogenic mushrooms by Mexican Indians. After contacting Schultes, Wasson organised an expedition to the Oaxaca region of Mexico the following year (see **Psilocybe**). In 1957 the Wassons published their first book, the monumental two-volume *Mushrooms, Russia and History*. Tragically, Valentina died soon after, on New Year's Eve 1958. Although an amateur scholar in the best sense of the word, Wasson became a research associate at Harvard and gained the respect of a number of eminent scholars in various fields, including Albert Hofmann, the chemist and discoverer of LSD, Roger Heim, the mycologist and Roman Jakobson, the great linguist. In 1963 Wasson began travelling in Asia, gathering information for what was to be his *magnum opus, Soma: Divine Mushroom of Immortality* (1968), published, like most of his books in a limited edition, highly sought after by bibliophiles and collectors. In *Soma* Wasson put forward the novel thesis that *Soma*, the mysterious hallucinogenic substance of the ancient Indians and Iranians, was the fly-agaric toadstool *Amanita muscaria* (see **Soma**, **Fly-Agaric**). As William Emboden, one of the world's leading experts on psychoactive plants, has put it, the mushroom was Wasson's muse.

According to the *General History of the Things of New Spain* by the sixteenth-century Franciscan missionary Bernardino de Sahagún, the Aztecs used a sacred mushroom known to them as *teonanacatl*, which means 'flesh of the gods'. Despite the fact that he explicitly describes it as a mushroom, his identification was challenged in the early twentieth century on the grounds that no psychoactive fungus was known to be used by the contemporary Indians of Mexico. It was suggested that, rather than being a mushroom, *teonanacatl* was actually the peyote cactus (see **Peyote**). Early in his career the renowned ethnobotanist Richard Schultes believed Sahagún's original identification to be correct. On linguistic grounds the mushroom thesis was supported by, among other evidence, the fact that the modern Mexican word for mushrooms is *nanacates*. Whilst travelling in Oaxaca, Mexico Schultes discovered that the local Mazatec, Chinantec and Zapotec Indians used mushrooms of the genus *Panaeolus* for their psychoactive properties, leading him to conclude that the Aztec entheogen called *teonanacatl* was one or more of the species of *Panaeolus*, which all have similar hallucinogenic effects. He later realised that other genera of mushrooms were also subsumed under this Aztec term, including *Psilocybe* species (see **Psilocybe**). The Indians of Oaxaca collected and dried the mushrooms before consuming them for divinatory and prophetic purposes. The effects of this fungus are described by Schultes:

> The doses which the Mazatec Indians prescribe vary with the size and age of the individual. Usually fifteen mushrooms are considered sufficient to induce the desired effect, but larger doses are reported. Overdoses of fifty or sixty mushrooms result in severe poisonings, whilst continued use of excessive quantities is said to produce permanent insanity . . . According to a number of descriptions from the Indians, the intoxication lasts about three hours. Shortly after ingestion of the mushrooms, the subject experiences a general feeling of levity and well-being. This exhilaration is followed within an hour by hilarity, incoherent talking, uncontrolled emotional outbursts and, in the later stages of intoxication, by fantastic visions in brilliant colours.

*Panaeolus campanulatus*, a small mushroom with a dark brown stripe and a yellowish-brown cap, was frequently employed by Mazatec diviners who made a living by using its powers to locate stolen property and give sundry advice to their clients. Diviners who habitually use this kind of mushroom in their work are reported to sometimes suffer from senility and premature ageing as a result of too frequently consulting the fungal oracle. These considerable occupational hazards were probably due to the accumulation of toxins from the mildly poisonous mushrooms. Nevertheless, the fungus was employed as a medicine and its use in the treatment of rheumatism shows a remarkable continuity in ethnomedical practice, as both the ancient Aztecs and the twentieth-century Mexican Indians used it as such. 'Mushroom drunks' among the native peoples of the Russian Far East are also reported to suffer debilitating symptoms because of their overindulgence with the fly-agaric (see **Fly-Agaric**). From rather closer to home comes an isolated account of a fungus being implicated in a 'drunk driver' case. This rather bizarre and unusual story was reported in the *Daily Telegraph* on 13 March 1937, in which it seems that a mushroom-intoxicated driver was prosecuted at the Clerkenwell police court in London.

Hallucinogenic species of *Panaeolus* or *Pholiota* have been identified as the fungi referred to in early Chinese accounts as *hsiao chün* or 'laughing mushrooms' and in Japan as *waraitake*, which also means 'laughing mushroom'. An amusing incident of accidental mushroom intoxication is included in an eleventh-century collection of Japanese folk stories entitled *Konjaku monogatari* ('Tales of Long Ago'), translated by James Sanford:

> Long long ago, some woodcutters from Kyoto went into the Kitayama mountains and lost their way. Not knowing which way to go, four or five of them were lamenting their condition when they heard a group of people coming from the depths of the mountains. The woodcutters were wondering suspiciously what sort of people it might be when four or five Buddhist nuns came out dancing and singing. Seeing them, the woodcutters became fearful, thinking things like, 'Dancing, singing nuns are certainly not human beings but must be goblins or demons.' And when the nuns saw the men and started straight toward them, the woodcutters became very frightened and wondered, 'How is it that nuns come thus out of the very depths of the mountains dancing and singing?'
>
> The nuns then said, 'Our appearance dancing and singing has no doubt frightened you. But we are simply nuns who live nearby. We came to pick flowers as offerings to Buddha, but after we had all entered the hills together we lost our way and couldn't remember how to get out. Then we came upon some mushrooms, and although we wondered whether we might not be poisoned if we ate them, we were hungry and decided it was better to pick them than to starve to death. But after we had picked and roasted them we found they were quite delicious, and thinking, "Aren't these fine!" we ate them. But then as we finished the mushrooms we found we couldn't keep from dancing . . .' the woodcutters were no end surprised at this unusual story.

Now the woodcutters were very hungry so they thought, 'Better than dying let's ask for some too.' And they ate some of the numerous mushrooms that the nuns had picked, whereupon they also were compelled to dance. In that condition the nuns and the woodcutters laughed and danced round together. After a while the intoxication seemed to wear off and somehow they all found their separate ways home.

Cases of both accidental intoxication by *Panaeolus* species and its recreational use have been reported from the eastern United States. It is not just hippies and others seeking psychedelic highs that deliberately used the mushrooms but also local farmers wanting to get 'drunk for nothing'!

The Taoists of ancient China seem to have made use of the fly-agaric mushroom (see **Fly-Agaric**) and often make reference to the 'Divine Mushroom of Immortality', an epithet used by Wasson in his book. The writings of ancient China are replete with many other references to psychoactive fungi and there is even a work called *On the Planting and Cultivation of Magic Mushrooms*. According to the account of Thao Hung-Ching, writing in AD 515, a respected young Taoist of the time named Chou Tzu-Liang died at the age of only twenty, apparently as the result of ingesting toxic fungi. There are frescoes decorating the Koguryo tombs of Korea (sixth and seventh centuries AD) that depict Taoist Immortals and their female consorts, known as Jade Girls, picking 'magic mushrooms'. *Fu-ling*, a parasitic fungus that grows on the roots of the pine tree – *Polyporus cocos* or *Poria* (*Pachyma*) cocos – is also considered to be an 'immortal medicine' in Chinese tradition. The Chinese Buddhist text called the Tripitaka (*Ta Tsang*) contains an account of a sage taking refuge in the mountains in order to meditate and consume mushroom elixirs. Yet, it would be simplistic to think that the Chinese attitude to psychoactive mushrooms was universally favourable. Wasson cites a twelfth-century Chinese official who berated the followers of the Manichaean religion (founded by the Iranian Mani, but once of some influence in parts of China largely through the efforts of Iranian and Central Asian travelling merchants) for consuming mushrooms as part of their religious observances. Wasson interprets this as an attack on the use of the fly-agaric as the same official states that the Manichaeans also ritually washed with urine.

Among both the Indians and Eskimos of Alaska and the Yukon chewing tobacco is mixed with fungus ash. The Eskimos of the Bering Strait would chop their tobacco finely on a wooden cutting board, then mix it with the ashes of a burnt fungus. The mixture was then kneaded like dough and shaped into pellets. If the ashes were still not mixed in thoroughly enough one of the women would chew it until, with the help of her saliva, the quid was ready. As with many other 'chewing' preparations (see, for example, **Betel**, **Coca**, **Pituri**) it was not really chewed at all but held in the cheek. An Eskimo man would often take the quid out of his mouth and put it behind his right ear. Interestingly enough, the Aborigines of Australia do exactly the same with their *pituri* quids (see **Pituri**). It has been suggested that the Aborigines do this because the 'drug' permeates the skin behind the ear (which is much thinner than most other parts of the body). At least in the Eskimo case, it may simply be done to store the quid temporarily when required, very much as a cigarette is put behind the ear until required. The fungi in question were important items in the traditional trading networks of this region.

Nor has this tradition died out. The use of 'chew-ash', as it is called in the Yukon, is still a popular habit. According to the Canadian mycologist Paul Kroeger, a community school teacher in the region, reported that children that used chew-ash in school were generally more sedate than other children in the class. Chew-ash is made by reducing a birch polypore fungus (*Phellinus igniarius* = *Fomes igniarius*) to ash and then mixing it with chewing tobacco and sometimes commercial tea leaves. Although both tobacco and tea are stimulants, the resulting mixture is said to act as a sedative, which seems to indicate some mildly psychoactive input from the fungus (although this species is not known to have such effects). Other variations on the chew-ash theme include the addition of alcohol to fortify the mixture. An old Indian trapper named Joe Henry (belonging to the Gwich'in people of the Dene Nation) was reported to heat tree fungi in old coffee cans over a fire and then mix the resulting ash with tobacco soaked in rum (whisky is also reported as an additive).

Known among the Yupik Eskimo of Nelson Island as *iqemik*, the bracket fungus *Fomes pinicola* was burnt and the ashes were then mixed with snuff, said to give it a real 'kick'. On the other side of the Bering Strait the Kamchadal people used a fungus to make a snuff. The Khanty (Ostyak) people of western Siberia made a snuff out of a birch fungus, and they still use the ashes of the poly-pore fungus, *Phellinus nigricans,* in the making of a chewing tobacco mixture that is used by both men and women. Both the North American Indians and the Siberians use a number of different kinds of fungi as sacred incenses to drive away evil spirits and to ritually purify themselves.

There are also reports of the use of psychoactive mushrooms by some of the native cultures of Melanesia. In 1936 Father William A. Ross described an outbreak of 'mushroom madness' among the people of the Mount Hagen region of the New Guinea Highlands in the following terms: 'the wild mushroom called *nonda* makes the user temporarily insane. He flies into a fit of frenzy. Death is even known to have resulted from its use. It is used before going out to kill another native, or in times of great excitement, anger or sorrow.' Other cases of the 'mushroom madness' are known, such as the bacchanalia of the Sina-Sina people which is called *kirin*. Wasson and Heim concluded that the 'mushroom madness' was not in fact caused by psychoactive fungi at all and that the answer to this strange social phenomenon lay in 'mythology not mycology'. Heim and Wasson were only in New Guinea for a short period and, as William Emboden has pointed out, one cannot expect that native people will talk openly to strangers about sacred plants and fungi. This opinion is supported by the account of Fitz Poole, an anthropologist who spent considerable time among the Bimin-Kuskusmin, a small New Guinea community that had a full-blown mushroom cult and, despite his exemplary skill as a field worker, was unable to discover which species of mushroom were used by the elders in their esoteric and therefore private rituals.

The male initiation cult of the Bimin-Kuskusmin is the vehicle for both storing and transmitting the essence of their cultural lore. It is a hierarchical organisation comprising twelve successive stages of initiation, a deeper level of esoteric knowledge being imparted at each one. The elders of the highest degrees have themselves passed through each of the initiatory ordeals of the lower ranks. Although a considerable number of psychoactive plants are used in Bimin-Kuskusmin ritual life, three types of substance are central to the workings of the cult: ginger, tobacco and hallucinogenic mushrooms. All three are sacred and are ritually tended to by sacrificing marsupials and rodents at the place of their growth. Both women and children are forbidden to approach these sacred substances. The first ten degrees represent the complete cycle of male initiation, whilst the eleventh and twelfth are the junior and senior grades of a ritual elder. Novices belonging to the first three grades are given ginger which, although it is not normally considered to be a psychoactive plant, does cause visual and auditory hallucinogens when taken (as it is among the Bimin-Kuskusmin) after fasting and whilst in a state of great expectation and fear. Initiates of the next six stages smoke sacred tobacco whilst the mushrooms are only used by those in the highest three grades. Thus, each successive stage involves taking a more potent psychoactive substance. Whilst an individual is allowed to use the sacred substance appropriate to his grade (or that of any lower grade) on no account is he permitted to try those of higher levels. During the states of trance induced by each of the substances the initiate is said to travel out of his body and, with the help of a guardian ancestor spirit, visit the ancestral world. If he makes this difficult journey successfully then he will gain the sacred knowledge appropriate to one of his station.

Each of these twelve journeys is seen as an ordeal, not only offering the reward of spiritual revelations but also demonstrating the initiate's growing ability to control his consciousness. As is so often the case with the ritualistic use of hallucinogens the ecstatic experience of the journey must first be prepared for by undergoing privations. Abstinence from sleep, food and water are increasingly enforced as an individual climbs the rungs of the initiation cult. The most extreme preparations are therefore those of the final grade of senior elder. He must go three nights without food or sleep and two days without water before taking the secret type of mushroom alone in the mountains at night. This mushroom is said to be so potent that it would poison even the senior ritual elders if it were taken outside the context of the final rite.

In Bali the native people are reported to cultivate the hallucinogenic fungus *Copelandia cyanescens* both for their own use and to sell to tourists and hippies. It contains the psychoactive psilocin and psilocybin and is far more potent than species of *Psilocybe* mushrooms (see **Psilocybe**). There are numerous other intriguing references to fungi in the works of early travellers, anthropologists, herbalists and botanists which strongly hint that many more mushroom cults await discovery. Leona Stukey Tucker wrote that the Ovimbundu people of Angola call a certain tree fungus *ova wuti* which means 'dream'; perhaps a reference to psycho-active properties. Despite its great diversity and rich fungal wildlife no mushroom cult has been found in the entire continent of Africa. Despite the fact that there have been quite a few finds of species of tinder fungus (punk) and puffballs and other fungi having medicinal properties at prehistoric sites (and on the body of the famous Ice Man discovered a few years ago in the Alps) in various parts of Europe, no comparable use of hallucinogenic or narcotic mushrooms has come to light. There are vague reports, such as Robert Graves' assertion that Portuguese witches in the twentieth century used the hallucinogenic *Panaeolus papilionaceus*, and accounts of the Basque witches collecting puffballs and other fungi, but hard historical and ethnographic data has not yet been forthcoming. An early eighteenth-century English source des-cribes an unidentified species as being: 'about half an inch broad, spiring a little at the top; of a whitish colour, with a long stalk, and of the bigness of one's little Fingger [sic]. This is also called the Foolls Mushroom.' A Fool's Mushroom would seem to point to a hallucinogenic species. The vast amount of European folklore compiled by Wasson and his wife on the fly-agaric and other mushrooms indicates that in many areas of the Continent there were taboos in place against the use of certain fungi, suggesting an ancient ritual role for them. Despite the great efforts of the Wassons, neither archaeological sites nor archival materials have yielded up sufficient proof of such a cult.

Research into the traditional use of psychoactive fungi is still very much an ongoing project and many more discoveries will doubtless be made.

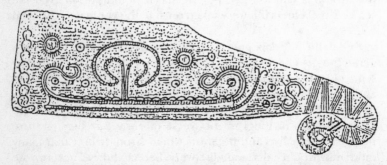

**BRONZE AGE RAZOR FROM SCANDINAVIA WITH 'MUSHROOM' MOTIF**

(See also: **Ergot**, **Fly-agaric**, **Puffballs**, **Amanita Pantherina**, **Psilocybe**.)

**Sources:** Ager and Ager 1980, Ellis 1946, Furst 1988, Graves 1976, Heim and Wasson 1965, Kroeger 1993a, Kroeger 1993b, Morgan 1995, Needham SCC 5, 6/1, Nelson 1899, Ott 1993, Poole 1987, Ramsbottom 1953, Reay 1960, Riedlinger 1990, Ross 1936, Saar 1991b, Salmon 1710, Sanford 1972, Schultes 1940, Schultes and Hofmann 1980a, Schultes and Hofmann 1980b, Tucker 1910, Wasson 1968, Wasson and Wasson 1957.

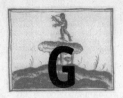

## GLUE SNIFFING see Inhalants

## GOOFBALLS see Barbiturates

## GUARANA

Guarana (*Paullinia cupana, P.* spp.) is a woody vine that grows in the central Amazon basin. The seeds contain both theobromine and caffeine. Caffeine is the more concentrated and the fresh seeds may contain up to 3.5 per cent caffeine; it is estimated to be three times the strength of coffee. An essential oil in the plant is reported to have minor aphrodisiac and psychoactive properties. Some other species of the genus are toxic and have been used in tribal societies as fish poisons. The plant is used by various Indian cultures of the region who use it as a stimulant, particularly when hunting, as its considerable caffeine content maintains a high level of alertness. It also has a number of medical applications, such as a cure for headaches and a treatment for diarrhoea and fevers. Among the Tupi Indians it has an important place in the practices of shamans. In one of their myths a female shaman named Omniamasabé was highly revered for her esoteric knowledge. Whilst in the forest she was made pregnant by the snake god Mboy and had a son from him. Her brother on hearing of this employed a shaman to kill his nephew. The shaman then took *ayahuasca* and transformed himself into a parrot. In this form he flew off and, managing to locate the boy, killed him. Omniamasabé, on finding her dead son, wept upon his body, which transformed him into the guarana plant. Shamans who wish to learn the arcane lore of Omniamasabé eat the fruits of the bush.

Guarana is now cultivated commercially and its seeds are used for making a popular carbonated soft drink. Powder and concentrate are also produced. Guarana has begun to make commercial inroads to the Western market, aided by growing public knowledge of, and interest in, Amazonia and its indigenous peoples. The marketing of one such product, 'Buzz Gum', relies heavily on its natural 'jungle' image.

(See also **Caffeine.**)

**Sources:** Erickson et al 1984, Rätsch 1992, Schultes and Hofmann 1980a.

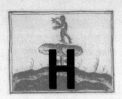

## HALLUCINOGENS

The name given to a group of psychoactive substances that cause visual, auditory and other sensory hallucinations. The term seems to have first been used by three physicians – Humphry Osmond, John Smythies and Abram Hoffer – and it first appeared in print in Donald Johnson's *The Hallucinogenic Drugs* (1953). Naturally occurring and synthetic substances that are usually designated as hallucinogens include 'magic mushrooms'(*Psilocybe* spp.), the fly-agaric mushroom (*Amanita muscaria*), LSD, peyote, ayahuasca, mescaline, the San Pedro cactus and species of *Datura*. Some researchers have found the use of this term unsatisfactory and prefer to designate the use of such sacred substances as 'entheogens' (see **Entheogen**). The psychoactive effects of the hallucinogens have been eloquently described by Albert Hofmann, the discoverer of LSD, in an unpublished lecture quoted by Christian Rätsch:

Hallucinogens distinguish themselves from all other psychoactive substances through their extremely profound effects upon the human psyche. They bring about radical psychological changes which are associated with altered experiences of space and time, the most basic categories of human existence. Even the consciousness of one's own corporeality and one's own self may be changed dramatically. Hallucinogens take us to another world, to a type of dream world which is nevertheless experienced as completely real, as even more intense and consequently in some ways more real than the ordinary world of everyday reality. At the same time, if the dosage is not too high, consciousness and memory are retained completely. This is a key distinction between these substances and the opiates and other intoxicants, whose effects are associated with an obscuration of consciousness.

**HAOMA** see **Soma**

**HARMEL** see **Peganum Harmala**

**HEMP** see **Cannabis**

**HENBANE**

There are about fifteen species of henbane (*Hyoscyamus* spp.) found in Europe, North Africa, western Asia, India, Central Asia and China. The most notable for both its traditional uses as a psychoactive plant and because of its recent cultivation as a source of medicinal drugs is black henbane (*Hyoscyamus niger*). Black henbane grows to between a foot and two-and-a-half feet and has sombre green-grey leaves. The flowers are white or faint yellow in colour with purplish veins and the seeds are dark grey. The plant has an unpleasant fetid odour which inspired two of its names in folk botany – stinking nightshade and stinking Roger. It flowers in July or August and the seeds are ripe in October. It grows on wasteland and near rubbish dumps and abandoned human habitations, or, in the words of an early herbalist, 'rude and untilled places'. The psychoactive alkaloids are present in all parts of the plant but more concentrated in the seeds and especially the roots. High doses can be poisonous. It contains the tropane alkaloids, the main one being hyoscyamine, but scopolamine (the main hallucinogenic agent) and atropine are also present.

Henbane has a soporific action, induces stupefaction, irrational behaviour and, in the words of William Salmon, 'abates acrimony'. Visual, auditory, olfactory, gustatory and tactile hallucinations (whether awake or asleep whilst under its influence), temporary loss of memory (users report difficulty in recalling the experience of intoxication in any detail), distortions of vision and hearing, profuse sweating and physical discomfort, sometimes involving the sensation that the body is breaking up or dissolving, intense pressure in the head, macroscopia (i.e. seeing objects as larger than they actually are), constant desire to move, lack of

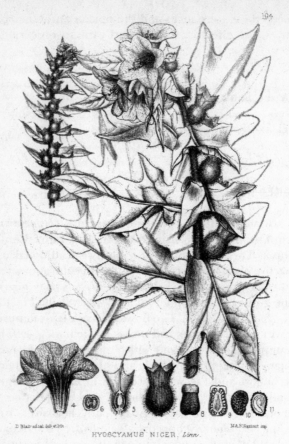

HYOSCYAMUS NIGER, *Linn.*

## HENBANE

consciousness of the external world and sensations of flight. According to Welsh folk belief if a child falls asleep near the henbane plant he or she may die. This echoes a similar belief concerning the related mandrake plant, the mere fragrance of which is said to cause deep sleep (see **Mandrake**). These two beliefs, whilst exaggerations, are based on truth for both plants have soporific and toxic effects.

To the Greeks it was known by a number of names, including Pythonion (perhaps because the drug was used by the Delphic oracle?), Adamas and Atomon. Henbane was also known as the Apollonian herb because its hallucinogenic properties inspired prophetic utterances and dreams. Pliny had this to say about henbane and its effects:

> All [kinds of *Hyoscyamus*] trouble the braine, and put men besides their right wits; beside that, they breed dizziness of the head . . . henbane is of the nature of wine, and therefore offensive to the understanding, and troubleth the head. However, good use there is, both of the seed it selfe . . . and also of the oile or juice drawne out of it apart . . . for my own part, I hold it to be dangerous medicine, and not to be used but with great heed and discretion. For this is certainly knowne, that, if one take in drinke more than four leaves, thereof, it will put him beside himself.

Among henbane's many medical applications in Greece was its use as an anaesthetic, a practice that was carried on to the Middle Ages (as was also the case with mandrake; see **Mandrake**).

The plant genus derives its name from *Hyoscyamus*, meaning 'hog's bean'. Some believe it was called this because it was poisonous to pigs (the source of the later European name 'swine's bane'). In the Semitic languages henbane is known as *sakiru* in Assyrian, *sakrona* in Aramaic, *shakhrona* in Syriac and *saykaran* in Arabic. In the Middle East it was known as *bang* (rendered as *bangue* or *bengi* by the seventeenth- and eighteenth-century physicians of Europe), and seems also to have been the hallucinogenic substance *mang* which played an important role in the religion of ancient Iran (see **Mang**). The English name henbell dates from around AD 1000 (bell referring to the shape of the flower). The name henbane comes from Anglo-Saxon roots and means simply hen bane (or poison). Other names, such as stinking nightshade and fetid nightshade, show how closely it was associated in folk botany with its sister plant belladonna (see **Belladonna**). Henbane has been known under a variety of other epithets, including henquale and castilago, and it was sold by apothecaries as Iusquiamus and Hyoscyamus.

According to the herbalist John Gerard: 'when the [henbane] flowers are gone, there commeth harde knobbie huskes, like small cups or boxes wherein are small brown seedes.' A type of prehistoric pottery known as 'grape cups' may perhaps be skeuomorphs of henbane's 'knobbie huskes' (for an explanation of the term skeuomorph and its use in interpreting prehistoric artefacts

see **Datura**). Henbane has been found in connection with prehistoric human habitations dating back to the Neolithic. In the
mid-1980s at Balfarg Riding School, Glenrothes, Fife in eastern
Scotland, an important group of Neolithic ritual enclosures
(including a stone circle) were excavated. Significant among the
archaeological finds were many broken pieces of pottery of the
type known as Grooved Ware (*c.*2800–2300 BC). Analysis of the
botanical residues preserved in the pottery fragments revealed the
presence of a number of plants, including henbane. Sherratt has
suggested that henbane may have played an important role in the
ecstatic rites of such Stone Age communities. At a Bronze Age
settlement site located in northern Serbia a large amount of
henbane seeds have been recovered and seeds were also found in
a Bronze Age grave at Leobersdorf in Austria. Black henbane was
a common weed around prehistoric settlements in Britain and
elsewhere in both the Bronze and Iron Ages.

The psychoactive properties of henbane were also recognised
and made use of in Asia. Li Shih-chen, writing in the sixteenth
century, notes that the seeds of henbane (Lang-tang) increase
stamina and aid communication with demons and other spirits. In
1561 a Chinese warlord offered wine to Kitan tribesmen who had
surrendered to him. Unaware that the wine had been laced with
henbane, they drank it and fell unconscious and were buried alive
by the warlord's troops. The Tungus people of Siberia make a
coffee substitute out of the roasted seeds of *H. physaloides. H.
reticulatus* is reportedly used traditionally in Afghanistan as a
hallucinogen and *H. niger* used transdermally (i.e. through the
skin, as with the witches' preparations which also contained black
henbane; see **Witches' Ointments**) in conjunction with the fly-
agaric mushroom. Henbane has been used in India as a form of
birth control; the seeds are mixed with mare's milk to make a
paste which is kept wrapped in a piece of wild bull's skin and then
worn by the woman. In Kashmir and Pakistan henbane is sometimes smoked with tobacco or cannabis.

Remains of the henbane plant have been found at ancient
Egyptian sites, such as the rubbish dump at the animal cemetery at
Saqqâra. It is also mentioned in the *Ebers Papyrus* (*c.*1500 BC).
Seeds of *H. muticus* have also been found in a burial site dating
from the New Kingdom. Henbane has been widely used by the
Bedouin people. The Bedouin of the Negev region of southern
Israel smoke a few henbane leaves to alleviate the symptoms of

shortness of breath, depression and nervousness. Although considered socially reprehensible among the Bischarin Bedouins of Egypt, the smoking of hallucinogenic henbane flowers (*H. boveanus*) with other herbs or tobacco is, nevertheless, known among them. The Khushmaan Ma'aza Bedouins have told visitors that they previously smoked the leaves of the same species for its intoxicating effects. The abuse of henbane by children in Turkey has also been reported.

The Vikings made use of henbane, as is made clear by the discovery of several hundred seeds in a female grave in north Jutland dated to the tenth century. This archaeological find suggests that henbane may have played a role in their funerary practices. In the tenth-century Anglo-Saxon *Leech Book of Bald and Cild* (the first 'modern' medical text in Western Europe) there is a medical preparation described as: 'a salve against the elfin race and nocturnal visitors, and for women with whom the devil hath carnal commerce.' The ingredients of this salve/ointment include henbane. The vessel containing the salve is placed under the altar where the ritual exorcism is to take place. Nine masses are to be sung over it and then the eyes and forehead of the patient are rubbed with the ointment whilst they are censed with incense and the sign of the cross is made over them. As henbane was an ingredient the salve would have been topically active, that is to say applying it to the skin would have caused psychoactive effects. This use of such an ointment in apparent harmony with the Christian tradition is particularly surprising as similar ointments containing henbane and other narcotic and hallucinogenic drugs were later used by European witches and, as such, seen as demonic in origin (see **Witches' Ointments**).

According to the sixteenth-century magician Henry Cornelius Agrippa, henbane is a plant that is under the astral influence of Jupiter, although it is also one of the constituents of the suffumigation (magical incense) of Saturn, according to the same author. Agrippa also gives recipes for two psychoactive suffumigations, the first, consisting of henbane, hemlock, smallage and coriander, when made, brings visions of spirits; the second, of sagapen, the juice of hemlock, henbane, black poppy and other herbs, makes spirits and strange shapes appear (he adds that if smallage is added, the spirits are chased away and the visions pass). The magical and medicinal uses of henbane often overlapped. In order to make a charm effective against gout it was said that henbane should be gathered when the moon is in the sign of Aquarius or Cancer just before dusk, with the warning not to touch the root but dig it up by using a bone. The collector then fashions the root into an amulet which when worn is believed to have the desired effect. There was once a widespread tradition in Europe that on St John the Baptist's Day (24 June) – a holiday replacing the pagan celebration of the summer solstice – henbane was burnt in stables to drive away evil spirits from livestock and from children, who would go in procession through the ritually purified stables.

Henbane also had numerous other medical uses. Excavators working under Dr Brian Moffat at the Soutra Medieval hospital near Edinburgh in Scotland (which flourished 1190–1460 and was run by Augustinian monks) unearthed a cache of 574 seeds of hemlock, opium poppy and henbane; the great majority of them were henbane, showing that it was an important medicinal plant, valued for its anaesthetic properties. In Italy it was called Priapeia and is said to have been used to treat priapism. The soporific effects of henbane could apparently be made use of by the insomniac bathing the feet in a decoction of the plant. An extract of henbane was also used by Anthony Störck in the 1760s to treat the mentally ill. Henbane was often added as an ingredient in the making of laudanum and other opium preparations. Henbane was not just used in medicine and magic in early Europe, it also had its hedonistic uses. The Old Germanic tribes put it in their beer and mead, which makes the 'strong ales' of today seem rather tame. In some of the bath-houses of early Europe – a kind of forerunner of the seedy sauna – henbane seeds were burnt on hot dishes as an erotic incense designed to encourage sexual abandon.

Henbane seems to have first reached the Americas through the Spanish. Because of its psychoactive powers, and, no doubt, due to its similarity to the indigenous datura, Californian and Mexican Indians have made use of it in the form of an infusion and also as an additive to their alcoholic drinks.

**Sources:** Abu-Rabia 1983, Bennett 1991, Braunschweig 1527, Bulleyn 1562, Camporesi 1989, Coles 1657, Gerard 1597, Goodman and Hobbs 1988, The Grete Herball 1526, Heiser 1969, Mabey 1996, Manniche 1989, Mehra 1979, Ott 1993, Radford and Radford 1980, Rätsch 1992, Rudgley 1995, Salmon 1693, Schenk 1956, Schultes and Hofmann 1980b, Sherratt 1996a, Störck 1763, Thorndike 1923–58.

# HEROIN

As the abuse of morphine and other opiates is inextricably linked to the history of heroin use, it is included here. Although heroin (known by a number of street names, such as junk, scag, smack and horse) is quite often smoked or snorted, the main way of administering the drug is by injection, using a hypodermic syringe. The needle can be put under the surface of the skin (a practice known as 'skin-popping') or intravenously ('mainlining', if into one of the main veins). The injecting of heroin results in near-instantaneous analgesic and euphoric effects. The user experiences a state of well-being and tranquillity and this accompanies a general depressing of the central nervous system, with a slowing of the pulse and breathing rate and a drop in blood pressure. As is the case with tobacco, initial use may cause nausea and discomfort. Opiates such as heroin are extremely addictive and regular users find they often need much higher doses to get the same feeling as novices. Chronic heroin addicts can inject extraordinary amounts of the drug that would kill an inexperienced user. The widespread misconception that smoking or snorting the drug means that the user side-steps the danger of becoming addicted is false. The opiate molecules ape the effects of naturally occurring chemicals in the brain which helps to explain why the desire to introduce them into the body in artificially high amounts is so strong. Somewhat perversely these substances are called endorphins, a word coined from the Greek words meaning 'morphine within'. Aside from the real possibility of addiction with all the problems that that entails, there are numerous other serious health risks involved with the use of the drug. Death can occur from taking an overdose of heroin or from injecting contaminated supplies of the drug which may contain a wide variety of potentially lethal adulterants. Other dangers include blood poisoning and, if using a dirty or shared needle, AIDS. As with any hypodermic injection, if an air bubble is injected death can be almost immediate. A number of drugs have been used with greater or lesser success rates in the treatment of heroin addiction, including methadone.

The stereotypical image of the modern user of opiates is that of the back-alley junkie. Whilst many heroin users are forced by their habit and their 'criminal status' into such lifestyles, this is too narrow a view. One of the side-effects of the invention of the

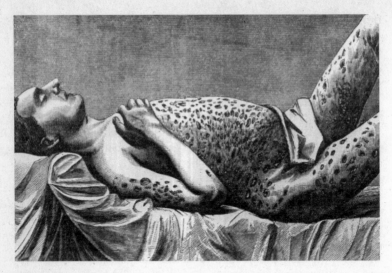

**MORPHINE ADDICT**

hypodermic syringe in 1845 was inadvertently addicting those who were too liberally injected with morphine on medical grounds. Thousands of troops returning home from the American Civil War were coming back into civilian life as addicts who had become used to regular shots of morphine. Marek Kohn, in a historical investigation of the early drug scene in Britain, cites a turn-of-the-century newspaper report of morphine use at a well-to-do ladies' tea party: 'The fashion, which is said to have originated in Paris, consists of the formation of what may be termed a morphine club. A number of ladies meet about four o'clock every afternoon, tea is served, servants are sent out of the room, the guests bare their arms and the hostess produces a small hypodermic syringe with which she administers an injection to each person in turn.'

Heroin was initially synthesised from morphine in 1898 and was actually thought at this time to be useful in treating morphine addiction. The name heroin was given to this novel substance by the pharmaceutical company Bayer, who produced a cough medicine that contained it. At first its addictive properties were not recognised and when US legislation just before the First World War effectively reduced the distribution of other opiates and of cocaine, heroin slipped through the net. One of the consequences was that many of those who were addicted to opium, morphine and other opiates became heroin addicts. It was only in 1924 that a federal law was passed making heroin an illegal substance. Having now become criminals, heroin users were pursued with considerable gusto by the authorities, and doctors were prosecuted in great numbers if found to be supplying addicts' needs. Much of the anti-heroin rhetoric of the time foreshadowed the War on Drugs that has dominated late twentieth-century official thinking. Heroin addicts (usually dubbed 'dope fiends') were portrayed as intertwined with politically destabilising forces such as anarchism and Bolshevism. The fact that the drug was synthesised by the Germans gave American propagandists during the First World War further fuel to fan anti-German feeling. After the war some attempts were made in the United States to give heroin addicts the opportunity to get detoxification treatment but, due to pressure from puritanical groups, this policy was seen as condoning or even propagating heroin use, and the clinics that had been set up soon closed down. This attitude must be seen in the light of contemporary events, particularly as in 1919 the Prohibition era had started. Under Prohibition the highly profitable drug trade (largely, of course, the dealing in alcohol which was then an illegal substance) built the criminal foundations for the later, even more profitable, narcotics business. In Britain the situation was completely different and, until the 1960s, heroin users were generally seen as medical patients whose problems were to be dealt with by doctors who could provide them with morphine and related drugs to monitor and hopefully to ease their condition.

Statistics concerning the distribution and use of heroin are notoriously inaccurate since both the majority of addicts avoid official surveillance like the plague and most governments are reluctant to advertise the extent of their drug problems. However, the estimates clearly show that the problem is on a very large scale; in 1985 there were said to be between 600,000 and 700,000 heroin addicts in the USA, about a third of them in New York City. Heroin addiction is a world-wide concern and, whilst the Communist world had, comparatively speaking, a relatively minor problem, the collapse of the Soviet Union and changes in policy in China has meant an increased availability and use of the drug in both regions. Reports also suggest a growing level of addiction in Pakistan and Latin America. With an inevitably high demand for the drug there is no shortage of willing suppliers. India and Turkey are key producers of the opium destined for the legitimate market in codeine, morphine and other much needed medical drugs. Turkish traffickers were also once one of the main suppliers to the black market, but they suffered a major setback when their inroads into Europe (and indirectly to the United States) via Marseilles were cut off with the defeat of the smugglers, as immortalised in the film *The French Connection*, starring Gene Hackman. The Golden Triangle (an area incorporating parts of Thailand, Burma and Laos) is still seen as the epicentre of the cultivation of the opium poppy for use in the international heroin trade. More recently the Colombian cocaine cartels have financed the widespread cultivation of poppies in their own region in order to rival their Asian counterparts. The heroin trade is seen by them as potentially far more profitable than the selling of cocaine, and with more direct access to the enormous North American market, it seems likely that they will meet with considerable success.

On the economics of the heroin trade, William Burroughs, ex-junkie and ground-breaking author of *The Naked Lunch* writes: 'Junk is the ideal product . . . the ultimate merchandise. No sales talk necessary. The client will crawl through a sewer and beg to buy . . . The junk merchant does not sell his product to the consumer, he sells the consumer to his product.' The blank, hermetically sealed and sessile world of the heroin addict is again captured succinctly by Burroughs:

Morphine alters the whole cycle of expansion and contraction, release and tension. The sexual function is deactivated, peristalsis inhibited, the pupils cease to react in response to light and darkness. The organism neither contracts from pain nor expands to normal sources of pleasure. It adjusts to a morphine cycle. The addict is immune to boredom. He can look at his shoes for hours or simply stay in bed. He needs no sexual outlet, no social contacts, no work, no diversion, no exercise, nothing but morphine. Morphine may relieve pain by imparting to the organism some of the qualities of a plant.

Elsewhere in the same work, based on his experiences with heroin use in a society which outlaws the drug and so condemns the addict to the status of a criminal, Burroughs wrote that 'there are no opium cults'. In fact there is evidence that prehistoric societies of the Mediterranean used opium in their cult practices (see **Opium**). Despite, or perhaps because of, heroin's image as the most evil and dangerous of all drugs, it has had a certain cult status in the music scene. Numerous rock songs have been written about the drug – 'Heroin' and 'I'm Waiting for the Man' by the Velvet Underground, 'Sister Morphine' and 'Brown Sugar' by the Rolling Stones and 'Golden Brown' by the Stranglers, to name but a few.

**Sources:** Abel 1980, Burroughs 1959, Kohn 1992, Tyler 1995, Zackon 1988, Zzaro 1977.

## HYPNOTICS

A class of psychoactive substances that William Emboden has described as: 'organic or inorganic chemicals causing . . . sedation, tranquillity, stupor.' The hypnotic group correspond to Louis Lewin's earlier class which he called Hypnotica. The narcotics (see **Narcotics**) can be described as a sub-class of the hypnotics.

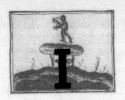

**IBOGA** see **Eboga**

**ICE** see **Amphetamines**

## INHALANTS

Inhalants are a group of volatile substances that are rarely produced for their psychoactive properties but can be abused for such purposes. Glue, petrol or gasoline, carpet cleaners, paint thinners, fire extinguishers, correction fluids and aerosols (such as hairspray, insect sprays and deodorants) are all used as cheap, legal but highly dangerous inhalants. Other substances such as ether, chloroform and nitrous oxide – all developed as anaesthetic agents – may also be categorised under the general heading of inhalants.

The effects of nitrous oxide go beyond its role as 'laughing gas'. Sir Humphrey Davy, who first realised its medical applications, described the effects it had on him:

> I felt all the links in my relationship with the outer world loosen and break. Trains of vivid, visible images rapidly crossed my mind. Another time I felt with indescribable pleasure the sense of touch increasing in my feet and hands. Dazzling perspectives enthralled me. I distinctly heard the most imperceptible sounds ... and no aspect of my condition could escape me. Little by little, the crisis becoming intense, I was completely cut off from my natural perceptions. I felt a physical and involuntary detachment that lifted me from my earthly cares and caused me to pass, through voluptuous transitions, into delicate sensations that, speaking candidly, were completely new to me. It seemed that, in

my privileged condition, everything was performed spon-
taneously and instinctively. Time, in other words, existed
only in my memory, and in a flash the most remote traditions
were revived in all their splendour.

The use and abuse of solvents and other volatile substances and
inhalants seems to go back to the time that they were first made,
largely for industrial purposes. Louis Lewin documented a case in
the 1920s of a German bandage-maker who sniffed benzine for its
hallucinogenic effects. The great blues singer and harp player
'Sonny Boy' (John Lee) Williamson (born *c.*1916 and murdered
on 1 June 1948) is said to have overindulged in the sniffing of shoe
polish. Petrol sniffing is indulged in, largely by adolescents, in
both urban and rural Australia. Among remote Aboriginal communities in the 'outback' the habit began, rather sporadically, in
the 1940s and 1950s and by the mid-1970s had become a significant social problem, although it was never undertaken by more
than a small minority. As with so many other inhalants, the side-
effects of its chronic abuse are serious and include seizures, brain
damage and even death. Petrol sniffing has none of the romantic
allure that leads people to use other psychoactive substances, it
has no real ceremonial to accompany it; it is simply the inhalation
of a brutally industrial fluid. Yet even with petrol the social
environment in which it is used connects it with cultural
traditions. The acquisition of X-ray vision and the ability to run at
extraordinary speeds are feats attributed to petrol sniffers. Both
these magical powers are among those attributed in Aboriginal
traditions to sorcerers and ritual elders.

Glue sniffing came to public attention during the late 1970s
when it was a drug of choice among young punks. Not only was
this a rejection of other drugs, those associated with the rather
turgid rock establishment, it also embodied the punk ethos, as
Richard Ives put it: 'Punk was about expropriating consumer
items and turning them into art, and glue fitted perfectly with that
kind of ideology. They took a mundane, ordinary, everyday
product that nobody thought about or had any feelings towards
and they got high on the stuff. They had hallucinations, they had
ecstatic experiences. They pulled a fast one against materialism.'
Glue sniffing played a role in the lifestyle of the punks from the
beginning; the first punk fanzine was called *Sniffin' Glue* and the
first Ramones album contains the anthem 'Now I Want to Sniff

Some Glue'. Although glue's complete lack of glamour was something that attracted the punks it is, more generally, perceived as a drug of the lowest status, its main users being children and young adolescents who cannot afford or get hold of other drugs.

The psychoactive effects of toluene (glue) include tactile, auditory and visual hallucinations, distortions in the perception of time, macroscopia and microscopia (i.e. seeing things as larger or smaller than they are respectively), euphoria, delusions, fear and marked changes in behaviour. The hallucinogenic experiences of one young glue sniffer are both innocently touching and yet disturbing: 'I take my toy soldiers, that's the best thing. I put them on the floor and they grow and talk to me, or they stay small and walk about on my hand. I had a toy ambulance and it grew to its proper size and two plastic men grew and became proper men and put me in the back to take me away because I was glue sniffing.' Glue and other inhalants are often taken by soaking a rag in the substance and then putting it in the mouth to get the full effect (this method is known as 'huffing') or putting the substance in a plastic bag and then holding the bag around the nose and inhaling ('bagging').

One cannot come further from the shamanic use of entheogenic plants to contact the spirits to the abuse of inhalants by adolescents whose phantasmagoric world is populated by UFOs and space invaders, Batman and Kung fu fighters drawn from TV programmes and computer games. The abuse of volatile hydrocarbon (butane gas) is largely undertaken by boys aged eight upwards. The psychoactive effects of butane are similar to those of toluene-based adhesives – auditory and visual hallucinations, macroscopia and microscopia, euphoria, anxiety and delusions (including the belief that one can fly, an effect which has caused injuries and even deaths). The statistics on fatalities caused by butane gas inhalation show that it is far more dangerous than many other drugs that have received a disproportionate slice of media attention. In the UK alone 398 people died from gas fuel abuse between the years 1988 and 1990; about a third of them were trying it for the first time. In the same period fatalities attributed to Ecstasy numbered less than ten. Gas fuel also caused way more deaths than either heroin or cocaine. Many of the fatal accidents happened when users sprayed the butane down their throats. As the highly compressed liquid from the canister rapidly expands it may get cold enough to freeze the larynx and result in the lungs being filled with fluid. This can cause death by drowning. Other butane-related deaths are caused by heart failure or by total lack of mental and physical co-ordination resulting in fatal falls or accidents involving cars or trains. Brain damage can also be caused by such substances.

Measures have been taken to limit volatile substance abuse in Britain. The 1985 Intoxicating Substances (Supply) Act makes it an offence for shopkeepers to sell substances with abuse potential to under-eighteens if they believe they are likely to be misused. Prosecutions under the Act have not been high and the effectiveness of such measures in significantly tackling the problem has been brought into question. The problems caused by the abuse of such substances in the Western world pale into insignificance when compared with the situation in the so-called Third World. According to Andrew Tyler:

> among the estimated 100 million street children worldwide, volatile-substance-sniffing is widely practised. It's done to stay alert to possible violence, to bring on sleep, to dull physical and emotional pain, or as a substitute for food. The products selected are the cheapest and most readily available: glues in shoemaking areas; solvents where there is nearby industry. In Uganda, street children gulp the fumes of aviation fuel and petrol. In Guatemala, as many as nine out of ten rough-sleeping youngsters are thought to be dependent on paint thinner and cheap glue. A South African survey of a group of their own young homeless showed high levels of brain damage, with the 'subjects' unable properly to think, speak, remember things, or physically co-ordinate their movements.

Of the various psychoactive substances the inhalants have the lowest status of all.

(See also **Ether**, **Nitrates**.)

**Sources:** Brady 1992, Evans and Raistrick 1987, Lange and Fralich 1989, Moreau de Tours 1973, Russell 1993, Sharp and Rosenberg 1992, Tyler 1995.

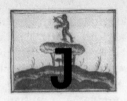

**JIMSON WEED** see **Datura**

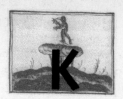

**K**

## KAVA

Kava is the name given by Pacific islanders to both *Piper methysticum*, a shrub belonging to the pepper family Piperaceae, and the psychoactive beverage made from it. *P. wichmannii* is now seen to be a wild variant of *P. methysticum* rather than a genuinely distinct species. *P. methysticum* is a hardy perennial which often grows up to three metres or more. The rootstock or stump contains the psychoactive substances. Its psychoactive constituents are called kavalactones and, despite claims to the contrary, there seem to be no psychoactive alkaloids in kava. The roots and stumps of kava are prepared by pounding, chewing or grinding them and soaking them in cold water. Drinking the resulting infusion has a soporific and narcotic effect. More specifically the user typically feels a state of mild euphoria and tranquillity. The muscles relax and the user remains in control; outbursts such as those precipitated by alcohol are alien to the kava experience. Some users report an increased mental clarity under its influence. As its effects go on its soporific qualities come to the fore and the user falls asleep. Occasionally drinkers may experience mild side effects such as double vision. Excessive drinking of kava has significant effects on the health particularly skin complaints and loss of appetite.

Unlike betel (also of the pepper family) which became a widely popular stimulant in the Pacific (see below and **Betel**), kava was not imported by man but rather discovered by him on his arrival in the region. Current research suggests that it may have first been domesticated less than 3,000 years ago in Vanuatu (which used to be called the New Hebrides), a group of islands in eastern Melanesia. The use of kava seems then to have diffused both westward to New Guinea and part of Micronesia and eastward into

Fiji and then Polynesia. The archaeology of the region has not, as yet, revealed much about the origins and early history of kava use. Part of a fossilised stem, which can only tentatively be suggested as belonging to the kava plant, was discovered at the Talepakemalai site on Eloaua Island north of the Bismarck Archipelago of Papua New Guinea. It was found in association with a highly decorated style of pottery known as Lapita. The Lapita peoples are thought to be the ancestors of the modern Polynesians and their pottery vessels to be early examples of bowls used in drinking kava. However, things do not fit that neatly together as Lapita artefacts have been found in areas outside the kava-drinking zone. Another theory (developed by the early anthropologist W.H.R. Rivers), which has largely been abandoned, is that kava-using people were displaced by incoming populations of betel-users who replaced the indigenous drug with their own in some regions of Melanesia. This is now seen as too simplistic and it fails to explain why some cultures in the region use both substances.

An indication of just how important kava cultivation has been in the Pacific is the sheer number of types which the indigenous people recognise. In Vanuatu alone natives are known to classify kava into 247 types! Kava was, and still is in many regions of the Pacific, an important medicine being used in the treatment of rheumatism, menstrual problems, venereal disease, tuberculosis and even leprosy. By putting kava leaves in the vagina, abortions were said to be provoked.

In the mythology and symbolism of the Pacific peoples kava has a distinctly sexual aura. The preparation of kava using the native equivalent of a pestle and mortar in Vanuatu and some Micronesian islands is seen as a symbolic form of sexual intercourse. In both Tonga and Fiji the legs of kava bowls are called breasts. Often the myths relating the origin of kava attribute its genesis or discovery to women, although drinking it is a male prerogative. For women to drink it is perceived to be 'unnatural' and a symbolic form of lesbianism. Yet, somewhat paradoxically, kava is widely recognised as an anaphrodisiac, i.e. reducing the desire for sex.

One of the traditional ways of preparing it was for the chewing of the kava to be performed by children or by a young woman (preferably a virgin). According to Lebot, Merlin and Lindstrom, who have written the definitive study of kava, the ceremony as conducted in Samoa: 'required the girl who chewed and infused the kava to sit cross-legged and bare-breasted on a mat behind the kava bowl, with flowers carefully arranged in her hair and her hips swathed in a grass skirt. This presented an image of beauty that added to the aesthetic dimension of kava preparation.' The practice of chewing kava appalled the missionaries, who effectively encouraged its replacement with the more 'genteel' method of grating it. The anthropologist Ron Brunton has noted that: 'from my own experience I suspect that there is little, if any, difference in the effects of kava prepared by the alternative techniques. I have drunk kava prepared by chewing and by grating on many separate occasions in Vanuatu, and with both I have experienced feelings of tranquillity, difficulty in maintaining motor co-ordinations, and eventual somnolence.'

Kava was also of great religious significance and was seen to connect the user with the ancestors and the gods. It was not merely an offering or sacrifice to the spirits but a way of gaining access to the spirit world. It is used in healing ceremonies and to obtain hidden or esoteric knowledge. Its use as a means of divination was widespread and in Hawaii *kahunas* (native 'priests') would, in a fashion akin to that of tea-leaf reading, read the bubbles on the surface of a kava brew to predict the sex of an unborn child or the cause of illnesses.

Often the effects of colonisation and Western influence all but eradicated the use of traditional psychoactive substances. Whilst there were persistent attempts to stamp out kava use in many areas of the Pacific, its use continues unabated. In Vanuatu, independent since 1980, kava use has actually increased and is supported by the authorities as a desirable alternative to alcohol. This is at least in part an economic strategy as it has resulted in both a drastic decrease in the importation of alcoholic drinks and a development of kava as a highly significant cash crop. Kava bars have sprung up in the Pacific islands providing a modern way to consume it in an informal and sociable setting. Whether or not kava makes significant headway in the world market remains to be seen. The recent interest of Westerners in natural products (witness the small but growing interest in the Amazonian guarana; see **Guarana**) may well facilitate its emergence as a popular alternative to other beverages. It is also sold through small outlets in the West as a 'legal high' but this market is likely to remain on a small scale.

**Sources:** Brunton 1989, Lebot, Merlin and Lindstrom 1992, Lindstrom 1987.

# KETAMINE

Ketamine is the only PCP analogue (see **PCP**) that can be produced legally and has only 5–10 per cent of the potency of PCP. At present ketamine is not a controlled substance in the UK under the Misuse of Drugs Act but its availability is restricted under the Medicines Act. Like PCP it originated as an anaesthetic but it has since become a major adulterant of Ecstasy. Its effects are also very similar to those of PCP, typically involving distortions in the perception of the body (feeling that the body and immediate environment is made of a spongy or rubbery substance), hallucinations and distortions of the perception of time, and out-of-body experiences. Ketamine can be taken in a number of ways: it is usually snorted, swallowed or smoked but can also be injected intravenously. Because of its link with Ecstasy, it has been given attention by the British media.

**Sources:** Carroll 1985, Dalgarno and Shewan 1995, Tyler 1995.

# KINNIKINNIK

Kinnikinnik is the name given by numerous native peoples of North America to smoking mixtures, some of which contain tobacco but all of which contain other plants. The most widespread of these smoking mixtures contains leaves of the bearberry (*Arctostaphylos uva-ursi*). The leaves of this plant are known to have psychoactive effects if eaten or smoked. The Quinault and Lower Chinook Indians of the Pacific north-west use both methods, and the effects are giddiness and loss of control of body movements. Elsewhere in North America smokers of kinnikinnik have become so affected by it that they have been seen to fall into fires and remain there until dragged out. Many native cultures in British Columbia, including the Coast and Inland Salish, the Kutenai and the Athapaskans of the interior, smoked bearberry leaves sometimes mixed with willow bark (*Salix* sp.) or yew leaves (*Taxus brevifolia*) before the European introduction of commercial tobacco. Among the Flathead Indians of Montana, the bearberry kinnikinnik was prepared by drying the leaves in an oven or a sweathouse. It was mixed with tobacco and sometimes with the dried bark of the red willow (*Cornus stolonifera*) or the dried roots of other plants. Other smoking materials included the flowers of Wooly Yarrow (*Achillea lanulosa*), used ceremonially by the Ojibwa Indians and Pearly Everlasting (*Anaphalis margaritacea*), smoked by the Potawatomi in order to chase away evil spirits. Well over fifty different species of plants other than tobacco are known to have been used by the North American Indians in the making of their numerous smoking mixtures. As most of them have never been systematically analysed for their possible psychoactive constituents it is unclear what effects they may have caused. Whilst the use of many of these alternatives to tobacco has died out, some are still smoked in traditional ceremonies.

**Sources:** Emboden 1976, Hart 1979, Knight 1975, Turner and Taylor 1972.

## KRATOM

Known as *kratom* and *biak Mitragyna speciosa,* this is a south-east Asian tree containing a number of psychoactive alkaloids in its leaves. Two of these alkaloids were new to science – mitragynine and mitraversine. Mitragynine is the most significant of the plant's alkaloids and has been compared to psilocybin (an alkaloid found in the so-called 'magic mushrooms'; see **Psilocybe**) and lysergic acid amine (see **LSD**). Its connection with such hallucinogens has, however, been played down by some researchers. The leaves can be smoked or chewed or prepared in the form of an infusion. Colonial reports from the 1830s cite its use by the natives of Malaya as an opium substitute. In Thailand the most common way of consuming it is to simply chew the fresh leaves or take it in the form of a powder, adding salt to prevent constipation. The so-called 'Thai Narcotic Book' (*Norakanphadung*) describes it as weaker than morphine and less harmful than cocaine, being more analogous to the chewing of coca leaves.

**Sources:** Jansen and Prast 1988, Rätsch 1992.

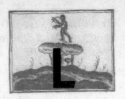

## LAGOCHILUS INEBRIANS

There are some thirty-five species of the *Lagochilus* genus that grow in Iran, Afghanistan and Central Asia. *Lagochilus inebrians* is a small shrub that grows on the steppes of Central Asia. It is made into a hallucinogenic tea by many of the native peoples of the region, including the Tatars, Turkmen, Tajiks and Uzbeks. These people collect the plant around October time and use the stems, leaves and fruiting tops to make the beverage and, as the plant has a markedly bitter taste, honey or sugar is usually added to it. Russian pharmacologists have been studying the plant since the Second World War and found it to have a number of medical applications, including the treatment of certain skin diseases and allergies, nervous problems and glaucoma. It is also used as a sedative.

**Sources:** Schultes 1977, Schultes and Hofmann 1980a, Schultes and Hofmann 1980b, Tyler 1966.

## LAUDANUM see **Opium**

## LAUGHING MUSHROOMS see **Fungi**

## LETTUCE

Species of lettuce (*Lactuca sativa* and *L. virosa*) were sacred plants to the ancient Egyptians and under the auspices of Min, the fertility god. Min was often depicted with an erect phallus and the milky exudation of the lettuce was identified with semen. For this reason lettuce seeds were used by the Egyptians as an aphrodisiac.

The Greeks, on the other hand, believed it to have anaphrodisiac effects, and for this reason it was used by the ascetic followers of Pythagoras. Lettuce seeds were used in European narcotic preparations and in the seventeenth century William Salmon noted that lettuce seeds are an effective anodyne and soporific. Its psychoactive qualities are due to lactucin, a morphine-like substance present in the sap. It was one of the constituents used by the European witches (see **Witches' Ointments**) and its leaves and roots are reportedly smoked by contemporary sex magicians for their aphrodisiac effects. It is not yet clear how the plant can be considered to both suppress and encourage erotic desire.

**Sources:** Manniche 1989, Rätsch 1992, Salmon 1693.

## LICHENS

Although there are reports of psychoactive lichens from Alaska these are yet to be substantiated. It has been suggested that the lichen *Gyrophora esculenta* is one of the agents of immortality of the Taoists.

**Sources:** Needham SCC 5/3, Schultes and Hofmann 1980b.

## LSD

The accidental discovery of the hallucinogenic effects of LSD by Albert Hofmann is one of the most famous, if not *the* most famous, incidents in the modern history of drug use. Before and during the Second World War Dr Hofmann was a research chemist for the Sandoz pharmaceutical company in Basle, Switzerland. For a number of years he had been involved in research on the parasitic fungus ergot (see **Ergot**) and had succeeded in synthesising a number of ergotamine molecules considered to have potential in the development of medicines. He named one such chemical that he had initially discovered in 1938 LSD-25, but at that stage had no idea of its psychoactive properties nor the amazing social consequences that it would have. On Friday 16 April 1943, whilst he was making up some more LSD-25, he drank a crystalline preparation of it in a glass of water. He felt slightly sick and, unaware that this was due to the substance in question, he presumed he was getting a cold and thought it best to go home to bed. But later as he lay in his bed the hallucinogenic effects unfolded before him in: 'an uninterrupted stream of fantastic images of extraordinary plasticity and vividness and accompanied by an intense kaleidoscopic play of colours.' Being almost certain that these extraordinary effects were due to LSD-25, he decided the following Monday to consume it again. Thus, that afternoon about 4.20 p.m., he took it again, this time with some assistants present. By around 5 p.m. he had embarked on a full LSD trip and decided to cycle home with an assistant acting as his minder. As Jay Stevens, author of *Storming Heaven: LSD and the American Dream*, the definitive work on the political and social history of the drug, has put it, this was no ordinary trip home: 'In Hofmann's mind this wasn't the familiar boulevard that led home, but a street painted by Salvador Dali, a funhouse rollercoaster where the buildings yawned and rippled.' In other words Hofmann was experiencing powerful hallucinations under the influence of LSD and when he finally got home he had an out-of-body experience in which he was looking down on what seemed to him to be his own dead body. Since these first experiments, Hofmann has treated LSD with respect and has not indulged in the recreational and often flippant use of the drug which was to reach its crescendo in the late 1960s.

During the Cold War the CIA and the United States Army ran covert and systematic researches into numerous psychoactive substances (including LSD) in order to ascertain their effects and their potential military and interrogatory uses. Jonathan Ott has described some of these highly dubious activities:

One fruit of this institutional paranoia was MKULTRA, an insidious domestic 'research' and spying operation run by the US Central Intelligence Agency (CIA), and similar 'non-conventional chemical warfare' studies conducted at the US Army's Edgewood Arsenal. In a program of research into interrogation drugs and illegal chemical warfare agents, LSD and other entheogenic drugs were given to at least 1,500 American military personnel and countless civilians. Some of the troops were coerced into 'volunteering' for the tests, and some of the civilians were given the drug without their consent or knowledge. One such dosing of a civilian employee of the CIA, Frank Olson, led to depression and suicide. The government kept secret the circumstances of the death ('national security' of course), but when a 'Freedom of Information Act' lawsuit forced public disclosure of the MKULTRA files, then President Gerald Ford was forced publicly to apologise to Olson's family. Canadian citizens subjected to psychological torture (including repeated doses of LSD) as part of this 'research' later sued the US government and were paid compensation. One civilian subject of the Edgewood Arsenal tests was killed by a massive overdose of MDA, an Army doctor commenting: 'we didn't know if it was dog piss or what it was we were giving him' . . . over 800 drugs, including LSD . . . were tested on prisoners in the federal government's Lexington, Kentucky 'Addiction Research Center Hospital' . . . when Sandoz Ltd. of Switzerland, owner of the patents on *Delysid* (LSD tartrate), refused to co-operate with the US government's desire to stockpile huge quantities of the drug for military purposes, the government ordered the Eli Lilly Company of Indiana to make the drug in violation of international patent accords. Yes, Eli Lilly Company and the CIA became the first illicit manufacturers of LSD, more than a decade before the drug was illegalised!

One of the lesser known prime movers in the history of LSD was the extraordinary and improbable millionaire businessman Al Hubbard, who was the president of the Vancouver Uranium Corporation. Having tried it himself, Hubbard felt a burning desire to proselytise on behalf of LSD and, although his motives were entirely different from those of the CIA, he was also a bulk buyer ordering forty-three cases from Sandoz in 1955. In the same year Aldous Huxley, who had first tried mescaline in 1953, was introduced to LSD.

The drug is intimately connected with the 'High Priest' of LSD, Timothy Leary, for it is he, above all others, who encouraged its widespread use. Whilst Hofmann was rightly cautious about the drug, Leary did everything in his power to propagate it. He held the rather simplistic belief that LSD and kindred hallucinogens were to be the focus of twenty-first-century religion. His prophetic tone soon drew the attention of the authorities, who were concerned that there was a counter-cultural plot to put LSD in the water supplies of New York ('Blow the Eight Million Minds of New York' was one of Leary's battle cries). However, bearing in mind the MKULTRA plot and other nefarious goings-on, it seems that such an idea was probably more likely to be implemented by the CIA than a motley army of hippies! To be fair to Leary, his initial over-zealous attitudes were later toned down.

LSD is a widely used drug and to most people the experience seems to be a purely recreational activity. However, there are those who have found it to be of great emotional and intellectual value. The film star Cary Grant took LSD after a long period of depression and felt that he had been reborn. His enthusiasm to share this experience with others was quashed by his agent who – no doubt correctly – thought it would result in a scandal. Michel Foucault, the inheritor of Jean-Paul Sartre's mantle as the unofficial president of the French intelligentsia, whilst visiting the United States in the 1980s, had his first LSD experience at Death Valley. It is reported that it had a profound effect on him and influenced the tenor of his later works.

**Sources:** Hofmann 1980, Leary 1970, Ott 1993, Stevens 1989, Tyler 1995.

## LYCOPODIUM

*Lycopodium selago*, often called club moss or wolf's foot, is common in the temperate forests of North America, thriving in damp and shady places. William Emboden states that: 'three of these stems, which are only a few inches tall, induce a mild hypnotic narcosis, eight result in total stupor or even a comatose state.' The Ojibwa Indians are known to have used another species (*L. complanatum*) as a stimulant, which suggests that the psychoactive constituents of *Lycopodium* species can cause radically different effects. In Peru a species of club moss is boiled as an additive to the hallucinogenic San Pedro cactus brew (see **San Pedro**). A species of club moss is used as a medicine by the Gimi people of New Guinea. In Western medicine spores of *L. calvatum* are still used for dusting sores, as a coating for pills and to lubricate suppositories.

**Sources:** Emboden 1976, Emboden 1979, Glick 1967, Rätsch 1992.

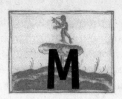

## MAGIC MUSHROOMS see **Fungi and Psilocybe**

## MANDRAKE

The mandrake is the most magically charged of all plants, with an enormous body of folklore from Europe and the Near East on its powers. Over twenty books have been written devoted solely to this peculiar plant and its properties.

The mandrake is a plant belonging, along with a number of other psychoactive plants such as henbane and belladonna, to the family Solanaceae. There are at least six species of *Mandragora*, the

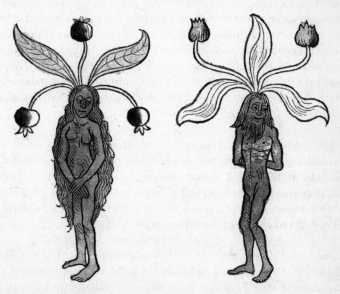

**FEMALE AND MALE MANDRAKES**

most famous of which is the mandrake (*Mandragora officnarum*). The early botanical name of the mandrake, given to it by Linnaeus, was *Atropa mandragora,* indicating that it was seen as having comparable properties to *Atropa belladonna* (see **Belladonna**). The mandrake should not be confused with the American mandrake or May apple (*Podophyllum peltatum*). The mandrake is a stemless perennial which grows to a height of about one metre. It has large wrinkled leaves and a thick root which is usually branched and up to a metre in length. The forking of the root is the plant's most characteristic feature; its similarity to the human form was seen by a great many cultures as demonstrating its great magical and medicinal potency. In Europe in particular it was seen as a panacea, or cure-all, rather as was ginseng in China, although the latter, whilst a highly versatile tonic, does not have the powerful psychoactive effects of the mandrake. The large bell-shaped flowers vary in colour from white or greenish yellow to violet. Its small berries give off a distinct fragrance.

The highly subjective nature of the sense of smell is nowhere better illustrated than in descriptions of the mandrake odour. William Turner (*c.*1508–68), Dean of Wells and author of a sixteenth-century herbal, wrote that the female mandrake fruit was 'well smellyng' and that of the male did 'smell pleasantly joyned to a certain grevousness'. William Salmon, a physician and druggist writing at the turn of the eighteenth century, described the smell of the female mandrake fruit as pleasing but less heady than that of the male. The famous Egyptologist Wallis Budge found the mandrake to have 'a foetid and somewhat nauseating smell'. Recent investigators of the mandrake in the wild have this to say of the fragrance:

> The odour of mandrake is unique. It is not perceived as a smell of classic fragrant flowers like rose, lily or jasmine. There is a hint of subtle danger in it. Intoxicating and addictive, it makes a powerful impression on one's memory and evokes images of unspoiled wilderness, desert wind, excitement of danger and romantic exaltation.

These researchers (Fleisher and Fleisher) suggest that the widespread and enduring folk belief in the aphrodisiac qualities of the mandrake is based on the erotically charged smell of the plant rather than any of its chemical constituents that could be extracted by chemical means. Modern laboratory researchers have to date failed to isolate any principles from the plant that have or could have significant aphrodisiac effects but belief in such effects still survive today in the Mediterranean and Near East. However, the fragrance of the fruit alone has been ascribed with soporific powers. Celsus advises that it be put under the patient's pillow to induce sleep, a remedy echoed by William Salmon. The mandrake grows in Mediterranean Europe, North Africa and western Asia as far as the Himalayas, often in stony places and areas of deserted cultivation.

The psychoactive constituents of mandrake are the tropane alkaloids, the major alkaloid being hyoscyamine. Scopolamine, atropine and mandragorine (also called cuscohygrine) are also present. Mandrake has been variously described as narcotic, aphrodisiac, hallucinogenic and hypnotic. It was used as an effective anaesthetic from early times but in higher doses it could cause deleterious effects and delirium. In toxic levels of intake death by respiratory paralysis has been reported. The root is the most potent part of the plant but the berries are also said to cause changes in consciousness. More fancifully some early herbalists believed that just smelling the berries could cause a marked drowsiness or even sleep (as detailed above).

The origin of the word mandrake is obscure. Some derive it from the Sanskrit *mandros* ('sleep') and *agora* ('substance'). Other commentators prefer a Sumerian origin (see below). Dioscorides gives the names Antimelon, Archinen and Morion. In the Old Testament the mandrake appears as *dudaim,* meaning 'love and fear'. The English name mandrake also appears in numerous other forms, such as mandrage, mandrag, mandragges, mondrake and mandragon (more than ten different spellings are known from Middle English alone); all derive ultimately from the Latin *mandragoras.* Due to its prominent role in folklore the plant gained numerous epithets – Satan's apple (in reference to the evil reputation of the berries); the Copts, the early Christians in Egypt, called it Satan's testicles (the berries being seen as similar in shape to the testicles, which of course also alludes to the aphrodisiac qualities attributed to the plant); apples of the fool (acknowledging its intoxicating properties); and love apple (because of its aphrodisiac qualities). To the Germans it was 'dragon doll' and *galgenmännlein,* 'the little man of the gallows' (for reasons given below). Other German names include *Dolkraut* and *Schlaffbeer* and it is now known in Germany as *Hexenkraut.*

The plant was widely used in the ancient Near East for its various properties. To the Sumerians the mandrake was known as *nam-tar,* literally 'plague god plant', and this is thought by some authorities to be the ultimate origin of the word mandrake. The ancient Egyptians featured the plant among the symbolic motifs that adorn the tombs of the pharaohs. The tomb of Rameses II of the nineteenth dynasty depicts the mandrake in conjunction with the narcotic water-lily (see **Water Lily**) and the opium poppy (see **Opium**). There is a legend in which the god Ra conquers the goddess Hathor by drugging her with mandrake beer. The ivory casket of Tutankhamun has depicted on it the picking of mandrake roots. The mandrake is mentioned twice in the Old Testament. In Genesis (30: 14-16) Rachel obtained mandrake fruit from Leah to assist her in becoming fruitful. In the Song of Solomon (7: 11-13) Shulammite invites her lover to go out into the country where the mandrakes grow. The soporific and anodyne effects of mandrake are known to have been used in Palestine to induce a deep narcotic trance in those being crucified. As mandrake was known as *morion,* it has been thought that the sponge that Jesus was offered as he was on the cross may have been a mandrake wine.

A number of dessicated specimens of mandrakes which have been 'carved' to make them human-like in appearance have been unearthed in the cities of Antioch, Constantinople and Damascus. This demonstrates in no uncertain terms that it is not just the use of the plant which is ancient, but also the desire to increase the magical potency of the root by altering its shape. The ancient Arabic name for it was *abu'lruh,* which has been translated as 'master of the breath of life' or 'lord of spirit'. This has led to the suggestion that in the pre-Islamic Arab world mandrake was an entheogen (see **Entheogen**) or perhaps even a god. As such with the coming of Islam the plant was demonised in a similar way to the fate of henbane and belladonna in Christian Europe. Thus, the plant was no longer 'lord of spirit' but *Tufah al-jinn* ('apples of the demon') or *Baydal-jinn* ('testicles of the demon'). Apparently the Arabs also called it the 'devil's candle' because it (or rather the glow worms that were attracted to its leaves) shone at night. The nocturnal glowing of the mandrake reappears as a theme in later European lore (see below). The later malevolent value of the plant to the Arabs is attested to by a surviving formula for a poison made from the decomposing root and numerous additives.

Mandrake lore has not disappeared in Asia but continues to be used across the continent, as it has been down the ages. It is an Armenian folk belief that the burning of the root drives evil spirits out of the house; inhaling the smoke is a cure for insanity. Among the Bedouin tribes of the Negev region of southern Israel the mandrake still plays an important role in folk medicine; the plant is considered sacred and it is forbidden to harm it. A barren woman who is seeking a cure will eat the ripe mandrake fruit immediately after her menstrual period whilst reciting verses from the Quran (Koran). The Egyptologist Wallis Budge said that the Cairo druggists regularly made up love philtres containing mandrake for newly-weds who hoped to have many sons. C.J.S. Thompson, who wrote a book on the mandrake in the 1930s, said that the carving of the roots for sale in the markets of Syria, Palestine and elsewhere in the Near East was still very much a thriving trade. In present-day Morocco *M. autumnalis* is used medicinally for its narcotic effects. In Indian folk medicine the root of *M. officinarum* is known as *Lakshmana*, which means 'possessed of lucky signs or marks'. It is used as an aphrodisiac and believed to assist conception. The roots of *M. caulescens* are used in magical rites in Sikkim in the Himalayas. Knowledge of the mandrake was passed to the Chinese by the Muslims no later than the thirteenth century, perhaps significantly earlier. No doubt the Chinese saw many parallels between the new plant and their beloved ginseng root.

Pythagoras is said to have called the root *anthropomorph* or 'tiny human being', an association which continued in later European lore with the idea of the homunculus. As is still common practice among native peoples of the world from Mexico to New Guinea, the ritual and magical operations that must be performed before uprooting or cutting a sacred plant were widely performed in the ancient world. Theophrastus of Lesbos (*c.*370–328 BC), the founding father of botany, describes the magical precautions that accompanied the digging up of the root in his *Enquiry Into Plants* (Book IX. viii): 'it is said that one should draw three circles round mandrake with a sword, and cut it with one's face towards the west; and at the cutting of the second piece one should dance round the plant and say as many things as possible about the mysteries of love.' In the *Jewish War* (Book VII. 180), written in the first century AD, Josephus writes the following about a plant he calls *Baaras* (or

*Barras*), which many believe to be the mandrake:

> Flame-coloured and towards evening emitting a brilliant light, it eludes the grasp of persons who approach with the intention of plucking it, as it shrinks up and can only be made to stand still by pouring upon it certain secretions of the human body. Yet even then to touch it is fatal, unless one succeeds in carrying off the root itself, suspended from the hand. Another innocuous mode of capturing it is as follows. They dig around it, leaving but a minute portion of the root covered; they then tie a dog to it, and the animal rushing to follow the person who tied him easily pulls it up, but instantly dies – a vicarious victim, as it were, for him who intended to remove the plant, since after this none need fear to handle it. With all these attendant risks, it possesses one virtue for which it is prized; for the so-called demons – in other words, the spirits of wicked men which enter the living and kill them unless aid is forthcoming – are promptly expelled by this root, if merely applied to the patients.

The human secretions referred to in the passage are menstrual blood and urine. In the subsequent mandrake lore of Europe the plant was said to spring up from the spilt semen of a hanged man. There are also ethnographic cases where semen is put on magical and psychoactive plants as, for example, among the Bimin-Kuskusmin of New Guinea, who treat hallucinogenic fungi in this way. Josephus' statement concerning the glowing of the plant (which also recurs in later, European, accounts) may not be pure fantasy, as in specific weather conditions chemical particles in the night dew and on the berries may emit a faint glow.

Dioscorides stresses the importance of mandrake wine as an effective surgical anaesthetic (which could also be administered in the form of a clyster), in fact, it continued to be used as such in Europe as late as the beginning of the eighteenth century, according to the testimony of the English physician William Salmon. William Emboden, a world authority on narcotic plants, says that the first ever volatile anaesthetic was a sponge boiled in a mixture of mandrake root bark, wine, lettuce seed (see **Lettuce**), and mulberry leaves. The sponge was held over the face of the patient. In his biography of the neo-Pythagorean Apollonius of Tyana, Philostratus describes the mandrake as a soporific drug.

Venus was sometimes known by the epithet Mandragontis on account of the plant's extraordinary reputation as an aphrodisiac. The Emperor Julian (AD 331–363) in a letter to Callixeine, a priestess of the goddess Demeter, uses the drinking of a draught of mandrake as a metaphor for dull-witted, but also makes reference to its aphrodisiac effects. Yet it also had its martial applications. I have illustrated elsewhere the use of the mandrake's solanaceous cousins *Datura*, henbane and belladonna in warfare and it is not surprising to find the mandrake's narcotic properties being put to similar use. In *The Stratagems* of Sextus Julius Frontinus (AD *c.*35–*c.*103), an early military classic, there is, in a chapter on ambushes, the following account:

> Maharbal [an officer under the command of Hannibal], sent by the Carthaginians against the rebellious Africans, knowing that the tribe was passionately fond of wine, mixed a large quantity of wine with mandragora, which in potency is something between a poison and a soporific. Then after an insignificant skirmish he deliberately withdrew. At dead of night, leaving in the camp some of his baggage and all the drugged wine, he feigned flight. When the barbarians captured the camp and in a frenzy of delight greedily drank the drugged wine, Maharbal returned, and either took them prisoners or slaughtered them while they lay stretched out as if dead.

Isidore, Bishop of Seville's (*c.* AD 560/570–636) mention of the anaesthetic use of mandrake in surgical operations gives us a historical link between its classical usage and the later European tradition. The use of a mandrake kept in a house as an amulet, or magical form of protection, is recorded in an English manuscript of the eleventh century. No doubt both indigenous traditions and Biblical precedent were behind the continuing belief in the mandrake as an aid to procreation. It was thought that the roots of the male and female mandrakes would assist a barren woman to conceive a boy or girl respectively. The anaesthetic properties of mandrake wine were made use of by those who were to be burnt at the stake or dismembered. By perverse irony, perhaps, some of the witches who were executed made final use of the very drug that was one of the most powerful hallucinogens used in the making of the psychoactive substances of witchcraft (see **Witches'**

**Ointments**). It is even more perverse to think that they may have shared the same anaesthetic to deliver them from their suffering as Jesus. To the alchemists and learned magicians of Europe, mandrake was classified as a plant under the astral influence of Saturn.

The ancient idea that the mandrake root was a 'little man' continued to have common currency in later European beliefs. There is a theme here which is common to many psychoactive substances and the 'little people' of fairy lore throughout the world. From the cultures of eastern Siberia we hear of the 'fly-agaric men', who appear to those who take the hallucinogenic fungi; Mexican Indians intimately link the *Psilocybe* mushrooms to the little people etc. That the psychoactive mandrake should be bound up with similar beliefs in Europe should not surprise us as it is so widespread a theme. An early herbalist, William Turner (*c*.1508–*c*.1568), describes carved roots in the form of little people as puppets or 'mammettes', which means idols, and is derived from the name Muhammad who was, to many in Europe at the time, seen as an idol of the Muslims. The Emperor Rudolf II who was deeply involved in the occult sciences and regularly entertained alchemists from all over Europe is said to have kept two roots himself that he tended to personally. These two mandrakes are preserved in a collection in the Curiosa of the Hradschin Castle in Prague. At her trial Joan of Arc was accused of having a mandrake fashioned in the form of a mannikin that she is supposed to have used as a talisman for attracting wealth, a charge that she denied.

The Reverend William Bulleyn (1500–76), who was also a physician, was an early critic of the belief that the mandrake was generated from the seed of a dead man: he dismissed it as 'an invention of Satan-inspired witches'. He goes on to attack the belief that the mandrake was a little man, blaming friars and superstitious monks for duping the populace into believing such nonsense. According to Bulleyn, witches of old used it to bewitch men into 'blind fantasies' or trances called Love, by which he states in no uncertain terms he means 'noisome beastly luste'.

Due to the scarcity of the genuine mandrake in Britain and other parts of northern Europe the bryony root (*Bryonia diocia*) was widely used as a substitute, and, in order to sell this as the real thing, charlatans would go to great lengths in manipulating its natural form. John Baptista Porta describes one dishonest, if highly ingenious method:

You must get a great root of bryony ... and with a sharp
instrument engrave in it a man or a woman, giving either of
them their genitories: then make holes with a puncheon into
those places where the hairs are wont to grow, and put into
those holes millet, or some such thing which may shoot out
his roots like the hairs of one's head. And when you have
digged a little pit for it in the ground, you must let it lie there,
until such time as it shall be covered with a bark, and the
roots also be shot forth.

John Gerard (1545–1612) was something of an iconoclast when it
came to plant lore, and the selling of false mandrakes was
something he felt compelled to attack:

the idle drones that have little or nothing to do but eate and
drinke, have bestowed some of their time in carving the
rootes of Brionie, forming them to the shape of men and
women; which falsifying practise hath confirmed the errour
amongst the simple and unlearned people, who have taken
them upon their report to be the true Mandrakes.

Some of the early British herbalists and botanists dismissed much
of the lore that surrounded the mandrake, deriding it as empty
superstition. John Gerard was scathing not only about the stories
of the dog being required to pull up the root safely (he says both
his servants and he uprooted many a mandrake without suffering
any ill effects) but also about its supposed resemblance to the
human form. The gallows superstition and even its aphrodisiac
reputation were also rejected by Gerard. Despite the attempts of
Gerard, Porta and others to remove some of the supernatural aura
that surrounded the plant, at least among the peasants demand
for the roots continued unabated.

In France the mandrake was known by the name *main de gloire*,
i.e. 'hand of glory' or *mandragloire* – seemingly a conflation of
*mandragora* and the name of a French fairy, *Magloire*. *Magloire* was
seen as an elf, a familiar spirit rather like the German *alruna*, and
also embodied in the form of a carved root of mandrake. Furthermore, in the lore of Brittany there is a tale concerning a nocturnal
spirit who appears with its fingers alight (the fishermen of the
region are also reported to have worn the mandrake root as an
amulet to protect them from the perils of the sea). By a further

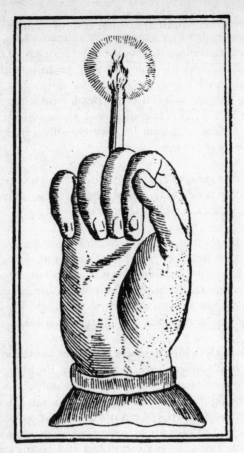

**THE HAND OF GLORY**

twist in the tangled lore of the mandrake, the hand of glory is also
the name given to the amputated hand of a dead man that was
used as a magical torch in committing acts of burglary (see
below).

The hand of glory is a popular theme in western European
folklore, appearing in accounts of witch trials, in sundry folk
beliefs and in the *grimoires* or written manuals of sorcery that
usually contained an indiscriminate mixture of cabalistic ritual
magic and a cluster of spells, recipes for magical potions and
beauty secrets. The *Picatrix*, a *grimoire* based upon an earlier Arabic
manual of magic (suggesting links to the ancient traditions of the

Muslim sorcerers), prescribes the use of mandrake in the preparation of magical compounds. In another such work, the *Grimorium Verum* (dating from the eighteenth century, but falsely bearing the date 1517), Sustugriel, a spirit subordinate to the demon Satanachia, is said to supply the magician with mandrakes. The great medieval scholar Albertus Magnus, author of *The Book of Secrets*, had gained a reputation as a magician on account of his fabulous learning and was also to gain a literary homunculus in the form of one Albertus Parvus ('Little Albert'). The French version, *Petit Albert*, went through over thirty editions and contains information on the preparation and use of 'the glorious hand'. The purpose of the hand of glory is: 'to stupefy those to whom it is displayed and to render them motionless, in such a way that they can no more stir than if they were dead.' The reader is instructed to take either hand of a felon hanging from a gibbet beside a highway, wrap it in a piece of a funeral pall and squeeze it dry. Afterwards it must be put in an earthenware vessel with zimat, nitre, salt and long peppers and then left for a fortnight before being dried in the sun during the dog days. If the weather is not hot then the prepared hand may be put instead in an oven and heated with vervain and fern. Next, a candle must be made from the fat of a hung criminal, virgin wax, sesame and ponie. The hand of glory acts as the candlestick. The author then states that if one lights it in any place that one goes in with this baneful instrument then the occupants shall remain motionless.

The actual use of such strange tools of the burglars' trade continued much longer than one might expect. A hand of glory was found, dropped at the scene of a failed burglary (the occupants awoke during the break-in) at the house of a Mr Napier of Loughcrew in County Meath, Ireland, on 3 January 1831; the incident was reported in the *Observer* newspaper on 16 January of the same year. An actual specimen of the hand of glory is preserved at the Whitby Museum in Yorkshire, England.

There is more than a name to link the hand of glory with the mandrake. Firstly, the hand is said to glow at night, an attribute of the plant according to a long established tradition (interestingly, the mandrake is called the 'devil's candle' in Sweden and *thjofarot*, or 'thieves root', in Icelandic). The hand is, like the plant, to be found at a gallows. As the mandrake is dried and mixed with other ingredients so too is the hand. The soporific effects of the hand mirror those of the narcotic mandrake. *Datura*, a cousin of the mandrake, is reported to have been used by thieves in India for the express purpose of rendering the victims senseless (see **Datura**) and it is quite possible that mandrake may have been put to similar use. The French writer Gérard de Nerval (1808–55), whose experiences with hashish are well-known, makes it the subject of his early novella *La Main Enchantée*, written in 1832 and originally entitled *La Main de Gloire*.

Yet it was not just the common burglar that made use of the plant. Lucrezia Borgia (1480–1519), later to become the Duchess of Ferrara, is said to have employed it as a poison. Machiavelli (1469–1527) wrote *Mandragola*, first published in Rome in 1524 and which some consider to be his best play, in which he dissects the corruption and sexual debauchery of Italian society. References to the mandrake and its powers are to be found in many of the plays of Shakespeare, including *Antony and Cleopatra, Henry IV Part Two, Henry VI Part Two, Romeo and Juliet* and *Othello*. It is also mentioned in other classic plays, including Marlowe's *Jew of Malta*, Webster's *Duchess of Malfi* and Jonson's *Masque of Queens*. In English heraldry the mandrake is rarely portrayed, an exception being the arms of Bodyham, which bears three mandrakes as symbols of the human body.

Belief in the myriad powers of the mandrake has by no means died out in Europe anymore than it has in Asia. Until recently Alpine climbers carried it as an amulet to protect them from bad weather. In mainland Greece and on the islands as late as the 1960s parts of the plant would be worn on a necklace by a barren woman in the hope that it would make her fruitful, and either the fruit or root would be put on her body during sexual intercourse with her husband to achieve the same end. Even into the twentieth century, women in Kent, England wore it on their person to overcome sterility. A report from 1925 states that London street traders sold it as a panacea for a penny a slice! It was also used as a homoeopathic remedy for gout. In 1966 BBC Radio broadcast an interview by Wilfred Pickles with a herbalist based in the Old Kent Road, London, who was advertising the root as a way to give up smoking. The belief in the dangers of digging up the root also survived into recent times. When a chemist from Wales died he bequeathed a mandrake plant to the local College Botanic Garden. Some of those who attended the uprooting expressed anxiety at the fate which might befall the intrepid college gardener. The gardener himself was unconcerned and completed the task without coming to any harm.

Belief in the demonic powers of the plant have been maintained. Anton Szandor La Vey, leader of the California-based Church of Satan (that once boasted Jayne Mansfield among its members), conducts his parodies of the Christian Eucharist with a chalice containing bourbon and mandrake root. Whilst the literary career of mandrake has declined since its Shakespearean roles, it nevertheless turns up in a number of minor works. *The Screaming Plant* by Hal Pink is the story of a man who plants mandrake seed in his cellar; in a triffid-like fashion it grows to menacing proportions and proceeds to kill a cat and drink its blood. It is finally killed by the novel's hero and a friend. Mandrake has also been used as a slang term for Mandrax (see **Methaqualone**).

**Sources:** Abu-Rabia 1983, Bennett 1991, Budge 1978, Bulleyn 1562, Collin de Plancy 1825–6, Ellis 1946, Emboden 1974, 1979, Fleisher and Fleisher 1994, Frontinus 1925, Gerard 1597, Grillot de Givry 1931, Guazzo 1929, Hansen 1978, Heiser 1969, Holzer 1974, Julian 1953, Josephus 1961, Kenk 1963, Mabey 1996, Manniche 1989, Mehra 1979, Monter 1976, Needham SSC 5/4 1980, Opie and Tatum 1992, Ott 1993, Rätsch 1992, Safford 1922, Seymour 1913, Theophrastus 1916, Thompson 1934, Thorndike 1923–1958, Turner 1568, Waite 1990.

## MANDRAX see Methaqualone

## MANG

Like *haoma* (see **Soma**), *mang* was a psychoactive substance of great importance in the pre-Islamic religions of the ancient Iranian peoples, and, like *haoma*, exactly what it was is a mystery. The archaic Iranian languages are very difficult to understand and it is therefore no surprise that the experts differ widely in their conclusions. Walter Henning, who was one of the greatest, if not the greatest, linguist to tackle the problems of these languages, insisted that *mang* was simply a poison. This conclusion is contradicted not only by the scriptures of the ancient Zoroastrian religion in which *mang* was used, but also by most subsequent scholars. Henning was simply unable to accept that the religion of Zoroaster (Zarathustra) could have involved the use of psychoactive substances for spiritual ends. Thus, his judgement was clouded by preconceived prejudice and he refused to see any meaningful link between the word *mang* and *bang* (*bhang*), the latter being known to refer to one or more hallucinogenic plants.

*Mang* is mentioned in a number of Zoroastrian holy books. The most complete account of its psychoactive effects and also of the reasons it was used are given in the *Arda Viraz Namag*, or *Book of Arda Viraz*, often called the Iranian 'Divine Comedy,' as the hero, like Dante, visits both heaven and hell and witnesses the punishments of the wicked and the rewards of the righteous. In another work, called *The Greater Bundahisn*, which expounds the Zoroastrian version of the creation of the world and mankind, the Evil Spirit Ahriman attacks the primal bull in a fit of destructive rage. The supreme God Ohrmazd relieves the bull's pain by giving it *mang* (IV.20). Clearly Henning's idea that it was a poison is completely out of the question as Ohrmazd would never have given it as a medicine if that were the case. Two later scriptures reveal how *mang* was given to King Vistasp, who, as a consequence of the visions he saw under its influence, converted to Zoroaster's doctrines and subsequently became his patron. With the formidable backing of the King the survival of the religion was assured. In the account of this incident given in the *Denkart (VII.4.85)*, the *mang* was mixed with *hom* (i.e. *haoma*) and Vistasp saw the full glory of paradise and the *Amesa Spentas*, or Bounteous Immortals. In the *Zardust Nama* a similar account is given in which the King, after drinking the mixture from a bowl (received from Ardvahist, one of the seven Zoroastrian 'archangels'), sees the celestial world. Both the *Arda Viraz Namag* (V.16) and the *Videvdat* (XV.14) describe such a psychoactive drink as *mang-i-vistaspan*, or '*mang* of Vistasp'.

These accounts show that *mang* was not identical with *haoma* (as some commentators have suggested) since the two are mixed together. As I said above, the word *mang* is connected to *bang* which derives from the Avestan (Avestan is the oldest Iranian language and of comparable importance to Sanskrit, both having an unknown common ancestor) *bangha*. Those who have suggested that *mang* was actually hemp (i.e. cannabis) have pointed out that the Sanskrit *bangha* (*bhang*) means 'hemp' or 'an intoxicating drink containing cannabis' and that the New Persian word *bang* also means 'hemp';

thus showing that both the ancient Indian and the modern Persian words refer to cannabis, and concluding therefore that the Middle Persian *mang* must also be the same drug. Whilst this is superficially convincing it is fatally flawed from both a linguistic and botanical point of view. The meaning 'hemp' was given to the New Persian word *bang* in the twelfth century; before that it referred to a different plant, namely henbane (see **Henbane**). The word for henbane occurs in related forms in other languages, such as the Armenian *bang* and the Arabic *banj*, the latter of which has the additional meaning of '*Datura*' (see **Datura**). Thus, the oldest connotation of *mang/bang* in the Iranian languages refers not to cannabis but to henbane. This is compatible with the known psychoactive effects of the two plants. We know from the Zoroastrian literature that *mang* has two particularly striking effects. First, it can send the user into a narcotic trance for a number of days (even allowing for the fact that Arda Viraz's trance may have been said to last seven days for symbolic reasons – seven being a holy number in Zoroastrianism – clearly an extended period is meant). Second, whilst in this physically dormant state the user experiences very powerful hallucinations and believes his spirit to have travelled to other worlds. Although cannabis can, in sufficient quantities, induce both hallucinations and narcotic states, it is not of the same potency in either of these spheres as henbane (or for that matter *Datura*). The known effects of henbane make it a far more likely candidate than cannabis to be the basis of the ancient Iranian entheogen (see **Entheogen**) *mang*. A further mystery may be attached to this linguistic puzzle. The New Persian word *mung* (which is apparently related to the word *mang*) means 'a black intoxicating grain'. Could this refer to some psychoactive fungus such as ergot (see **Ergot**) that contaminated the rye crops of Europe?

**Sources:** Belardi 1979, Boyce 1975, Flattery and Schwartz 1989, Mackenzie 1971, Vahman 1986.

## MDMA see **Adam** and **Ecstasy**

## MESCAL BEANS

Mescal beans is the name given to the psychoactive seeds of *Sophora secundiflora*, a small tree or evergreen shrub. Its natural habitat is Texas, New Mexico and parts of Mexico. The pods contain 1–8 seeds which often remain on the plant for several seasons. They are usually maroon or orange-red in colour, although a distinct form (*S. secundiflora* forma *xanthosperma*), known only from Texas, produces a yellow variety. The principal alkaloids contained in mescal beans are cytisine, N-methylcytisine and sparteine, all of which belong to the quinolizidine (or lupine) group of alkaloids. Despite the use of mescal beans by native Americans pursuing the vision quest, none of these alkaloids are known to have hallucinogenic properties. Depending on the amount consumed and the means of preparation, mescal beans can cause a wide variety of effects, ranging from vomiting, head-aches and nausea to intoxication, stupor and even death. Mescal beans are usually consumed in a decoction and, among the Chiricahua and Mescalero Apache they were used as a potent additive to *tulbai* or *tiswin*, a fermented maize beverage. A number of the Plains Indian people also gave the beans to their horses both as a stimulant and a medicine.

Mescal bean use is of considerable antiquity and may, in fact, be the oldest known psychoactive plant (if it is actually psychoactive) used in the Americas. At least sixteen prehistoric cave and rock-shelter sites spread across Texas, New Mexico and Mexico have been found to contain palaeobotanical remains of *S. secundiflora*. Some of these sites are between 8,000 and 7,000 years old. There is, however, no definitive proof that, at this early date, they were used for their purported psychoactive properties. The discovery of a loincloth with mescal beans decorating its fringe at a site in Val Verde county in Texas proves that they were used for their ornamental value at a very early date, but this does not rule out their other potential uses in medicine and ritual practices. In historical times some thirty different native American peoples have made use of mescal beans – almost all for their decorative value – and less than half have used it for its psychoactive effects. The epicentre of the ceremonial use of mescal beans was among the Caddoan and Siouan-speaking peoples of the southern and central Plains. The Wichita Indians were instrumental in dissemi-nating the mescal-bean ceremonial society. Connections with the subsequent spread of the peyote cult are unclear. Some researchers view the peyote cult as growing out of the mescal-bean cult (and then replacing it), whilst others think the links between the two were insignificant.

**Sources:** Adovasio and Fry 1976, Boyd and Dering 1996, Bye 1979, Merrill 1977, Schultes and Hofmann 1980a.

## MESCALINE

In the 1890s the German chemist Arthur Heffter isolated a number of alkaloids from the peyote cactus (see **Peyote**), one of which he named mescaline. This hallucinogenic substance soon attracted interest in medical, artistic and intellectual circles. Probably the most influential user of mescaline was Aldous Huxley, the famous writer of *Brave New World*, who came from one of the most distinguished intellectual families in England. An English doctor named Humphrey Osmond, who pioneered the psychiatric use of hallucinogens, gave Huxley mescaline on 4 May 1953. Huxley, who was in his late fifties at the time, was overwhelmed by the experience and felt compelled to expound his visionary experiences with it in two short texts, *The Doors of Perception* (said to be the inspiration for the name of Jim Morrison's group The Doors) and *Heaven and Hell*, which have since become among the most widely read classics of 'drug literature'.

Not all those who read Huxley's works on the mescaline experience were sympathetic. R.C. Zaehner, an Oxford Professor of Eastern Religions and Ethics, after reading *The Doors of Perception*, decided to try mescaline himself. Whilst under its influence he strolled through the grounds of the Oxford colleges and experienced humorous insights of a trivial nature, but no more than that. He concluded that mescaline did not produce the transcendent effects claimed by Huxley, and furthermore that the use of psychoactive substances was both artificial and deeply 'anti-religious'. This is a remarkable conclusion coming from a man who had dedicated his whole academic life to the study of Indian and Iranian religious traditions (he wrote weighty tomes on both Hinduism and Zoroastrianism), both of which used the psychoactive *soma* plant (see **Soma**) in their archaic religious rites! He was thus describing the Eastern Religions as anti-religious! Zaehner was later to become a vociferous critic of Timothy Leary and the growing use of LSD and other drugs in the counter culture of the 1960s.

For some inexplicable reason there is a certain snobbery

attached to the use of mescaline; many of those who have (or think they have) taken it compare it favourably with LSD. This is probably due to its comparative rarity rather than any qualitative difference in the actual experience. Although many experienced 'druggies' believe that they have taken mescaline it is, in fact, extremely rare that it reaches the underground drug market, although there are numerous street concoctions purporting to be the genuine article.

**Sources:** Huxley 1954, Huxley 1956, Ott 1993, Stevens 1989, Tyler 1995, Zaehner 1957, Zaehner 1972.

## MESCAL BUTTONS see Peyote

## METHAQUALONE

Methaqualone was first synthesised in India in 1955 by M.L. Gujral and soon afterwards was put on the market in Japan and Europe as a supposedly non-addictive hypnotic in the form of a sleeping pill. In 1960 it was sold by the Boots company under the names Melsed and Melsedin and by Marck as Renoval. In 1965 methaqualone in combination with an antihistamine was marketed as the sedative drug Mandrax by Roussel laboratories. By 1965 methaqualone was the most commonly prescribed sedative in Britain; it was also becoming a popular drug of abuse, earning it the street names mandies and mandrake. It was also a commercial success in the United States (where it was called Quaalude by the William H. Rover company); in 1972 it was the sixth best-selling sedative on the market. As has so often been the familiar pattern with the life-stories of sedatives, methaqualone was originally believed to be non-addictive, with no significant side effects. Thus, it replaced barbiturates on a large scale, with the expectation that it would be a harmless alternative to the now discredited panacea barbiturates. Predictably problems came to light with methaqualone and it was withdrawn from the British market at the beginning of the 1980s. In its heyday it was not a controlled drug but in 1971, with its well-established reputation as a drug of abuse (somewhat ironically it gained the slang name 'Dr Jekyll and Mr Hyde', which describes perfectly the social transformation the drug went through – from being a respectable member of the medical arsenal to an anti-social street drug) it came under the UK Misuse of Drugs Act. The US followed suit in 1973, classifying it as a Schedule II drug, that is to say a drug with a significant existing rate of abuse, with dependency problems but with limited but legitimate medical applications. These acceptable medical uses had been rejected by 1984 when it became a Schedule I substance.

Fatal overdose with methaqualone is usually due to lung, liver, kidney or heart failure.

**Source:** Carroll and Gallo 1985.


**MORNING GLORY** see **Ololiuqui**

**MORPHINE** see **Heroin**

**MUSHROOMS** see **Fungi**

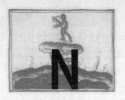

## NARCOTICS

Narcotics are, strictly speaking, a distinct class of psychoactive substances that cause states of stupor, sleep and calm. Opium and its derivatives, such as heroin and morphine, are the narcotics *par excellence*. Narcotics may be seen as a sub-division of the hypnotics (see **Hypnotics**). To drug enforcement organisations narcotics means something rather different, for they refer to various 'hard drugs' – particularly heroin and cocaine – as narcotics. Cocaine is, in terms of its psychoactive effects, a stimulant rather than a narcotic. Furthermore, many of the older generation of researchers (such as Richard Schultes, Weston La Barre and William Emboden) have used the term narcotics as a general all-encompassing rubric for all psychoactive substances.

## NATIVE AMERICAN CHURCH OF NORTH AMERICA

So rapid was the spread of the peyote cult (see **Peyote**) across the Plains of North America that by 1906 there was a loose inter-cultural network of peyote-using native peoples known as 'Mescal Bean Eaters', with members from Oklahoma in the south to Nebraska in the north. In 1909 this group, seeking to incorporate white patterns of religious organisation, called itself the Union Church. In 1918, with the assistance of James Mooney (a researcher into the peyote cult among the Kiowa Indians), the Native American Church, as it was then known, was officially incorporated in Oklahoma. It became a national organisation in 1944 with the name The Native American Church of the United States, changing once again eleven years later to The Native American Church of North America to accommodate the peyote users north of the border in Canada (among them the Cree, Blackfoot and Coast Salish peoples). The official acceptance of the Native American Church (and the legal right of its members to consume peyote) was a long and hard battle. Many prominent anthropologists campaigned on behalf of native people, including Franz Boas, Alfred Kroeber, Weston La Barre and Ares Hrdlicka.

**Sources:** La Barre 1989, Ott 1993.

## NEO-AMERICAN CHURCH

Based on the model of the **Native American Church of North America** (see above) the Neo-American Church, a white organ-isation, sought to obtain the rights that the native Church had; namely the right to consume peyote for religious reasons. The Neo-American Church has been ridiculed and condemned for being a very pale imitation of a genuine religious group and for having rather different motives for taking peyote. Weston La Barre, who began his lifelong professional interest in the cultural uses of psychoactive plants, has been one of its most outspoken critics, attacking them in no uncertain terms:

> I defend the Native American Church among Amerindian aborigines; but I deplore the 'Neo-American Church' among Caucasoid Americans who pretend to follow their 'religion' through the use of mescaline [the psychoactive alkaloid derived from the peyote cactus; see **Mescaline**] as a 'sacrament'. Ethno-graphically the latter is a wholly synthetic, disingenuous and bogus cult, whose hypocrisy (one would suppose) honest young people would discern and despise; indeed, to it could properly be applied the old missionary cliché against peyotism as the 'use of drugs under religious guise'.

In his turn La Barre has been criticised by Jonathan Ott for such attitudes, Ott accusing him of: 'pure, unalloyed discrimination . . . racial and religious discrimination . . . [the] sacramental use of entheogens is as much a part of Caucasian heritage as it is a part of New World Indian heritage.'

**Sources:** La Barre 1989, Ott 1993.

# NEW GUINEA, PSYCHOACTIVE PLANTS OF

In *Plants of the Gods* by Richard Schultes and Albert Hofmann, one of the most important surveys of the global use of psychoactive substances, there is a map of the world showing the distribution of many such substances. Australasia and Oceania are left entirely blank. Concerning this apparent lack of cultural interest in hallucinogens and other psychoactive substances the authors write:

> curiously, no hallucinogenic plants are known to have been employed by the aboriginal populations of Australia and New Zealand. Nor has the use of any hallucinogen been reported from the Pacific Islands, although plants with hallucinogenic principles are known to exist in the flora of Polynesia ... it is in the New World that the number and cultural significance of hallucinogenic plants are over-whelming, dominating every phase of life among the aboriginal peoples.

Whilst it is undoubtedly true that the Amerindian peoples do use an extraordinary number of psychoactive substances, it is also the case that the great majority of ethnobotanists and anthropologists interested in such plants and their uses have tended to concentrate their field researches in the western hemisphere, particularly in the Amazon region and Mexico. Richard Schultes has certainly done more than any other individual to inspire and train other researchers to work in these regions and the results speak for themselves. However, since most research has been conducted by North Americans among American aboriginal cultures the rest of the world has tended to be overlooked and understudied. Whilst there do not seem to be many psychoactive plants used by the Australian Aborigines in New Guinea and the nearby islands, the case is rather different. There are numerous reports of the use and effects of such plants but many of them tend to be passing references by individuals usually concerned with other aspects of native life; nevertheless it is clear from the examples given below that there is a very extensive use of such substances in this area that have barely been investigated.

The Wopkaimin people, a Mountain Ok people of inner New Guinea (and close neighbours of the Bimin-Kuskusmin, whose ritual life is based around the entheogenic use of mushrooms and tobacco) eat the nuts of an unidentified species of mountain *Pandanus*. It is a woody, palm-like plant, some 500 species of which grow throughout the tropics from West Africa to eastern Polynesia in large quantities. The Wopkaimin eat it, precipitating what has been dubbed the 'Karuka madness', an altered state of consciousness that lasts some twelve hours and is characterised by excitability, restlessness and violent behaviour. The Chimbu people of New Guinea have also been reported to use an unidentified species of *Pandanus* for its psychoactive properties (which are due to the presence of the hallucinogenic DMT). During the season when the fruits are ripening the Chimbu eat large amounts of raw *Pandanus* nuts and are said to go 'mad'. The nuts of a palm (*Archontophoenix* sp.) and the leaves of another plant (*Pueraria phaseoloides*) have been used for their psychoactive effects in West Nakanai, New Britain as reported by an ethnobotanist named Floyd in the early 1950s.

The seeds of *Castanopsis acuminatissima*, a tree which is known as *kawang* in the Banz region of New Guinea, are steamed and eaten by the native people of the region as a way of experiencing similar effects to those of the 'mushroom madness' (see **Fungi**). The mushrooms in question often grow at the base of this very tree. Among the Gimi people of the New Guinea Highlands the bark known locally as *kikisira* (from an unidentified species of *Bubbia*) is smoked in a mixture with tobacco and is reported to cause a dream-like state of consciousness utilised during magical healing ceremonies. The Gimi are also reported to use another bark (from *Himantandra belgraeveana*) to induce trance states. The Gunantuna make use of the pollen of a plant called *baibai* or *bebai* (*Cycas circinalis*) for its narcotic properties. On the islands of the Torres Straits, which lie between the New Guinea mainland and Australia, a *maidelaig*, or local magician, would eat the immature leaf shoots of *budzamar* (*Cycas* sp.) when he wished to enter a 'wild state'. Magicians of the same region also eat the roots and leaves of another plant they call *kara* (*Capparis* sp.) for its similar psychoactive effects, and *kubilgim* (*Diospyros* sp.) is believed to transform a novice into a fully-fledged magician. *Kaempferia galanga* is reported to be used for its effects in two areas of New Guinea; in the Fore region it is used as a hallucinogen and in the Morobe region for its ability to cause pleasant dreams.

This list is by no means exhaustive. Fitz Poole, an anthropologist who has studied the entheogenic (see **Entheogen**) cult of the Bimin-Kuskusmin people of inner New Guinea (see **Fungi**), records the use of numerous additional magical plants used by these people, some of which may also be psychoactive. Peter De Smet has compiled a list of some forty psychoactive plants used by New Guinea peoples in addition to their use of betel, tobacco, alcohol, kava and mushrooms. It seems clear that if more research on the use of psychoactive substances in this region of the world is undertaken then the full extent and significance of them in the cultures of New Guinea will be realised.

See also **Betel**, **Fungi**, **Kava**.

**Sources:** De Smet 1985, Glick 1967, Haddon and Seligmann 1904, Heim and Wasson 1965, Hyndman 1984, Poole 1987, Powell 1976, Rudgley 1993, Schultes and Hofmann 1980b.

## NICOTIANA see Tobacco

## NICOTINE see Tobacco

## NITRITES

Nitrite inhalants such as amyl, butyl and isobutyl nitrite have been used medicinally since the middle of the nineteenth century. Nitrites are esters of nitrous acid and are very volatile liquids. Although amyl nitrite is a prescription drug in the United States, the substance is best known by the name 'poppers' (the name derives from the popping sound made when a pearl of amyl nitrite is opened) as a recreational drug. Inhalation of the drug causes an immediate but short-lived high (hence their other street name of 'rush') but some report having felt an uncomfortable pressure in the head whilst using it. It has a reputation as an aphrodisiac based on the belief that it can maintain erections and relax the anal sphincter, thus making it popular in the homosexual community. These supposed attributes of amyl nitrite are not corroborated by scientific findings. There is, however, research that suggests that the use of nitrites may make the user more prone to HIV infection. In America analysis of various brands found some to contain toxic additives such as kerosene and hydrochloric acid.

**Sources:** Lange and Fralich 1989, Tyler 1995.

## NUTMEG

Nutmeg and its sister spice mace both come from the nutmeg tree *Myristica fragrans*. This tree grows thirty to forty feet high and its seed is nutmeg. The nutmeg tree grows in the Molucca Islands and elsewhere in Indonesia. It is now cultivated commercially in the West Indies, especially Grenada, for its spices. The international trade in nutmeg seems to have originated with Arab traders and it was unknown in the classical world. The early European spice trade was remarkable for the sheer ferocity of the European nations that struggled with each other for control of this lucrative market. The apparently insignificant nutmeg that is found in almost every kitchen today was once fought over by competitors from Venice, Genoa, the Netherlands, Portugal and England. In the stampede most of the native inhabitants of the Banda Islands in the Indonesian archipelago (the source of the nutmeg tree) were wiped out.

Nutmeg has been considered to be a useful medicine in a number of Asian societies. Among the Arabs it has been used to treat digestive problems and also been valued as an aphrodisiac; the Indians used it to combat asthma and heart complaints and still use it as a sedative. Nicholas Culpeper (1616–54), the famous English herbalist, attributes to nutmeg the capacity to induce sleep and delirium. William Salmon, on the other hand, said that the oil of mace or nutmegs, if rubbed on the genitals, excited sexual passion (thereby echoing the Arabs' use of its aphrodisiac qualities). Nutmeg also was seen as having magical properties and is one of the ingredients of a magical perfume described in the most famous of all the grimoires, or black books of the sorcerers, *The Key of Solomon the King*. The use of nutmeg as a magical medicine continued far into the twentieth century in England. The belief that carrying nutmeg in the pocket could cure various complaints has been recorded from various parts of the country. In Yorkshire it was considered as the best way to relieve rheumatic pain, in Lincolnshire it was said to cure backache and in Devon it was eaten to clear up boils. Elsewhere it was used by gardeners as a prophylactic measure against the occupational hazard of backache. As late as 1966 a Hampshire coalman who suffered from lumbago was told to carry nutmeg, and when he did so he swore he never suffered from it again. Nutmeg was also believed to be lucky in gambling. A newspaper article from the mid-1960s reported that an individual sprinkled nutmeg powder on their football pools coupon and, on the advice of a gypsy, left it for twenty-four hours before posting it.

Nutmeg's intoxicating properties have long been known in Europe but it never seems to have been a culturally significant psychoactive substance and most early reports concern its accidental rather than intentional ingestion for use as a drug. Its more prominent role in modern times has not been due in the main to an increased desire for it as it has a very lowly status in the hierarchy of drugs, owing to its uncomfortable side effects such as nausea and stomach cramps. Rather it has been a substitute for other substances that for one reason or another were unavailable or unaffordable. Thus prisoners, soldiers, seamen and struggling musicians were among its users. A jazz musician who played regularly with the legendary saxophonist Charlie Parker (known as 'Bird') recalled that: 'Bird introduced this nutmeg to the guys. It was a cheap and legal high. You can take it in milk or Coca-Cola. The grocer across the street came over to the club owner and said, "I know you do all this baking because I sell from eight to ten nutmegs a day." And the owner came back and looked at the bandstand and there was a whole pile of nutmeg boxes.' In 1946, before his conversion to Islam, Malcolm X used nutmeg whilst in jail when his supplies of marijuana ran out. In his autobiography he wrote: 'I first got high in Charlestown [prison] on nutmeg. My cellmate was among at least a hundred nutmeg men who, for money or cigarettes, bought from kitchen worker inmates penny matchboxes full of stolen nutmeg. I grabbed a box as though it were a pound of heavy drugs. Stirred into a glass of cold water, a penny matchbox full of nutmeg had the kick of three or four reefers.' When the authorities became aware of such uses of nutmeg it was removed from many prison kitchens.

Although nutmeg has been demoted to a 'pseudo-hallucinogen' by many authorities, a self-experiment by Paul Devereux, a writer on the alignments of prehistoric sites, seems to indicate that its psychoactive effects can nevertheless be quite dramatic. In July 1989 Devereux took two level teaspoons of ground nutmeg and then went to bed, sprinkling nutmeg essential oil on his pillow and sheets. He began to feel the minor discomforts often associated with nutmeg use – mild nausea, irritation of the skin and so on. When he had been asleep for a few hours he had a dream in which he was travelling down a tunnel and flying at ever increasing speeds. He became fully conscious when in full flight and travelled over a landscape. During the flight he passed close to a tree and snatched at its leaves, feeling 'the pull of the branches and the foliage digging into my hand'. In other words the tactile sense was fully operative. He decided to terminate the journey by retracing his path and arriving back at his starting point, and opened his eyes. His hallucinations were thus both visual and tactile but he experienced no auditory or olfactory sensations during the experience.

**Sources:** Balick and Cox 1996, Culpeper 1805, Devereux 1992, Opie and Tatem 1992, Salmon 1693, Weil 1979.

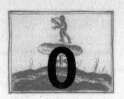

## OLOLIUQUI

*Ololiuqui* was the name given by the Aztecs to the morning glory (*Turbina corymbosa,* also known as *Rivea corymbosa*) or more particularly to its psychoactive seeds. *Ololiuqui* may also have been a name given to other plants too but not *Datura,* as was once thought by some botanists. The Aztecs also made use of another morning glory with psychoactive properties (*Ipomoea violacea = I. tricolor*) which they named *tlitliltzin.* Both contain ergot alkaloids, of which the most prominent are lysergic acid amide (ergine) and lysergic acid hydroxyethylamide. Although closely related to LSD these plants have, in addition to their hallucinogenic effects, a marked narcotic effect not experienced with LSD. The Aztecs used the morning glories to procure visions (or 'satanic hallucinations', as an early Spanish commentator put it), as aphrodisiacs and as medicines. One such medicine combined the forces of *ololiuqui* with those of *Datura* and peyote. The use of *Turbina corymbosa* has continued into modern times in Oaxaca, southern Mexico among the Mazatec, Mixtec, Zapotec and Chinatec Indians who use it in their medical systems and also as a clairvoyant means of locating lost or stolen property.

A bastardised form of the Aztec word, 'oliukqui', is reported by an official narcotics agency document (dated 1963) to have been used as a slang term for cannabis. The compilers of this anonymous work may have been misled by their informants. It seems more likely that it is a reference to the use of psychoactive morning glory seeds derived from widely available horticultural varieties as an alternative to LSD.

**Sources:** Anon 1963, Ott 1993, Rätsch 1992, Schultes and Hofmann 1980a, Schultes and Hofmann 1980b.

## OPIUM

The opium poppy (*Papaver somniferum*), being the source of both the indispensable pain-killer morphine and the most notorious of all street drugs, heroin, is at once a universal boon and a universal bane. From prehistory to the present it has played a central role in human life and its future, for better or for worse, seems to be guaranteed. Opium is the congealed juice of the poppy. It is extracted from the plant by cutting slits into the surface of its capsule and then collecting the juice once it has coagulated.

Despite considerable research into the origins of opium cultivation and use, it is still not clear exactly when and where it started. However, it appears to have been first domesticated about 8,000 years ago somewhere in the western Mediterranean region. Its use was widespread in Neolithic (New Stone Age) Europe, as the numerous finds of poppy seeds in various countries attests. Its archaic ritual use as a psychoactive substance can be inferred from the discovery of numerous opium poppy capsules at a prehistoric burial site in southern Spain dated to around 4,200 BC. There is every reason to believe that it continued to be cultivated and used as both a medicine and an entheogen right through into the historical period.

In the ancient Egyptian tomb of Kha at Deir el-Medina a pot was found, still containing some of its contents. This residue was subjected to scientific analysis at a laboratory in Genoa. Extracts of it were injected into a frog and a mouse and both animals fell into a deep sleep. The substance was found to be morphine and the opium from which it had been taken was about 3,000 years old and still active! It appears that there was an ancient trade in opium and that Egypt received its supplies from Cyprus. This has been demonstrated by the discovery of Bronze Age Cypriot pottery in ancient Egypt. Some of this pottery belongs to a type known as Base-ring juglets. In the early 1960s Robert Merrillees drew attention to the fact that the form of the Base-ring juglets seemed remarkably similar to the opium poppy and suggested that these artefacts were in fact skeuomorphs (see **Datura** for an explanation of this term) of the opium poppy and that they were containers for transporting opium. Later chemical analysis of the organic residues on samples of this pottery by John Evans revealed the presence of opium. Recently, however, the accuracy of this analysis has been questioned. Yet the case still remains highly persuasive.

Among the finds from the archaeological site at Kition in Cyprus were artefacts that seem to have been used for smoking opium. In temples belonging to the Late Bronze Age period (Late Cypriote III) a number of ivory objects were found and dated to the period *c.*1220–*c.*1190 BC, one of which has been identified by the excavators and other experts as an opium pipe; another is a cylindrical vase identified as a ritual vessel for smoking opium. The ivory pipe is just under 14cm in length and tapers slightly from one end to the other. It is embellished with curved and zigzag lines. At the smaller end there is an opening which was made to create a passage which goes approximately a third of the way down the length of the pipe. This is joined by another opening made in the top of the pipe; this latter opening still bears the signs of burning. At the broader end there is a diagonal passage leading from the end itself to an opening at the top which is a suspension hole. At this end another hole was started but never finished and is presumably an unsuccessful attempt to make the suspension hole. The cylindrical vase is of a similar form to a vessel found in Crete, which has also been identified as an object used in the ritual smoking of opium, most likely as an integral part of the worship of a fertility goddess. Mark Merlin states in his *On the Trail of the Ancient Opium Poppy* that opium probably first arrived in Greece during the first phase of the Late Helladic period (*c.*1600–1450 BC). Mycenaean signet rings have been found that show a female deity holding what seem to be opium poppies, a motif that may be the source of later Classical Greek depictions of Persephone holding opium poppies. The opium poppy was important throughout the Greek and Roman worlds,

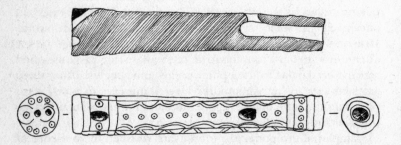

**PREHISTORIC OPIUM PIPE FROM CYPRUS**

and it is even reported that the Neo-Platonist philosopher Plotinus was an opium addict.

Whilst Greek and Roman medical traditions undoubtedly influenced the use of opium in the rest of Europe, the other countries clearly had their own ancient lore to draw upon, having used it themselves since Neolithic times. It seems that the psychoactive and perhaps the addictive properties of opium were not unknown in earlier times. A fourteenth-century manuscript entitled *Papal Garland Concerning Poisons* includes an assertion that opium causes mental disturbance. The Paracelsian physician Oswald Crollius (*c.*1560–1609) noted that in his master's *Archidoxes* there is a description of a specific anodyne based upon opium. Paracelsus (1493–1541), the great alchemist and physician of the sixteenth century, not only did more to popularise the use of opium in medicine than any of his contemporaries but he was also the first to make laudanum – a mixture of opium and alcohol. Laudanum (also known as ledanum and labdanum in early writings) was to remain popular right into the twentieth century and is still made on a small scale in the UK and available for doctors to prescribe, although few are aware of the fact. There were innumerable preparations of opium in the seventeenth and eighteenth centuries: William Salmon lists about 170, including Quercetan's Extract (which was a mixture of opium and mead), Crollius's Extract of Opium, Extract of Opium with Henbane, Paracelsus's Specifick Anodyne, Nepenthe of Sala, Liquid Laudanum of Joel Langelot, Laudanum Starkii (a laudanum preparation of George Starkey usually identified with Eiraneus Philalethes, the alchemist) and Laudanum Liquidum Helmontii (i.e. a preparation of John Baptista van Helmont, 1577–1644). In his work *Oriatrike* van Helmont is highly sceptical of the efficacy of opium for treating mental disturbances because it does not cure the patient at all but artificially induces a narcotic stupor to calm the 'waking nightmares' of the afflicted individual. In Victorian England opium was a part of daily life and was almost universally used to pacify babies and children. It was particularly popular among child carers who routinely used it to dope their charges. No doubt many childminders and nannies today would reach for the laudanum bottle if they were allowed!

Western erotomania projected itself on to the East during the eighteenth and nineteenth centuries, as the following tale of opiate aphrodisiacs shows: 'there is an Electuary prepar'd by the

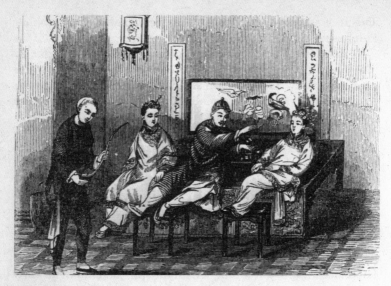

**CHINESE OPIUM DEN**

Indians of Opium, which the Chinese make use of to excite venery; by the use whereof they are so enraged with a libidinous Fury that the Whores are not able to endure their furious assaults and encounter.' Towards the end of the nineteenth century opium use came to be more critically examined and in an entirely unfounded xenophobic onslaught against the Chinese opium became no longer an unquestioned part of daily life but an 'evil' and 'foreign' drug. Opium addiction may have declined as a consequence but the even more addictive morphine and heroin took its place (see **Heroin**).

**Sources:** Bisset et al 1994, Evans 1989, van Helmont 1662, Karageorghis 1976, La Barre 1980, Manniche 1989, Merlin 1984, Merrillees 1962, Parssinen 1983, Salmon 1693, Sherratt 1991, Thorndike 1923–58, Williams 1947.

## OSTEOPHLOEUM

*Osteophloeum platyspermum* is a scarce primary forest tree found in the Amazon, belonging to the Myristicaceae. It is used by the

Quichua people (who call themselves Runa) of Ecuador as a hallucinogen. The red sap of the tree is heated with pieces of the bark, allowed to cool, then drunk by Runa elders for its psychoactive powers. The elders informed visiting ethnobotanists that they drank it 'to see phantoms and ghosts' and to contact the world of the spirits. Excessive doses can be fatal. The psychoactive constituents contained in the sap are tryptamines.

**Sources:** Bennett and Alarcón 1994.

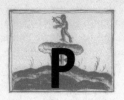

## PANAEOLUS see Fungi

## PCP

Phencyclidine (commonly known as PCP) was first synthesised in 1926. In the mid-1950s the pharmaceutical organisation Parke, Davis and Company began to investigate its potential as a human anaesthetic. The drug, in expectation, was given the trade name Sernyl (the name is said to be derived from serenity), but this was an epithet that was to become wildly inappropriate. Initial researches with the drug's effects on animals demonstrated its action on the CNS (central nervous system). In low to moderate doses it acted as a stimulant whilst higher doses had a depressant effect. The company ran into problems in 1957 when it was tested for the first time on human subjects. Worrying side effects such as hallucinations, mania, delirium and disorientation made them realise that it was inappropriate for use as a human anaesthetic and they finally abandoned their goal in 1965. As an anaesthetic agent phencyclidine was then relegated to the realm of veterinary medicine. Its psychoactive effects were investigated for their use in treating psychiatric disorders and, in the process, its properties became clearer. The human guinea-pigs consistently reported radical transformations in the perception of their own bodies. The tests revealed that the subjects experienced altered consciousness of the boundaries of the body and the dissociation of body parts, both sensations reported in cases of sensory deprivation. PCP was shown to interfere with the normal discrimination of internal stimuli in the body.

Only two years after PCP was dropped by Parke, Davis and Company it began its career as a street drug in the 1967 'Summer of Love' under a variety of local names, and was often sold under the pretence that it was cocaine, LSD or THC (THC is the psychoactive principle of cannabis; see **Cannabis**). By 1968 it was available in the form of pills in a number of major American cities, including New York (as 'hog'), Philadelphia (as 't-tabs'), Chicago (as 'THC') and Miami (initially as 'PeaCe pills' and later as 'THC tabs'). Use of the drug seems to have spread significantly in the years 1973 to 1975, partly because of its availability in forms suitable for smoking and snorting; both methods allowing users to control the dose more efficiently than the pills had permitted. PCP can also be taken intravenously, vaginally and rectally. In the mid-1970s PCP was still something of an unknown quantity in the drug scene and, as such, a negative mystique grew up around it, giving its users a reputation for daring.

By the mid to late seventies PCP use was sufficiently common for it to attract the interest of the media and government agencies. When a relatively unknown drug suddenly gains prominence the initial reactions to it are often highly distorted and even hysterical. The PCP case is no exception. Through media hype and a lurid concentration on exceptional reports of its use by aberrant individuals PCP became inextricably linked with extreme violence. The myth was thus born that simply by taking PCP an individual would become prone to commit all kinds of monstrous attacks. In 1978 at special hearings organised by the Select Committee on Narcotic Abuse and Control of the US House of Representatives one senator called PCP: 'one of the most dangerous and insidious drugs known to mankind.' Whatever the dangers of the drug, violent behaviour does not appear to be among them. Ethnographic and sociological studies of PCP users do not support such a view. Most of the users interviewed expressed surprise that PCP was associated with violence at all.

The use of PCP is particularly common among young adolescents, many of whom leave it behind them by the age of seventeen or eighteen. A user from Miami makes an analogy between the recreational use of the drug and watching television (which Terence McKenna has, not without some justification, described as one of the most dangerous drugs known to man!): 'It's as though life is like television and you're going through it on one channel and you suddenly discover that you can change the channels. Kind of like watching the 11.00 o'clock news and switching back and forth.' Based on information obtained in numerous interviews with 'dusters' (regular PCP users; the name comes from the street name 'angel dust'), researchers have produced a four-fold classification of dose levels and stages of the altered states of consciousness induced by the drug. When a user is 'buzzed' they have taken a stimulant dose which does not interfere with everyday tasks or the ability to work whilst under its influence. Being 'wasted' means that body co-ordination is affected, out-of-body experiences are frequent, as is the sensation of walking on a spongy surface. When a user has taken a higher dose and is incoherent and basically immobile but still conscious they are said to be 'ozoned'. An overdose is the final stage and involves loss of consciousness, according to most users not considered to be life-threatening. Taking Valium is a commonly used way of counteracting the effects of PCP. Like amphetamines (see **Amphetamines**) regular overindulgence with PCP can have debilitating effects, such as loss of appetite, weight loss and constipation. It can also be dangerous if taken during pregnancy; studies show that such use may result in premature birth to under-weight and under-size babies. PCP does not appear to result in permanent damage to the cells or internal organs of the user's body.

There are numerous varieties of PCP, ranging from purer crystalline forms (white in appearance and known simply as 'crystal') to adulterated low-quality products (such as 'rocket fuel': moist, yellowish and said to increase the likelihood of a bad trip). From Chicago it is reported that a green form of PCP was sold especially for St Patrick's Day! PCP is also smoked in marijuana joints (known as Krystal Joints or simply KJs). In addition to all these kinds of PCP there are some thirty PCP analogues on the street.

**Sources:** Beschner and Feldman 1979, Carroll 1985, Cleckner 1979, Feldman 1979, James and Andresen 1979.

## PEGANUM HARMALA

The shrub *Peganum harmala* (commonly known as harmel or Syrian rue) grows in arid regions across Eurasia from the Mediterranean in the west to Pakistan and India up to Mongolia and as far east as Manchuria. Five other species of *Peganum* are found in Asia, the south-west of the United States and Mexico. *P. harmala* seeds have hallucinogenic properties as they contain ß-carboline alkaloids, including harmaline and harmine.

In both India and Pakistan the seeds are used as a narcotic. In an Indian pharmacopaeia the plant is assigned various properties – an aphrodisiac when taken orally, a treatment for asthma and in higher doses it is used in abortion. In direct contrast to this latter usage is the ritualistic burning of the seeds in a room where a baby has just been born, a practice that is known from both north-western India and Pakistan. In the Punjab the seeds are also burnt at wedding ceremonies. In the Hunza region in the north-western corner of Pakistan shamans inhale the smoke given off by the burning seeds to communicate with spirits. A similar use is reported from Morocco where clairvoyant states are induced by smoking the seeds in conjunction with cannabis. In Bukhara in Central Asia inhaling the smoke was practised for its euphoric effects. The plant's psychoactive effects (in the form of both the smoke of its burning seeds and infusions made from the seeds) are also widely known in rural Iran. On account of its psychoactive effects and its wide use in Iran and Central Asia it has been suggested that *Peganum harmala* was the ancient entheogen *haoma/soma* (see **Soma**).

**Sources:** Flattery and Schwartz 1989, Hassan 1967, Rätsch 1992, Rudgley 1993, Schultes 1977, Schultes and Hofmann 1980b.

## PETROL SNIFFING see **Inhalants**

## PEYOTE

Peyote (*Lophophora williamsii, L. diffusa*) is a small spineless cactus found in the desert regions of Texas and Mexico. The heads of the cacti are cut off and used for their psychoactive properties by a number of Indian peoples. Because of their button-like shape they are often called peyote buttons or mescal buttons (not to be confused with mescal beans; see **Mescal beans**). Peyote is eaten raw or dried and sometimes in the form of a tea. It contains numerous alkaloids, including the powerfully hallucinogenic mescaline.

Remains of the peyote cactus dating back several thousand

years have been discovered by archaeologists excavating rock shelters in the Texas and Mexico border region. Rock art from the sites that dates from 4200–2950 years ago depicts recurrent images that bear a striking resemblance to those used by the Huichol Indians of Mexico up to the present day (for the Huichol see below). The prehistoric images of particular significance show a close metaphorical link between the peyote and the deer (in Huichol ritual life the two are seen as synonymous), depictions of peyote on deer antler tines (peyote collected by the Huichol is attached to antler tines carried by the shaman and the antler/ peyote connection also features in their mythology), and finally deer and dots – thought to represent peyote – pierced by arrows (the Huichol shaman ritually stalks the peyote and shoots it with an arrow). These three remarkable parallels that reach across the millennia strongly imply that the peyote ceremonies of the Huichol are essentially repetitions of rituals that have been performed for some 4,000 years.

In more recent times there have been three basic types of peyotism – the Mexican rituals, the transitional form of the Mescalero Apache and rites of the Plains Indians. Of the various Mexican Indian peoples who traditionally consumed peyote it is the ritual use of it by contemporary Huichol Indians that is thought by anthropologists to most closely resemble the Mexican rite as it would have been performed in pre-Columbian times. Two anthropologists, Peter Furst and Barbara Myerhoff, worked closely with the Huichol *mara'akame* (shaman-priest) Ramón Medina Silva and accompanied him on the annual peyote pilgrimage to Wirikuta, the geographical and mythical homeland of the Huichol, situated over 300 miles away from his community. The pilgrimage may be undertaken any time in the dry season between October and February. In December 1966 both anthropologists accompanied seven *peyoteros*, or peyote pilgrims, on their sacred journey. Pilgrims may be of either sex; and children, even infants, are encouraged to make the journey as their purity is considered beneficial to the whole party. Before their arrival in the sacred country the pilgrims must confess their sexual sins, for which they are forgiven. As the pilgrims approached the edge of the sacred land their leader Ramón located the cactus and ritually stalked it (see prehistoric paintings discussed above), then shot two arrows into it. Then he gave out pieces of the peyote to all the pilgrims, who ate it reverently. At this stage of the pilgrimage the amounts of peyote given out were not a dose sufficient to cause hallucinations. However, the pilgrims felt a great sense of communal ecstasy. In the later consumption of peyote on the pilgrimage hallucinations would be experienced by both the leader and his fellow pilgrims. Yet it was the visions of the *mara'akame* that were the most important; only he was able to communicate with deities and receive esoteric knowledge.

The sense of communal well-being that the peyote pilgrimage engendered in traditional Mexican societies was certainly not mirrored in the spread of the use of the cactus to the Apache. In fact, almost in direct contrast to the Mexican rituals, the use of peyote among the Mescalero Apache seemed to bring to the surface many tensions and discordant elements inherent in the community. Before the arrival of peyote around 1870, Mescalero spiritual authority lay squarely in the hands of shamans (or medicine men) who by entering into ecstatic trances were an elite with special access to the spiritual realm. But with the appearance of peyote, community members could, without having the training that the shamans had, go into altered states of consciousness with the help of the hallucinogenic properties of the cactus, in the process destabilising the traditional pattern in which such access was restricted to shamans. Peyote use became a great source of communal conflict and was seen not as a sacred plant but a social evil. Despite its rejection by the Mescalero Apache the peyote cult continued to find eager converts among the Plains Indians, so much so that an inter-cultural organisation was built around the sacred aura of the cactus (see **Native American Church of North America**). The Plains peyote rite has been practised as far north as Alberta and British Columbia. It is based on the ceremony as developed by the Kiowa and Comanche peoples.

Antonin Artaud, who, whilst travelling in Mexico, took peyote with the Tarahumara Indians, had this to say about the great differences between the psychology of whites and Indians:

A European would never allow himself to think that something he has felt and perceived in his body, an emotion which has shaken him, a strange idea which he has just had and which has inspired him with its beauty, was not his own, and that someone else has felt and experienced all this in his own body – or else he would believe himself mad and people would probably say that he had become a lunatic. The Tarahumara, on the contrary, systematically distinguishes between what is his own and what is of the Other in everything he thinks, feels, and does. But what makes him different from a lunatic is that his personal consciousness has expanded in this process of internal separation and distribution to which Peyote has led him and which strengthens his will.

Artaud wrote these words whilst being given detoxification treatment in France, having spent part of the previous year in Mexico. He had made the pilgrimage to the Tarahumara to, in his own words, 'regain a Truth which the world of Europe is losing'. He was still reeling in the wake of his failure to imprint his artistic vision on the European theatre, something which was only to occur fully after his death. Artaud, an opium addict and intermittent inmate in the asylum, regularly crossed the line between genius and madness and was unable to remain in the confines of the Western world view; he was thus lost in a limbo from which he hoped the experience of participating in the Mexican peyote ceremony would release him. To the communal ecstasy of the Indian peyote experience Artaud sadly remained an outsider. For him: 'With Peyote MAN is alone, desperately scraping out the music of his own skeleton, without father, mother, family, love, god, or society. And no living being to accompany him. And the skeleton is not of bone but of skin, like a skin that walks. And one walks from the equinox to the solstice, buckling on one's own humanity.'

Artaud was not the first member of the European intelligentsia to experiment with peyote, although he was one of the few to take it among native people. The psychologist and sexologist Havelock Ellis was one of the first to try it. He took three peyote 'buttons' on Good Friday 1896, alone and in the peaceful surroundings of his apartment. His visions were dramatic and aesthetically pleasing with none of the sombre and painful tones of Artaud's experience. Ellis introduced peyote to a number of poets, including W.B. Yeats. In 1914 the Greenwich Village socialite Mable Dodge performed a peyote ceremony based on the rituals of the Kiowa Indians, thus imitating the Indian use of this entheogen as was later to be done by the Neo-American Church with its psychoactive derivative mescaline (see **Neo-American Church**).

**Sources:** Adovasio and Fry 1976, Artaud 1976, Boyd and Dering 1996, Bye 1979, Ellis 1898, Furst 1972, La Barre 1989, Myerhoff 1974, Schultes and Hofmann 1980b, Stevens 1989.


## PHENCYCLIDINE see PCP

## PIPES

It is impossible to do justice to the history of the smoking-pipe in a few hundred, or even a few thousand, words. For the pipe is the commonest kind of object of all that is intimately connected to the consumption of psychoactive substances, with the sole exception of the drinking vessel. Whilst pipes are most readily associated with the smoking of tobacco a great many other substances have been taken in this fashion, cannabis and opium to name but two. One of the earliest known pipes was found in Cyprus. It is over 3,000 years old and was used for the ritual smoking of opium (for further details see **Opium**).

Before the arrival of tobacco in eastern North America (see **Tobacco**) about 2,000 years ago a number of other plants – alone or mixed together – seemed to have been smoked in pipes by native peoples (see **Kinnikinnik**). In the eastern Woodlands region of North America the earliest pipes are in the form of simple stone tubes (about 1000 BC), although it is not universally accepted that they were pipes at all and they may have been 'sucking tubes' used in native medical practices. It is only with the discovery of later forms of such artefacts (with mouthpieces) that they can clearly be classified as smoking pipes. Out of these simpler forms came an extraordinarily rich variety of highly ornate pipes which highlight the importance of smoking among the cultures of the region. The most significant of these belong to the Hopewell cultures of Ohio (100 BC–AD 200). The Hopewell pipes were typically made of stone and are called effigy pipes as they are made in the form of various mammals, birds, amphibians and other creatures. Their ceremonial function is obvious and some were designed for communal use and weigh several pounds.

The legendary calumet or 'peace pipe' of the North American

Indians was used on important social and ceremonial occasions, including treaties with the Whites. Father Louis Hennepin, writing in 1679, described the Iroquois use of such pipes:

> It is nothing else but a large Tobacco-Pipe made of Red, Black or White Marble: the Head is finely polish'd, and the Quill, which is commonly two feet-and-a-half long, is made of a pretty strong Reed or Cane, adorn'd with Feathers of all Colours, interlac'd with Locks of Women's Hair. They tie to it two Wings of the most curious Birds they find, which makes their *Calumet* not much unlike *Mercury's* Wand, or that Staff Ambassadors did formerly carry when they went to treat of Peace. They sheath that Reed into the neck of Birds they call *Huars* [loons] which are as big as our Geese, and spotted with Black and White; or else of a sort of Ducks who make their Nests upon Trees, tho' Water be their ordinary element, and whose Feathers are of many different Colours. However every Nation adorns the *Calumet* as they think according to their own *Genius* and the Birds they have in their Country.

Among the most famous and celebrated Amerindian pipes are those made of argillite by the Haida Indians of the Queen Charlotte Islands off the west coast of Canada during the nineteenth century. These were not in fact used by the Haida themselves or by anyone else since they were not actually smokable. They were an early (and artistically remarkable) form of tourist art, designed to bring in much needed revenue.

Elsewhere in the world other cultures also invested much time and effort in making smoking apparatus, although the complex symbolism of the American Indian pipes remains unsurpassed. The typical traditional Chinese tobacco pipe consists of three parts: a small round bowl (often made of white copper or a specifically Chinese alloy called tootnague, made of copper, zinc, nickel and iron), a stem (of bamboo, ivory or a hard wood such as ebony) and a mouthpiece (of ivory, jade or glass). It is from the designs of the Chinese tobacco pipes that the subsequent opium pipes were developed, with an intermediate phase of smoking the two substances together. Human ingenuity seems to be inexhaustible when it comes to finding ways to make smoking-pipes. In the early 1950s the Italian anthropologist Lidio Cipriani visited the Andaman Islands, an isolated group of islands in the

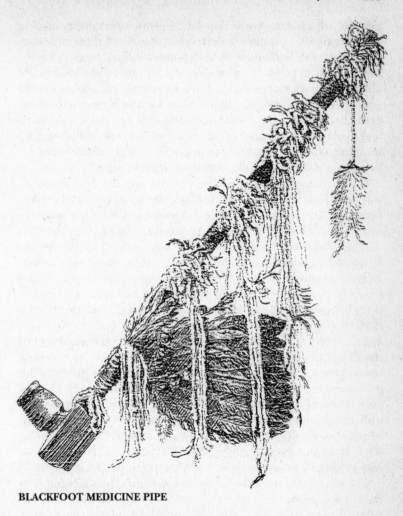

**BLACKFOOT MEDICINE PIPE**

Bay of Bengal inhabited by so-called Negrito people or Asian 'pygmies'. He found that they used giant crab-claws as pipes (crab-claw pipes are also known from Arnhem Land in northern Australia. One should not too readily assume that there must be a direct historical link between these crab-claw pipes, they are simply a suitable type of object for using as a smoking-pipe that is readily available in the immediate natural environment. Similar uses exist elsewhere, for example, among some of the native peoples of eastern North America lobster claws were used as smoking-pipes). Cipriani believed that the use of these pipes was very old on the Andamans, as he reported finding examples at the lower levels of archaeological deposits on one of the islands. He also notes that tobacco had only been recently introduced on the Andamans. If his rather vague claims for the antiquity of these crab-claw pipes were to be substantiated by more systematic archaeological investigations then one of two possibilities springs to mind. Either tobacco was available much earlier than he believes or other plants were smoked in these pipes.

Called the *narghileh* or *hookah* in India and the Islamic world, the 'hubble-bubble pipe' in Europe, the water-pipe is an Asian invention for smoking tobacco by passing it through water in order to cool it for a more pleasant smoke. The native Americans had no tradition of water-pipes. The word *hookah* or *hukka* is an Urdu word taken from the Arabic *hukka*, meaning 'casket' (alluding to the water container part of the pipe). *Narghile* comes from the Persian *nargile*, which in turn is derived from the Sanskrit term for coconut, *naragila*. Associated with the latter term is the Persian *qalyan*, from an Arabic root meaning 'boil' or 'bubble'. *Qalyan* refers to the pottery water-bottles that are a component of the Persian water-pipes. The first pictorial evidence for this kind of smoking apparatus comes from Safavid Persian paintings of the seventeenth century. Rather suprisingly, considering the general association of the water-pipe – and, indeed the pipe in general – with men, these paintings show both sexes using the apparatus. African water-pipes made of gourds, horn and pottery may be local examples imitating the Persian and Arabic prototypes or may belong to a more archaic type that developed far earlier.

The water-pipe seems to have entered China from Central Asia via Gansu province in the far west of the country. To some authorities on the subject (such as Berthold Laufer), the Chinese water-pipes (*shui yen tai*) represent the pinnacle of achievement both technologically and aesthetically. One of their specialities was a particularly compact form, specifically designed to be portable. The origins of the water-pipe are obscure; some authorities like Joseph Needham believe that the *narghile* cannot possibly be earlier than the introduction of tobacco from the New World, namely the first half of the sixteenth century. He has suggested that the model on which they might have been based when they first developed in China may have been the tradition among peoples of southern China and Vietnam of consuming wine from a communal vessel through tubes (made from cane, bamboo or straw) at festivals and other formal social occasions. Such drinking vessels are, of course, known from other parts of the world, for example the famous spouted *porrón* of Spanish culture. The water-pipe has an important place in the history of science as the prototype of the chemical gas bubbler or Woulfe bottle.

Needham is almost certainly right to see indigenous traditions of drinking as behind the design of the water-pipe. However, it does seem to be an error to think that such pipes were the invention of Asian peoples unfamiliar with smoking materials who simply needed to adapt drinking vessels in order to smoke the novel substance tobacco that first reached them in the sixteenth century. The discovery near Lake Tana in Ethiopia of the thirteenth- or fourteenth-century remains of pottery water-pipes with traces of cannabis in them shows that the use of cannabis in water-pipes preceded their use as tobacco-related paraphernalia. The history of the water-pipe is therefore not quite what it appeared to be, i.e. the invention of a tobacco-smoking apparatus out of a tradition of drinking alcohol. Braziers of one form or another have been used in Asia (and parts of Europe) for inhaling cannabis smoke for about 5,500 years (see **Cannabis**). When alcohol use spread from the urban centres of the Near and Middle East into cultural zones already using cannabis one of the results was the invention of the water-pipe. It was only later that the same basic type of equipment was used to smoke tobacco. Other plants may also have been smoked in water-pipes before the introduction of tobacco. In areas such as western Siberia where both tobacco and alcohol are relatively recent one can see the most rudimentary form of the water-pipe used far from the epicentre of such equipment. Among the Khanty (formerly known as the Ostyak) people of the region there are reports that the mouth was filled with water and then the smoke from a dry pipe inhaled as the water was swallowed.

Unlike the famous 'hubble bubble' and its variants, earth smoking-pipes are little-known. Roughly made, often in a makeshift fashion, their use has been most prevalent in two disparate regions of the world, southern Africa and Central Asia (there are also reports of their use in the New World). Despite their modest place in the history of the pipe they nevertheless demonstrate the inexhaustible ingenuity of humankind in finding a way to smoke psychoactive substances. The collection of actual specimens of earth-pipes in conjunction with descriptions of their use in numerous travellers' accounts led Henry Balfour, a past curator of the Pitt Rivers Museum in Oxford, to classify both the Asian and African pipes into common types.

The two fundamental types are those that were made by shaping the earth at the surface level of the ground and those made below the surface. The first type was made by mixing earth with either water or urine (if the former was not ready to hand) into a mound. Before the pipe-to-be was either dried in the sun or baked, a smoking 'bowl' was fashioned out at the top and a plant stem or stick pushed into the body of the mound as far as the base

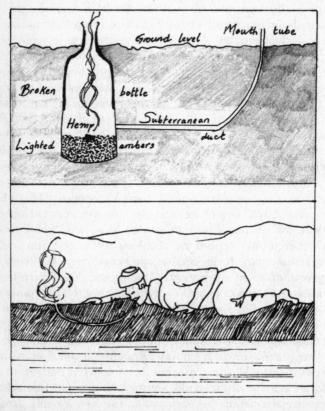

**THE METHOD OF SMOKING AN EARTH-PIPE**

of the bowl. When the pipe was dry the stem was removed in order to leave an open duct running from the bottom of the bowl to an opening at the side of the mound. A straw, or other available hollow tube, was then used to inhale the smoke generated by the burning substance in the bowl (in Africa both cannabis and tobacco were smoked in this fashion). Among the 'Bushmen' of the Kalahari desert the cannabis smoker would fill his mouth with water whilst inhaling, thus showing that in some instances the earth-pipe acted as a substitute for the genuine water-pipe. The size of this kind of earth-pipe varied enormously: in one particular example from Africa, clearly the work of a genuine aficionado, the duct was made by building up a mound around a spear-shaft!

At the other extreme the dried and finished earth-pipe would be detached from the ground in order to provide the user with a portable smoking instrument. African examples of this portable variant have been collected with the charred seeds of cannabis still remaining in the bowl. The advantage of the portable earth-pipe is not simply that it allowed the smoker to pursue the habit in different locations (which is particularly desirable in the roaming lifestyle of the hunting peoples of the Kalahari) but also that there is no need for the smoker to lie flat on the ground to use the pipe, which is hardly the most comfortable way to enjoy a smoke. Portable clay-pipes were also made in Africa which were not strictly earth-pipes but seem to derive from the mound-construction type. The other principal type of earth-pipe – that was made under the surface of the ground – was obviously not portable. It was used by men, women and children. All the key features of this type are shown in the accompanying illustration based on a communal African ground pipe used by Kaffirs for smoking opium or cannabis. A hole is dug in the ground and a broken bottle (with both neck and base removed) is placed in it with the top protruding slightly above ground level. Smouldering embers are put into the hole directly beneath the bottle and the substance to be smoked is placed on them. A subterranean duct leads from the 'bowl' and surfaces nearby; a mouth tube is then attached to that end of the duct in order to draw through the smoke. Other variants of the chthonic pipe contained water in the duct in imitation of a water-pipe.

There are a number of accounts in the writings of European travellers concerning the use of earth-pipes by Asian peoples. Descriptions of the way that such pipes were made clearly show parallels with the African traditions. E. Lovett describes a pipe built up on the surface of the ground and used to smoke a mixture of dried camel dung (Tibetans have been known to smoke yak dung with tobacco and the Plains Indians of North America to smoke bison dung and tobacco) and the leaves of an unspecified tree by the people of Kashmir who: 'built up with their hands, of the red, loamy material forming the kind of delta banks, in places where the streams ran more level, little elongated mounds ... these little mounds were from 5 to 6 inches long, about 2 inches wide at the base and about $1^1/_2$ inches high and, forming as they did a mere elevation of the clay bank, were really pipes of which the whole world may be said to form a part.'

As the earth-pipe has been shown to have sometimes acted as a substitute for the preferred water-pipe in Africa, so too is this the case in parts of Central Asia. Tekke Turkomans of the Merv oasis in western Turkestan are known to have used a *yer-chilin*, or earth-pipe, for smoking tobacco whilst travelling in circumstances not permitting the use of their beloved *kalian*, or water-pipe, and, like their African counterparts, are known to have held water in the mouth whilst smoking. The underground earth-pipe is known to have been used by poor men and women of Bokhara around the turn of the century for smoking the dried leaves of the apricot tree as a tobacco substitute. The antiquity of the earth-pipe can only be guessed at and it would be a mistake to interpret it simply as a crude forefather of the sophisticated designs of the water-pipe. In many cases it seems clear that earth-pipes were smoked when, for economic or other practical reasons, water-pipes were unavailable. That earth-pipes have been widely reported from two widely disparate regions of the world – southern Africa and Central Asia (including the mountainous areas of northern India) – led Balfour to suppose that there must have been at some time a diffusion of the practice from one area to the other. However, it is also quite possible that, despite the strong similarities between the earth-pipes of the two regions, this is an instance of independent innovation.

**Sources:** Balfour 1922, Cipriani 1966, Du Toit 1975, von Gernet 1995, King 1977, Knight 1975, Laufer 1924b, Needham SSC 5/4 1980, Sherratt 1994, Turner and Taylor 1972.

**PIPER BETLE** see **Betel**

**PIPER METHYSTICUM** see **Kava**

## PITURI

*Duboisia hopwoodii* is a shrub that grows in the arid interior of Australia and is found in all mainland States except Victoria. The plant contains both nicotine and d-nor-nicotine, an alkaloid first identified from *D. hopwoodii* in 1935. D-nor-nicotine is four times as toxic as nicotine. Levels of both alkaloids vary considerably from plant to plant. Chemical analysis has shown that one individual plant may contain fourteen times the amount of alkaloids found in another. Depending on dosage it is either a stimulant or a narcotic. *Pituri* is the Aboriginal name for preparations made from the plant *Duboisia hopwoodii*. Pituri, picheri, bedgery, etc were variations of this word that many travellers in the Australian outback gave to the Aboriginal of chewing mixtures, or quids, of either *D. hopwoodii* or the various species of tobacco that grow in Australia (for the latter see **Tobacco**). This has led to considerable confusion and the term *pituri* should be reserved only for mixtures made from *Duboisia*. Although mainly used by Aborigines, a few Whites, Chinese and Afghans (the latter of whom came to Australia with the camel to help 'open up' the desert interior of the continent) also made occasional use of *pituri*.

The earliest known reference to this psychoactive substance comes from an entry in the diaries of the Burke and Wills expedition, which refers to the giving of *pituri* by Aborigines to members of the expedition in May 1861. Wills wrote that: 'it has a highly intoxicating effect when chewed even in small quantities. It appears to be the dried stem and leaves of some shrub.' In order to make a *pituri* quid, about a tablespoon of leaf and stem from the shrub was either ground or chewed to break it up. As lime is added to betel or coca (see **Betel**, **Coca**) so the quid also had an alkali added to it. This has the effect of releasing the nicotine in the plant, thus increasing its psychoactive properties. That the Aboriginal users of *pituri* selected one of the most alkaline plants known to man to do this job (*Acacia salicina*) seems to indicate systematic experimentation on their part rather than fortuity. The Aboriginal use of quids made of tobacco also involved the releasing of nicotine by the same device. *Pituri* quids were usually a little bigger than a cigarette and brown-grey in appearance.

Despite its widespread natural occurrence, the shrub seems only to have been used in certain regions centred in the Mulligan-Georgina River Basin area of Queensland. Whilst it was used as an effective hunting poison (it was put in water holes frequented by kangaroos and emu and had the effect of making these animals intoxicated to the point where they became highly uncoordinated and thus easy to capture), its most important role was as a much-desired psychoactive substance for human use. The consumption of and trade in *pituri* was controlled, like many other aspects of traditional Aboriginal social life, by male elders. Under the supervision of these elders the plant was manipulated in a number of ways to ensure a potent supply of *pituri* was obtained. The older branches were subjected to fire to make way for new shoots which contain higher concentrations of nicotine. A fine description of a *pituri* 'laboratory' in the bush is given by Aiston:

> the secret of preparation was jealously guarded by the old men; the younger men were only allowed to accompany the party to the water nearest to the small clump of trees that were deemed to be the only true *pituri*. Here the younger men and the women stayed and prepared the bags to hold the prepared *pitcheri* and gathered food for the old men who did the harvesting. The old men went on to the trees, made a camp and built big fires. When these were burning down sufficiently they picked branch tips of the *pituri* bush, each about twelve inches at most in length. These were placed in a hole formed by raking out the fires down to the hot sand [and] were left to cook for at least two hours. When the steamed *pitcheri* was considered to be sufficiently cooked the sand was raked off and it was placed on a pirra to cool and dry. When thoroughly dry, it was beaten with the edge of a boomerang to break it up; all big twigs were picked out and the clean twigs bagged . . . the great secret lay in the length of time that was needed for the steaming and this was not taught the men until their beards were grey. When they were a 'little bit Pinnaru', that is, when the grey first showed in their hair and beard, they might be allowed to accompany the old men to the picking ground, and would be allowed to fill the bags with the prepared *pituri*, but the actual cooking

was done out of their sight. Sometimes, if the ground was hard, a hole was dug and the fire built in that, sometimes the fire was made close to a sandhill, and the sand was raked down from above. The method varied but the result was the same; too much steaming made the resulting 'cook' brittle and tasteless, too little made it musty.

There is little or no evidence that *pituri* played any role in native religions, rather *pituri* was used for its stimulant qualities in a number of practical ways – to increase work capacity, to suppress hunger, to assist in long journeys by foot and so on. Also, like other stimulants throughout the world, *pituri* was the focus of social gatherings and, as such, was an important substance in Aboriginal culture. One nineteenth-century observer describes its use:

in the social rites of these natives at their 'Big Talk' and feasts. The *pituri* quid . . . is ceremoniously passed from mouth to mouth, each member of the tribe having a chew from the pin'aroo, or head man, downward. This singular wassail cup never fails to promote mirth and good fellowship, or to loosen the tongues of the eloquent . . . there is a curious mode of greeting on Coopers Creek. When friends meet they salute with 'gaow gaow' (peace peace) and forthwith exchange *pituri* quids which, when well chewed, are returned to their owners' ears!

Other witnesses of such social events showed their complete lack of respect for their Aboriginal hosts, in some cases displaying their own mindless bigotry as the following account shows: 'it is a comical sight to see half a dozen nude niggers squatting on their hands gravely passing this, no doubt to them, delicious morsel from one to another, each chewing it in turn until the effects begin to appear in their staring eyes and . . . stupid look . . . I can only compare it to the appearance of an "habitual opium consumer" after indulging in his favourite drug.' This ignorant observer was, however, making a good point in some ways by comparing the effects of a potent nicotine experience with those of opium. Both morphine and nicotine are extremely addictive drugs and the extraordinary traditional trade in *pituri* must, in part at least, have been driven by the physiological needs of its consumers. It is reported that the possessor of the plant could buy anything that they desired – wives, husbands and all manner of goods. Major expeditions were undertaken by the Aborigines to obtain supplies of the plant: journeys of hundreds of miles for this express purpose were made without hesitation, even crossing the territories of hostile tribes along the way. The initial processing of the plants was done near to the place where they were gathered and then each man would carry up to 70 lbs of the drug home in special net bags or in the skins of wallabies. On their return the *pituri* dealers would keep some for their own people and trade the rest with neighbouring communities who were equally eager to obtain supplies. It has been estimated that the area that *pituri* was traded in was more than 300,000 sq km. The source of the *Duboisia hopwoodii* plants was kept secret both from White outsiders and other native people. The *pituri* trade was monopolised by those clans whose ancestors first discovered the properties of the plant and the way to prepare it for use. In stark contrast to most forms of exchange in tribal societies, the drug was not circulated through existing inter-community ties but traded on 'the open market', a very unusual kind of economic process among peoples who, at that time, still followed a very traditional hunting-and-gathering lifestyle.

In certain ways it is possible to view the Aboriginal tending of *Duboisia hopwoodii* as a tentative step towards agriculture. As Pamela Watson puts it:

the need to provision their society with a socially accepted means of altering consciousness meant that Aborigines developed means for intensified control over *Duboisia hopwoodii* plants, including discrimination between plants, on the basis of their phytochemistry; adoption of a particular technique to increase the proportion of preferred sections of the plant; specialisation of tasks in harvesting and curing the plant; and development of a complex curing process. This raises questions about the origin of agriculture. This is always viewed as the origin of food production ... [but] hunter/ gatherers appear to gain little, if anything, in terms of improved life styles or improved diet by their change in methods of procurement ... [but there is] an alternative: drug use, rather than food procurement, may have been the incentive for some early agriculture.

A similar suggestion has been made for the origins of agriculture in the Near East, particularly at Stone Age Jericho, by Andrew Sherratt: 'one might speculate that the first cultigens there were not cereals but something more valuable and negotiable: and a prime candidate would be one of the range of medicinal and narcotic plants whose products might be carried on the person.' He suggests mandrake, henbane, belladonna or *Withania* as possible trading plants. There is some evidence concerning tobacco cultivation in the New World that corroborates such views. Tobacco was one of the earliest plants cultivated by South American Indians (from about 6000 BC) and some North American Indian peoples such as the Blackfoot, indifferent to agriculture as a whole, grew their own tobacco.

The Aboriginal use of *pituri* seemed to die out partly because of the traumatic effects of colonisation (in the process of which the knowledge of *pituri* preparation was lost) and because the psychoactive substances brought in by the Whites took its place – particularly tobacco, alcohol and opium. Another psychoactive species, *Duboisia myoporoides*, is found in New Caledonia and contains the tropane alkaloids scopolamine and hyoscyamine.

**Sources:** Aiston 1937, Davis 1983, Peterson 1979, Sherratt 1996b, Watson 1983.

## POPPERS see Nitrites

## PROZAC

A phenomenal financial success, the anti-depressant drug Prozac was first developed in 1972 in the research laboratories of the pharmaceutical giant Eli Lilly & Co. After a pilot year on the Belgian market, it was launched in the United States in 1987. By 1993 sales had soared to $1 billion a year and Prozac established itself as the best-selling drug of its kind ever. Prozac differs from earlier drugs as it is the first of the group of compounds called selective serotonin reuptake inhibitors (SSRIs). It is mainly prescribed for those with clinical depression but it is also used in the treatment of drug abuse and compulsive eating disorders.

Praised by some as a 'wonder drug', it is supposed to have no significant side-effects and is not fatal in overdose. Barbiturates and other now defunct products were also hailed as wonder drugs with no side effects; history has shown it to be otherwise. Whether the same fate awaits Prozac remains to be seen. Already there are reports that a number of side-effects (including nausea, anxiety, insomnia and violent behaviour) do occur as a consequence of its use. Much publicity has surrounded the conflict between Eli Lilly and the Church of Scientology over the Prozac issue. According to the Scientologists – who are usually on the receiving end of bad publicity – the drug can cause not only suicide but also homicide. Despite this storm of controversy the drug encapsulates what the psychiatrist Dr Peter D. Kramer has called 'cosmetic psychopharmacology'. Residents of Hollywood (where else?) now give their pets Prozac when they think their poor animals are suffering from anxiety or depression.

**Sources:** Fieve 1994, Kramer 1994, Tyler 1995, Wurtzel 1994.

## PSILOCYBE

The *Psilocybe* are the hallucinogenic mushrooms most widely used for recreational purposes. Most users call them 'magic mushrooms' or 'Liberty Caps'. Psychoactive *Psilocybe* species are found almost the world over, including Europe, from Greenland to Tierra del Fuego at the most southerly tip of South America, in New Guinea, Australia, and New Zealand (both the north and south islands). There are estimated to be as many as eighty hallucinogenic species containing the psychoactive alkaloids psilocybin and psilocin (which are also found in species belonging to four other genera of mushrooms – *Conocybe*, *Panaeolus*, *Stropharia* and *Copelandia*). In sufficient quantities these mushrooms can cause visual, auditory and other hallucinations and profound changes in the perception of time and space (see the account of María Sabina below).

There is little evidence for the historical use of *Psilocybe* mushrooms in Europe, although the archaeologist Jeremy Dronfield has suggested that their use by the Neolithic builders and decorators of the Irish megaliths may have been responsible for the hallucinogenic imagery on these monuments, much of which still remains today. In fact, despite the near cosmopolitan distribution of the 'magic mushrooms', their traditional use has

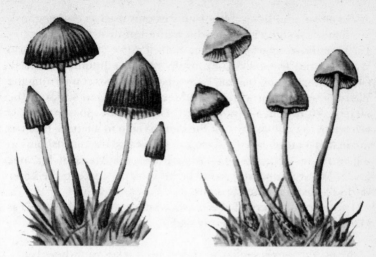

**PSILOCYBE**

yet to be demonstrated outside of the Americas. There are a number of types of ancient artefacts that indicate the antiquity of mushroom use in this part of the world. Mushroom-shaped stone artefacts (some of them incorporating toad designs) have been found in considerable numbers at sites in Guatemala dated between 100 BC and AD 300. Gold effigies from Colombia (AD 100–350) depict objects that have been interpreted as mushrooms. They are depicted in Mexican art dating from AD 300 and also feature in Aztec iconography. The most spectacular such representation in Aztec art is the sixteenth-century statue of Xochipilli, 'Prince of Flowers'. The pedestal is decorated with numerous mushroom caps identified as the hallucinogenic species *Psilocybe aztecorum*, which is known solely from the region around the volcano Popocatepetl where the statue was discovered. The body of Xochipilli is adorned with floral motifs of other psychoactive plants, including tobacco and morning glory (see **Ololiuqui**).

It was not known that the contemporary Indians of Mexico had maintained the cult of the mushrooms until earlier this century. In the thirties the anthropologist Robert Weitlaner obtained specimens of the mushrooms, which were subsequently investigated by the ethnobotanists Blas Pablo Reko and Richard Schultes (the latter correctly identifying them not as *Psilocybe* but as *Panaeolus*, another genus of mushrooms used as entheogens). Weitlaner's daughter attended a native mushroom ceremony in 1939 but did not partake of them herself. After the Second World War the trail was picked up again by the ethnomycologist R. Gordon Wasson and his wife Valentina (for details concerning the Wassons see **Fungi**), who visited Mexico in 1953 to seek out the sacred mushrooms after Robert Graves had pointed out a reference to the existence of the cult to them in a letter. This was the first of a number of field trips that revealed the mushrooms to the world at large. In 1955 Wasson met the Mexican Mazatec healer María Sabina who was to be his spiritual guide in the inner world of the sacred mushrooms.

The sacred powers of the mushrooms are not open to all, as María Sabina has so eloquently said:

the mushroom is similar to your soul. It takes you where the soul wants to go. And not all souls are the same. Marcial [her second husband, a violent and drunken man] had taken the *teo-nanácatl* [sacred mushrooms], had had visions, but the visions had served no purpose. Many people of the sierra have taken it and are taking it, but not everyone enters into the world where everything is known. Also Ana María, my sister, began taking them together with me, had the same visions, talked to the mushrooms, but the mushrooms did not reveal all their secrets. The secrets that they revealed to me are enclosed in a big Book that they showed me and that is found in a region very far away from their world, a great Book. They gave it to me when Ana María fell ill ... and seemed almost near death. So I decided to return again to the *teo-nanácatl*. I took many, many more than I had ever taken before: thirty plus thirty. I loved my sister and was ready to do anything, even to make a very long trip, just to save her. I was sitting in front of her with my body, but my soul was entering the world of the *teo-nanácatl* and was seeing the same landscape that it had seen many other times, then landscapes that it had never seen because the great number of mushrooms had taken me into the deepest of the depths of that world. I was going ahead until, at one point, a *duende*, a spirit, came toward me. He asked a strange question: 'But what do you wish to become, you, María Sabina?'

I answered him, without knowing, that I wished to become

a saint. Then the spirit smiled, and immediately he had in his hands something that he did not have before, and it was a big Book with many written pages.

'Here,' he said. 'I am giving you this Book so that you can do your work better and help people who need help and know the secrets of the world where everything is known.'

I thumbed through the leaves of the Book, many written pages, and I thought that unfortunately I did not know how to read. I had never learned, and therefore that would not have been of any use to me. Suddenly, I realised I was reading and understood all that was written in the Book and that I became as though richer, wiser, and that moment I learned millions of things. I learned and learned . . . I looked for the herbs that the Book had indicated to me, and I did exactly what I had learned from the Book. And also Ana María got well.

I didn't need to see the Book again because I had learned everything that was inside it. But I again saw the spirit that gave it to me and other spirits and other landscapes; and I saw, close by, the sun and the moon because the more you go inside the world of *teo-nanácatl*, the more things are seen. And you also see our past and our future, which are there together as a single thing already achieved, already happened. So I saw the entire life of my son Aurelio and his death and the face and the name of the man that was to kill him and the dagger with which he was going to kill him because everything had already been accomplished. The murder had already been committed, and it was useless for me to say to my son that he should look out because they would kill him, because there was nothing to say. They would kill him, and that was it. And I saw other deaths and other murders and people who were lost – no one knew where they were – and I alone could see. And I saw stolen horses and ancient buried cities, the existence of which was unknown, and they were going to be brought to light. Millions of things I saw and I knew. I knew and saw God: an immense clock that ticks, the spheres that go slowly around, and inside the stars, the earth, the entire universe, the day and the night, the cry and the smile, the happiness and the pain. He who knows to the end of the secret of the *teo-nanácatl* can even see that infinite clockwork.

On top of all her other suffering María Sabina was later imprisoned because she had inadvertently attracted the attention of unwelcome hippies who had heard about the mushrooms through the publications of Wasson and others. Wasson was deeply distressed at how his own sincere and respectful interest had indirectly had the consequence of causing additional suffering to María Sabina. But the hippies were not the first to profane the sacred mushrooms: that was done by the CIA. In 1955 the CIA had sought Wasson's co-operation, having become aware of initial publications concerning the hallucinogenic mushrooms. Their interest was in the possible military applications of the fungi. Wasson refused. The CIA would not take no for an answer and so successfully planted one of their operatives, James Moore, on the next expedition that Wasson had organised. It was only in 1979, when certain covert CIA activities were revealed, that Wasson learnt that Moore had played this role.

**Sources:** Dronfield 1995, Furst 1988, Halifax 1979, Ott 1993, Schultes and Hofmann 1980a, Schultes and Hofmann 1980b, Wasson et al 1974, Weil 1977.


## PSYCHEDELICS

Psychedelics is a name given to psychoactive substances with hallucinogenic effects. The word psychedelic was coined by Humphry Osmond and announced in a letter to Aldous Huxley as part of a discussion on how best to designate the drug mescaline. Huxley had suggested the word 'phanerothyme' in a rhyming couplet:

> To make this trivial world sublime,
> Take a half a gramme of phanerothyme.

Huxley derived this new word from the Greek and thought it should mean 'soul-manifester', although Jonathan Ott has shown that it actually means a drug that makes strong emotions manifest. Osmond was not keen on Huxley's term and had his own idea:

> To fathom Hell or soar angelic,
> Just take a pinch of psychedelic.

Huxley's word has disappeared almost without a trace whilst psychedelic remains a widely used term. The term became intimately associated with LSD and the counterculture of the 1960s largely through the liberal use of the term by Timothy Leary and his associates. It continues to be used in the counter-culture as the most common term for hallucinogenic drugs (as, for example, in the works of Terence McKenna), but most researchers of psychoactive substances prefer the term 'hallucinogen' (see **Hallucinogens**) or, more recently, 'entheogen' (see **Entheogen**), as the term psychedelic is too closely connected with the specifically modern Western use of such substances.

**Sources:** McKenna 1992, Ott 1993, Ott 1996.


## PUFFBALLS

Puffballs is the name commonly given to a group of fungi that includes the genera *Lycoperdon, Bovista* and *Calvatia*. The human use of puffballs can be traced back to the Neolithic (New Stone Age) period. Thirteen fruit bodies were found at the archaeological site of Skara Brae on the Orkney Islands off the coast of Scotland and have been radio-carbon dated to about 2,000 BC. Specimens have also been unearthed at other early sites in the British Isles, such as the discovery of *Bovista nigrescens* at Lochlee in Ayrshire during the 1870s. These puffballs were identified by Mordecai Cooke, an early mycologist and writer on psychoactive substances. The site of Vindolanda in Northumberland (dated AD 85–125) yielded three specimens of *Bovista nigrescens* and two specimens of *Calvatia utriformis*. What these various prehistoric and early historical communities were using puffballs for is unknown. Some puffballs are eaten and they have also been used traditionally to treat wounds in India, Europe and in North America; certain species seem to have psychoactive properties.

As R. Gordon Wasson and his wife pointed out in *Mushrooms, Russia and History,* their monumental work on the folklore of fungi, the puffball has more folk names attached to it than any other fungus by far. There are more names in the English language for puffball than any other kind of mushroom.

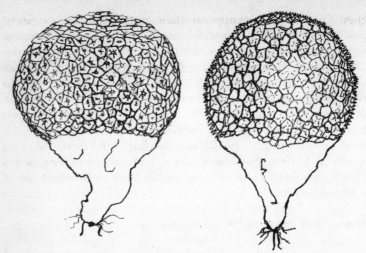

**LYCOPERDON MIXTECORUM (LEFT) AND LYCOPERDON MARGINATUM (RIGHT)**

Throughout Western Europe puffballs have demonic and scatological associations. The puffball is also called fuzzball, pixie-puff, fistball and puckfist. Puckfist means an 'imp's silent fart' (the releasing of the spores in the form of a dust cloud by the puffball being the inspiration for this scatological metaphor). In the French, Dutch and Danish versions of this the offender is not the imp but the wolf (the generic name of a type of puffball, *Lycoperdon*, also means 'wolf's fart' in Latin), whilst to the Basque people the puffball is the 'ass's fart'. As the Wassons note, the wolf, the ass, the pixie and puck are all linked in European lore with the devil. Later, and rather more discreet, names given to the puffball continue this tradition, such as the Russian 'devil's pepperpot' and the English 'devil's snuffbox'. In English the puffball was also given the name 'blind man's ball' on account of the belief that the spores were harmful to the eyes. This is corroborated by Francis Bacon who reported that, according to the medical opinion of his time, the dust that the puffball releases is bad for the eyes. Modern research has shown that inhaling puffball spores can cause a lung disease called *Lycoperdonosis*.

Among the Blackfoot Indians puffballs the size of golf balls were hung on the necklaces of men for their fragrance. The Blackfoot Indians call puffballs 'fallen stars' or 'dusty stars' and they feature prominently on their traditional *tipi* (wigwam) designs. The origin of these designs is a subject of Blackfoot myths. The Blackfoot were known for their considerable astronomical knowledge and had a number of star myths in their repertoire. In one of them, named 'Dusty Stars' (also called 'The Twin Brothers, or Stars' and 'The Origin of the Four-Tail Lodge'), a stranger visits a Blackfoot camp and teaches a man called Smart-Crow a new ritual and songs. The stranger also says:

> the punk which you use to make fires is made of bark, and does not kindle quickly; take puff-balls instead, for they are much better. They are the Dusty Stars. You are to paint these stars around the bottom of the lodge. At the top of the lodge you are to paint the Seven Stars on one side and the Bunch Stars on the other. At the back of the lodge, near the top, you must make a cross to represent the Morning Star. Then around the bottom, above the Dusty Stars, you shall mark the mountains. Above the door, make four red stripes passing around the lodge. These are to represent the trails of the buffalo.

Because the puffballs were known as fallen stars they also feature in these myths as the offspring of a woman and a star. In addition to the role that they play in Blackfoot mythology, puffballs are also burnt as incense to keep away ghosts. This may suggest that the Blackfoot were aware of the psychoactive properties of some puffballs which are known to have anaesthetic effects (see below). Also, the rubbing of spores of a *Lycoperdon* species by the neighbouring Flathead Indians of Montana on the eyelids and cheeks of children to cause sleep (in stark contrast to the European belief that this is dangerous to the eyes) may suggest a knowledge of the puffball's soporific properties.

Among the Tarahumara Indians of Mexico, puffballs (*Lycoperdon* sp.) are feared because of their association with sorcerers, who are said to employ them for causing sickness and to make them invisible to their victims. The Mixtec people of Oaxaca, Mexico use two species of puffballs which appear to have psychoactive effects. *Lycoperdon mixtecorum*, which the Mixtec Indians call *gi'i wa*, meaning 'a fungus of the first quality', causes the consumer of it to experience a soporific state in which auditory hallucinations are experienced. The voices heard are, according to the Indians, able to reply to questions that are posed to them, which suggests this puffball was valued in divinatory practices. *Lycoperdon marginatum*, the other puffball used by the Mixtec, has similar effects, although its native name *gi'i sawa* ('fungus of second qualities') suggests that it may be less potent. The amateur ethnomycologist Adrian Morgan reports from his own consumption of it that another fungus, an earth ball (*Scleroderma citrina*) causes a strong narcosis fifteen minutes after ingestion of half a specimen. He reports some visual disturbance, giving way to a deep sleep lasting two hours.

It has been a widespread practice in bee-keeping to put a smouldering puffball underneath a hive in order to sedate the bees, such a usage being mentioned by the famous herbalist John Gerard (1545–1612). Whilst this tranquillising effect has been explained away as due simply to an excess of carbon dioxide, the possibility that the puffball may have psychoactive properties cannot be dismissed. For puffballs have been used successfully in operations as anaesthetic agents. The Reverend Hugh Macmillan describes such little-known effects in a botanical work of the mid-nineteenth century:

the common puff-ball deprives the patient of speech, motion, and sensibility to pain, while he is still conscious of everything that happens around him ... when slowly burnt, this fungus has long been employed for stupefying bees, and thus robbing their hives of the honey with impunity. Experiments, with the same species, have also recently been made on dogs, cats, and rabbits, and similar effects have invariably been found to ensue. When the fumes of the burning fungus are slowly inhaled, they gradually produce all the symptoms of intoxication, followed first by drowsiness, and then by perfect insensibility to pain, terminating, if the inhalation be continued, in vomiting, convulsions, and ultimately in death.

**Sources:** Bacon 1627, Bye 1979, Emboden 1974, Hart 1979, Macmillan 1861, Morgan 1995, Munro 1879, Pegler et al 1995, Ramsbottom 1953, Schultes 1977, Wasson and Wasson 1957, Watling 1975, Watling and Seaward 1976, Wissler and Duvall 1909.

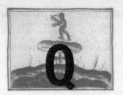

## QAT

*Qat* (*Catha edulis*) is an evergreen shrub that grows over a very large part of the African continent from South Africa to Ethiopia. Although the centres of cultivation are in the East Africa countries (Kenya, Somalia and Ethiopia) it is also reported to grow in Afghanistan and Turkestan. The plant is still said to grow wild in some mountainous regions in East Africa. It is used as a mild stimulant, more akin to tea or coffee than stronger psychoactive substances, despite its portrayal as a potentially dangerous drug by some Western medical and media reports. The main psychoactive alkaloid of *qat* is cathinone.

The first Islamic source that is thought to refer to *qat* comes from the work of al-Biruni in the middle of the eleventh century AD. According to al-Biruni the plant comes from Turkestan, which suggests, if he is indeed referring to *qat*, that the plant was taken there and cultivated some time before this. Krikorian has suggested that *hajis* (pilgrims) may well have brought the plant with them on their return from Mecca. Not all Muslims were immediately enamoured by *qat*. A fourteenth-century source recalls a rather amusing – and apocryphal – story of how the plant failed to inspire enthusiasm when first taken to the Yemen. When a Muslim from Abyssinia espoused the properties of the plant to the Yemeni sovereign he made much of its ability to lessen the appetite for food, drink and sex. The king is said to have replied: 'And what other pleasures are there in this base world besides those? By Allah, I will not eat it at all; I only spend my efforts on those three things. How am I going to use such a thing which will deprive me of the pleasures that I get from them?'

This contempt for *qat* is certainly not reflected in contemporary Yemen where *qat* houses abound. In these establishments coffee, tobacco and *qat* are consumed by men and it is one of the most important social forums for Yemenis. *Qat* is also widely consumed in Somalia, Kenya and Ethiopia. Although the market for *qat* is presently limited to this part of the world, on a local scale its cultivation is big business. At the beginning of the 1980s the Somali government estimated about 200,000 of its people were employed in the cultivation and distribution of *qat*. In addition to its role as a social stimulant, the plant is also used in traditional Islamic medicine. According to the *abjad* system of sacred numerology (each letter of the Arabic alphabet has a particular number attached to it; by adding up the numerical values of the letters of any word mystical relationships with other words and things are discovered), *qat* adds up to 501 and therefore the plant was believed to have that number of medicinal uses.

The use of *qat* first came to the attention of Europeans towards the end of the seventeenth century but, unlike other exotic stimulants such as tea, coffee and chocolate, never caught on. This may be largely due to the fact that the stimulating effects that are obtained from the leaves do not remain psychoactive; within two days they begin to disappear. It is now sold as a 'legal high' in the UK but the market for it is undoubtedly small. However, Andrew Tyler has predicted that the extraction of cathinone from *qat* may well result in it being used by illegal drug manufacturers to adulterate amphetamines and cocaine.

**Sources:** Kalix 1991, Krikorian 1984, Tyler 1995, Weir 1985.

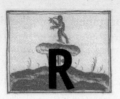

## RHODODENDRON

In the early part of the nineteenth century the German linguist Julius Klaproth, whilst travelling in the northern Caucasus, described how the nominally Christian local people used a rhododendron species for its apparent narcotic and hallucinogenic properties: 'the Ossetians often visit . . . caves to intoxicate themselves with smoke from the *Rhododendron caucasicum* which plunges them into sleep: the dreams that ensue are considered omens.' The species in question is now known as *R. ponticum*. It has been suggested that the psychoactive fruit of a tree mentioned by the Greek historian Herodotus as being used by the Massagetae people may be the same plant. He says that inhaling the smoke of the burning plant intoxicates like wine. The Greek historian of the fourth century BC, Xenophon, related in his *Anabasis* the mass poisoning of an army by the toxic honey which was derived from the nectar of *R. ponticum*.

**Sources:** Ott 1993, Sherratt 1996a.

## ROSEMARY

In Europe wild rosemary (*Ledum palustre*) has been implicated in the berserker frenzies of the Vikings. The Tungus people of Siberia were neighbours of many tribes using the hallucinogenic fly-agaric mushroom, although they chose not to use it, preferring instead *L. palustre* and *L. hypoleucum*. The dried leaves of these plants were burnt on a fire or in a frying pan and the smoke inhaled for its narcotic effects during shamanic healing sessions. A similar use is reported among the Gilyak, another Siberian people. Among the Kwaikutl Indians of British Columbia another species of the genus (*L. groenlandicum*) was used for its inebriating qualities.

**Sources:** Brekhman and Sam 1979, Ott 1993, Rätsch 1992.

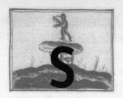

## SAFFRON

The pharmacology of saffron (*Crocus sativus*) has not been systematically investigated but it is known to have soporific and narcotic effects similar to those of opium. It can be very dangerous and is even reported to be deadly in the case of children. Notwithstanding, saffron has been attributed with healing powers since ancient times and was known to the Greeks as the Blood of Hercules. In the traditional medical systems of both India and the Islamic world it was seen to have aphrodisiac properties. Saffron was known as a euphoriant to the English herbalists, one of whom, William Coles, believed this property of the plant was the origin of the saying for one who was happy, namely that he or she 'hath slept in a bagge of saffron'. It was also one of the plants used in the making of the psychoactive ointments used by witches (see **Witches' Ointments**).

**Sources:** Coles 1657, Rätsch 1992.

## SALAMANDER

Salamanders have been used in medicine for at least 2,000 years. Parts of the common salamander were used in Greek medicine and, according to Dioscorides (first century AD) it is useful in the treatment of skin diseases and ulcers. At this time it was preserved in honey for use at a later date. The European alchemists extracted substances from all kinds of animals in their search for novel medicines and magical preparations. The seventeenth-century alchemist John Hartman recommends that rotten teeth will be encouraged to come out by rubbing them with a powder that is made of water lizards (by which he means either salamanders or newts) disembowelled and calcined in an oven. The salamander is particularly prominent in alchemical texts (in which some of the many discussions of dragons probably refer to this particular amphibian) and the illustrations that adorn them. It is possible that the alchemists extracted psychoactive substances from salamanders but this remains to be clarified. Paracelsus, one of the most respected of all alchemists, warned his readers that the salamander was to be treated with extreme caution: 'you cannot meddle with it without great danger, for the poyson of it is most deadly.' The modern investigation of salamander secretions has shown that they contain steroid alkaloids. The alkaloid samandarin is a powerful neurotoxin that has local anaesthetic properties but can also cause convulsions and death.

**Sources:** Crollius 1670, Gunther 1959, Habermehl 1981, Paracelsus 1656.


## SAN PEDRO CACTUS

The San Pedro cactus is the name given to psychoactive species of the genus *Trichocereus* (*T. pachanoi*, *T. peruvianus*) which comprises about thirty species, mainly found in the Andes. It is a large columnar cactus that grows up to heights of twenty feet and it contains mescaline, as does the well-known peyote cactus (see **Peyote**). The San Pedro cactus has also been found to have other psychoactive alkaloids. The mescaline seems to be most highly concentrated in the skin, which can be peeled, dried and made into a powder for consumption. The usual native preparation of the cactus involves boiling slices of the stem for a number of hours and then, once cooled, the resulting liquid is drunk. Sometimes the San Pedro is used in conjunction with other psychoactive plants, such as coca, tobacco, *Brugmansia* and *Anadenanthera*. The hallucinogenic properties of the cactus have been exploited by a number of native Indian peoples, especially those of the Andean regions of Bolivia, Peru and Ecuador. It is known by a number of names in the area of its traditional use, including *aguacolla*, *cardo*, *cuchuma*, *gigantón*, *hermoso*, *huando* and, of course, San Pedro.

Like many other of the entheogenic substances used in the aboriginal religions of the Americas, the use of the hallucinogenic San Pedro cactus is ancient and its use has been a continuous tradition in Peru for over 3,000 years. The earliest depiction of the cactus is a carving which shows a mythological being holding the San Pedro. It belongs to the Chavín culture (*c.*1400–400 BC) and was found in an old temple at Chavín de Huantar in the northern highlands of Peru, and dates about 1300 BC. A particularly surprising discovery was made by a Peruvian archaeologist named Rosa Fung in a pile of ancient refuse at the Chavín site of Las Aldas near Casma; namely what seem to be remnants of cigars made from the cactus. Artistic renderings of it also appear on later Chavín artefacts such as textiles and pottery (ranging from about 700–500 BC). The San Pedro is also a decorative motif of later Peruvian ceramic traditions, such as the Salinar style (*c.*400–200 BC), the Nasca urns(*c.*100 BC–AD 500) and pottery of the Moche period (*c.*100 BC–AD 700). It has also been proposed that a recurrent snail motif in Moche art represents a mescaline-soaked snail which has partaken of the San Pedro. If this is the case then the snail may be added to the list of animals having psychoactive properties (see **Animals**).

Not surprisingly, considering their general contempt for native life and particularly the use of psychoactive plants, European missionaries were very negative when reporting the use of the San Pedro. Yet a Spanish missionary, cited by Christian Rätsch, grudgingly admitted the cactus' medicinal value in the midst of a tirade reviling it:

> it is a plant with whose aid the devil is able to strengthen the Indians in their idolatry; those who drink its juice lose their senses and are as if dead; they are almost carried away by the drink and dream a thousand unusual things and believe that they are true. The juice is good against burning of the kidneys and, in small amounts, is also good against high fever, hepatitis, and burning in the bladder.

An account of the cactus by a shaman is in radical contrast to this rather contemptuous view:

> the drug first . . . produces . . . drowsiness or a dreamy state and a feeling of lethargy . . . a slight dizziness . . . then a great

'vision', a clearing of all the faculties . . . it produces a light numbness in the body and afterward a tranquillity. And then comes detachment, a type of visual force . . . inclusive of all the senses . . . including the sixth sense, the telepathic sense of transmitting oneself across time and matter . . . like a kind of removal of one's thought to a distant dimension.

The entheogenic status of the cactus remains as strong today as it always was. Not only do its uses in shamanic trances and healing sessions continue but it is also used to combat more recent problems such as alcoholism. The peyote cactus used widely by the North American Indians is also considered a medicine against alcoholism and this parallel is all the more striking as both cacti contain mescaline.

**Sources:** Ott 1993, Rätsch 1992, Schultes and Hofmann 1980a, Schultes and Hofmann 1980b, Sharon and Donnan 1977.

## SATURNIAN/SATURNINE HERBS

In medieval and later European occult thinking the doctrine of signatures ruled supreme. If an attribute of a plant or animal resembled some other phenomena in the natural world there was thought to be a hidden correspondence between the two. Most psychoactive plants were deemed to be under the celestial or astral influence of the planet Saturn (including henbane, the opium poppy and the mandrake; see **Henbane**, **Mandrake**, **Opium**). Of the seven planetary suffumigations (i.e. magical incenses) given by Cornelius Agrippa, one of the leading occult philosophers of the sixteenth century, only that pertaining to Saturn is clearly psychoactive. It consists of the seed of black poppy, henbane, the mandrake root, the loadstone and Myrrh, mixed with either the brains of a cat or the blood of a bat. The toad was also considered to be under this planet's influence (see **Toad**).

**Sources:** Agrippa 1651, Rudgley 1993.

# SCIRPUS

*Scirpus* is a grass-like plant with underground tubers that has been used traditionally as a hallucinogen in Mexico. Although its psychoactive constituents are at present unknown, some species of the genus as well as plants from related genera contain harmala alkaloids. Eating the tubers causes the consumer to go into a deep sleep followed by vivid hallucinations in which brilliant colours are perceived. An unidentified species of *Scirpus* is used by the Tarahumara Indians, who know it as *bakana, bakanoa* and *bakanawa*. The tuber is considered by them as an important medicine for treating various physical and psychological disorders. There are important rituals that must be performed before the plant can be used. Offerings of food must be placed by it and songs sung to it. Abusing or mistreating the plant in any way is believed to cause sickness or even death. According to the Tarahumara its entheogenic properties include the power to transport the user's spirit to distant places and communicate with the spirits of dead relatives. Its effects are seen as unpredictable and care must be taken to prevent users leaping recklessly into a fire. A number of species of *Scirpus* have been used in traditional medical practices of North American Indians but, apart from the case of the Tarahumara, no psychoactive effects have been reported.

**Sources**: Bye 1979, Ott 1993, Schultes and Hofmann 1980a, Schultes and Hofmann 1980b.

# SCOPOLAMINE

Scopolamine is a tropane alkaloid (see **Tropane alkaloids**) found in belladonna, henbane, datura, mandrake and other plants in which it occurs in amounts capable of producing powerful hallucinogenic effects. From 1902 scopolamine was administered along with morphine as an analgesic for use in childbirth. It was widely used but later dropped as it was implicated as a causal factor in an abnormally high rate of infant mortality. Scopolamine has been given to mental patients as a sedative. Like mescaline and harmaline, scopolamine was used as a 'truth drug' in certain criminal court cases. According to Burroughs the Russians experimented with scopolamine as an aid to interrogation: 'The subject may be willing to reveal his secrets, but quite unable to remember them. Often cover story and secret information are inextricably garbled.' There is scientific research that indicates that scopolamine may impair human serial learning. Scopolamine is also known in the scientific literature as hyoscine.

**Sources:** Burroughs 1959, Heiser 1969, Ott 1993, Schenk 1956.

## SCOPOLIA

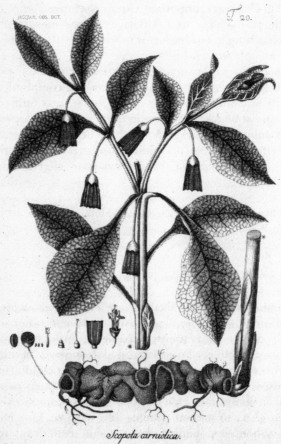

*Scopola carniolica.*

**SCOPOLIA**

*Scopolia carniolica* is one of the less well-known psychoactive plants of the Solanaceae family that includes belladonna, mandrake and henbane. Like these plants it contains the hallucinogenic tropane alkaloids scopolamine and hyoscyamine and other psychoactive substances. In Romania it was used as a substitute for the much-prized mandrake when the latter was unavailable. It is a native of central and eastern Europe and has a long history of use in folk medicine and magic. It is particularly associated with baneful sorcery and was one of the plants used in the witches' ointments (see **Witches' Ointments**). It also played a more positive role in eastern European societies when it was used to incite sexual desire during bacchanalian festivals. Scopolia is also reported to have been used in Chinese medicine.

**Sources:** Evans 1979, Ott 1993, Rätsch 1992.

## SCOTCH BROOM

Scotch broom is known to botanists as either *Genista canariensis* or *Cytisus canariensis* and, although it is an Old World plant in origin (its specific name derives from its abundance in the Canary Islands), it was introduced into Mexico. It has been used as a shamanic entheogen by the Yaqui Indians who prize its seeds for their hallucinogenic properties. Its flowers also appear to be psychoactive, as the Yaqui reportedly stored them in a sealed container for ten days before drying them and then smoking them in cigarettes. When smoked the flowers are said to increase mental awareness and perception of colour. Chemical analysis of the plant has so far failed to account for these psychoactive effects and the alkaloid cytisine which has been found to be present is known for its toxicity but not for hallucinogenic qualities. Although its magical use is often thought to be limited to the New World, the German ethnobotanist Christian Rätsch has suggested that it may have been employed as such by the Guanches, who were the original indigenous people of the Canary Islands. The same writer also reports that it was used in Europe as an ingredient in the making of aphrodisiac beverages. Modern practitioners of sex magic smoke its flowers together with cannabis to heighten the effects of their erotic rituals.

**Sources:** Emboden 1979, Ott 1993, Rätsch 1992, Rudgley 1993, Schultes and Hofmann 1980a, Schultes and Hofmann 1980b.

## SOLANUM

*Solanum nigrum*, commonly known as nightshade (not to be confused with deadly nightshade; for which see **Belladonna**) was used by the witches of both ancient Greece and medieval Europe. It is also a sacred plant in the Voodoo and Santería religions. The alkaloid solanine which is found in the plant is fairly toxic and is also found in green potatoes. It can cause headaches, fever and even hallucinations. Although the psychoactive effects reported for solanine are accompanied by highly unpleasant side effects, this may nevertheless explain the use of the plants in New World cults of African origin and in the ancient witchcraft traditions of Europe. Bedouin tribes of the Negev region of Israel use another plant of the genus (*Solanum luteum*) as a cure for toothache but are careful not to swallow it as it is seen as a dangerous poison. A South American species, *S. hirtum* is used by the Yanoama people as a substitute for tobacco.

**Sources:** Abu-Rabia 1983, Ott 1993, Rätsch 1992, Richardson 1988.

## SOLVENTS see Inhalants

## SOMA

The Indo-Iranians were an ancient people who had their homeland somewhere in Central Asia. About 4,000 years ago they split into two distinct groups. One group, the Indo-Aryans, moved south to the Indus Valley; the other became the ancient Iranian peoples. Both preserved a vast body of religious oral literature which was only later written down. This scriptures are the *Rig Veda* and the *Avesta*, of the Indians and the Iranians respectively. Both works describe rituals in which a plant with hallucinogenic properties was consumed. The plant was called *soma* by the Indians and *haoma* by the Iranians. Although some of the descendants of these peoples still perform their rituals, the identity of the sacred entheogenic plant has been lost and non-psychoactive substitutes are now used in place of the mysterious *soma/haoma*. In addition to the various non-psychoactive plants that have been used as *soma* substitutes in both the Zoroastrian and Hindu traditions, a great number of candidates for *soma* have been put forward by Western investigators over the last two hundred years. Among the suggestions of more or less convincing candidates have been cannabis, *Ephedra*, a fermented alcoholic drink, Syrian rue, rhubarb, ginseng, opium and wild chicory.

Most of these suggestions have been summarily rejected for reasons I will not go into here. Scholars had become rather bored with the whole question as it seemed to many of them an unanswerable one. However, the whole debate was rekindled by R. Gordon Wasson during the late 1960s when he proposed a new candidate for *soma* – the fly-agaric mushroom (see **Fly-Agaric**). The arguments he put forward are complex and since I have discussed them at length in an earlier book, *The Alchemy of Culture: Intoxicants in Society* (1993), published in the United States as *Essential Substances: A Cultural History of Intoxicants in Society* (1994), suffice it to say that many distinguished orientalists and other scholars accepted his thesis. In the late 1980s another highly plausible candidate was proposed by David Flattery and Martin Schwartz. Unlike Wasson, who had largely concerned himself with the Indian sources, they concentrated on the Iranian evidence. They suggest that Syrian rue (*Peganum harmala*; see **Peganum harmala**) was far more likely a candidate since its hallucinogenic effects are well-known in the Indo-Iranian homeland even today. Their arguments are highly persuasive and convincing.

However, just as Syrian rue seemed to be taking the place of the fly-agaric mushroom as the most likely candidate for *soma*, archaeological evidence emerged from Russian excavations in the Kara Kum desert of Turkmenistan that set the cat once more among the pigeons. In this area, known to the ancients as Margiana, the Russians uncovered a number of sites of monumental architecture dating from the second millennium BC One of these sites, Gonur South, consists of a fortified complex of buildings, a number of private dwellings and a fort. Within this complex there is also a large shrine (known to have been used as a sacred fire temple) consisting of two parts: one clearly used for public worship and the other, hidden from the gaze of the multitude, an inner sanctum of the priesthood. In one of these private rooms were found three ceramic bowls. Analysis of samples found in these vessels by Professor Mayer-Melikyan revealed the traces of both cannabis and *Ephedra*. Clearly both these psychoactive substances had been used in conjunction in the making of hallucinogenic drinks. In the adjoining room of the same inner sanctum were found ten ceramic pot-stands which appear to have been used in conjunction with strainers designed to separate the juices from the twigs, stems and leaves of the plants. In another room at the other end of the shrine a basin containing remains of a considerable quantity of cannabis was discovered, as well as a number of pottery stands and strainers that have also been associated with making psychoactive beverages.

The excavators believe that, given the considerable size of the fortress, the shrine may well have been dispensing the entheogenic drink to worshippers from all over Margiana in the first half of the second millennium BC. The shrine at the later site of Togoluk 1 (probably dating from the mid-second millennium) seems also to have been used to make hallucinogenic drinks as a similar pottery strainer has been found there, although traces of psychoactive plants have not been detected. The shrine at a third settlement, Togoluk 21, dated to the late second millennium, contained vessels which revealed remains of *Ephedra* again, but this time in conjunction with the pollen of poppies. An engraved bone tube from the same shrine was also found to contain poppy pollen.

These sites also yielded up other artefacts that give tantalising clues as to what sort of rituals took place in these Bronze Age shrines. Designs on a cylinder seal depict a drummer, an acrobat and two men with the heads of monkeys. The rituals that took place under the influence of the psychoactive drinks seem to have involved the participants wearing animal masks. The discovery of these sites in the eastern Iranian cultural region allows archaeologists to reach certain conclusions. First these temples, which were on the scale of contemporary Mesopotamian ones, show that the eastern Iranian region had its own architectural traditions on a grand scale and that it was not merely a 'cultural backwater'. Second, that the sites in Margiana precede the previously discovered fire temples of later Iranian tradition (in some cases by a whole millennium) and should be seen as their prototypes. Third, that the discovery in the shrines of the remains of opium, cannabis and *Ephedra* in ritual vessels that are dated between 2000–1000 BC show that *soma* in its Iranian form *haoma* may be considered as a composite psychoactive substance comprising of cannabis and *Ephedra* in one instance and opium and *Ephedra* in another. This identification of *haoma* has an archaeological background which neither the fly-agaric nor Syrian rue can match, unless such evidence comes to light. Despite the considerable efforts made to discover the botanical identity of *soma*, it may be that this is one mystery that will never be satisfactorily solved.

**Sources:** Flattery and Schwartz 1989, Rudgley 1993, Sarianidi 1994, Wasson 1968.

## SOPHORA SECUNDIFLORA see Mescal beans

## STIMULANTS

Stimulants are psychoactive substances that cause physical and/or mental stimulation. The more potent stimulants include amphetamines and cocaine (see **Amphetamines** and **Cocaine**) but the most commonly used stimulants are much milder and act as the fuel of everyday life (see **Betel**, **Coca**, **Coffee**, **Qat** and **Tea**). The milder stimulants are used by almost everyone, the young and the old, the rich and the poor, the drug-addict and the teetotaller. In almost all cultures few social occasions – formal or informal – seem complete without the mutual consumption of tea, coffee, betel or whatever is the most popular stimulant of the society in question. The introduction of a new and exotic stimulant can have great cultural significance, as in the case of the European conversion to two new substances during the seventeenth and eighteenth centuries, highlighted by Camporesi: 'Coffee and chocolate became the liquid emblem of a new society that was pulling in two directions – highly strung yet lazy, keen yet listless, industrious yet hedonistic, a late sleeper yet an early riser.'

Stimulants have, in the world religions, been largely saved from the diatribes against other types of psychoactive substances, particular venom being reserved for the hallucinogens. That the milder stimulants neither impair the workings of the rational faculty nor the physical capacity to work (and may actually improve mental and physical performance) meant not only the tacit acceptance of them by the religious authorities but their actual use by Christian monks, Jesuits, Buddhist nuns and monks and Muslim clergymen.

**Sources:** Camporesi 1994, Rudgley 1993.

**SWEET FLAG** see **Acorus calamus**

**SYRIAN RUE** see **Peganum harmala**

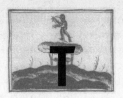

## TEA

The tea plant (*Camellia thea*, also known as *Thea sinensis*) is, along with coffee, the most widely consumed caffeine-bearing beverage. According to Chinese legends tea was discovered in remote times; the historical evidence shows that it was certainly known by the third century AD. It had long been the stimulant *par excellence* of the Chinese, Japanese and Tibetan peoples and is intimately associated with spiritual as well as secular persuits. According to Buddhist legend the sage Bodhidharma meditated so rigorously that he attained a permanently awakened state, so that he ceased to have any use for his eyelids, which fell to the ground. From his eyelids the tea plant grew. This legend is clearly a reference to the stimulating properties of tea as an aid to maintaining attention during meditation.

Tea was greatly valued by both the Taoists and the Buddhists, not only for such properties but also for its medicinal value. The Chinese believe that it is a tonic that can even promote longevity. China's tea ceremonies were far less formalised than their Japanese counterparts but both show an equal love and appreciation of tea. The Muslim peoples of Central Asia are great tea-drinkers but do not generally extol its spiritual virtues.

The gentle and serene art of tea in the Far East is hardly matched by its more prosaic role in Western societies. Nevertheless, despite its entirely secular role, the Western tea party embodies all kinds of social messages to do with class, status and etiquette. Western tea rituals began in the eighteenth century and became intimately associated with the essentially feminine sphere of the domestic parlour. As Woodruff Smith puts it: 'the centrality of women in the ritual of tea – at once ministering to the needs of the family and receiving the deference that their roles demanded – constituted a substantial difference from the masculinity of the coffeehouse ... topics and the manner of conversation were limited by the presumed sensibilities of ladies, and the women (especially the presiding woman) were expected politely to ensure that transgressions of this rule were immediately brought to the attention of the transgressors. In other words, women acted out roles as "civilisers". No doubt a thorough ethnographic investigation of the phenomenon today would yield results but most anthropologists would rather risk malaria or frostbite in some remote corner of the globe than face the terrors of regular attendance at suburban tea parties.

(See also **Caffeine**.)

**Sources:** Blofeld 1985, Goodman 1995, Rudgley 1993, Smith 1995.

## TEONANACATL see Fungi

## THORN APPLE see Datura

## TOAD

That the venom of certain toads contains hallucinogenic compounds has been discovered, or more likely rediscovered, only fairly recently. The venom of the Colorado River toad (also known as the Sonoran desert toad and found only in Mexico, Texas and Arizona), *Bufo alvarius*, contains high concentrations of the powerful hallucinogenic tryptamine 5-MeO-DMT, which is about four times the strength of DMT. 5-MeO-DMT is also present in the snuffs made by South American Indians from the plants *Virola* and *Anadenanthera peregrina* (see **Anadenanthera** and **Virola**). Scientific articles on the venom of this particular toad that were published in the 1960s seem to have been the impetus behind the self-experiments conducted by individuals seeking new drug experiences. A scarce underground classic entitled *The Psychedelic Toad of the Sonoran Desert* provides detailed instructions for collecting and consuming the venom. The author says that the venom should be extracted from the toad by squeezing the various glands which are located on its limbs and most importantly the parotoid glands on its neck. The viscous and

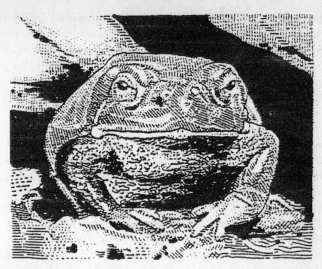

**BUFO ALVARIUS**

milky-white fresh venom (0.25–0.5g of venom can be extracted from a single toad) is then dried and smoked. The dried venom remains as potent as when it was fresh for at least two years. Andrew Weil and Wade Davis, who are both academics with considerable expertise in the field of psychoactive substances, have smoked the venom themselves. They note that within seconds of inhaling the smoke intense visual and auditory hallucinations are experienced for a period of about five minutes, while after-effects linger on for about an hour. They reported no side-effects during or after using the venom. A journalist named Larry Gallagher went to Arizona, somewhat cynically as he himself was happy to admit, to experience the effects of the venom. He vividly describes the powerful effects:

> Before I finish exhaling, I can feel myself disappearing. To say 'I' experience extreme hallucinations would be to miss the point. There is no perception of a 'me' experiencing anything: no visions, no memories, no fear, no pleasure or pain, nothing to hold onto and no one to do the holding. In its place is the most overwhelming cyclone of energy ever to rip through my brain, and it lasts for an eternity.
>
> On the way back in is an awareness of breathing, a wheezing inhalation followed by a roaring moan of exhaust

that spooks a few of the observers. Gradually I begin to realise that this human accordion is me. With each gasp I am sending out a life's worth of weariness and pain. After what I am told is five minutes I am able to open my eyes and speak again . . . then I lean over and cry my guts out into the dust . . . although my faculties gradually return over the course of the evening, my powers of cynicism do not.

Gallagher had taken the venom under the supervision of White Dog, a self-styled white shaman who took his name from his spirit familiar that appeared to him in a peyote vision. White Dog is one of a small number of devotees who conduct ceremonies around the smoking of toad. Such devotees call their cult 'The Church of the Toad of Light' and treat the venom as a sacrament.

Because the venom of *Bufo alvarius* contains traces of bufotenine, a Schedule I illegal substance in the United States, toad users can and have been prosecuted. The first state to contemplate outlawing toad-licking was South Carolina and one of the local politicians involved suggested a punishment of sixty hours of public service in a zoo would be appropriate! In 1994 a forty-one-year-old Californian scout-leader was arrested for having the venom in his possession and his four pet toads (named Peter, Brian, Franz and Hans) became wards of the state! Toad venom is poisonous if taken orally and the misguided craze for 'toad-licking' (which became a minor fad reported in the American media and even featured in episodes of *LA Law* and, perhaps less surprisingly, in the *X-Files*) can cause seizures. A case involving less drastic symptoms is recorded in 'Confessions of an Amphibian Abuser', the amusingly entitled introduction to Adrian Morgan's *Toads and Toadstools*. Morgan took two newly drowned female toads that he had found on the outskirts of London and pulverised a mixture of poison glands and skin in a mortar. After the resulting substance was dried he took some of it as a snuff. In his notes written at the time of the experiment he recorded the following effects – local anaesthesia of the nose and teeth, profuse sweating, and mild psychoactivity in the form of 'trails' following in the wake of moving objects and increased intensity of the perception of colour. He also notes that the snuffing of the venom had definite stimulant effects, both mental and physical. The overall effects were over in about an hour and the subject fell into a deep but short sleep. The effects recorded by

Morgan are more the symptoms of mild poisoning than a full-blown hallucinogenic experience. The stimulant effects mentioned above may explain why a toad skin preparation was used by some Chinese athletes competing in the 1992 Olympics in Barcelona.

There are indications that other species of toad have venom that is hallucinogenic. Jonathan Ott, one of the leading American experts on psychoactive substances, notes that an individual with whom he was in contact smoked the venom of the Marine toad (*Bufo marinus*) and reported similar effects to those caused by the Sonoran toad. There is interesting historical material from various parts of the world to suggest that toads were used for their hallucinogenic properties long ago. Some scholars believe that the Maya people used the toad for its psychoactive effects; Davis and Weil have suggested that it was not *Bufo marinus* that was used in ancient America (as had previously been suggested as the most likely species to have been so used) but probably *Bufo alvarius*, because they question whether the former is genuinely hallucinogenic at all (although there are recent reports to the contrary; see above). Toad poisons are well-known to the Chinese and even feature as an ingredient in seventeenth-century bomb-making manuals (Leonardo da Vinci was also interested in using the toad for the very same military application). There are hints that the Chinese may also have been aware of the psychoactive properties of the toad. Its flesh was considered by some ancient Taoists as aiding the quest for longevity and immortality. The use of dried-toad venom is still part of traditional Vietnamese medicine, the venom of *Bufo melanostictus* being used to treat children with high fever.

Toads have played an important role in the folklore and mythology of Europe since prehistoric times. Often such beliefs have connected the toad with various kinds of fungi epitomised by the English term toadstool, which refers to a number of mushrooms deemed inedible or poisonous (but also covering a number of psychoactive species, including the fly-agaric; see **Fly-Agaric**). This conjures up an image of a toad squatting on a mushroom but this kind of figurative stool may not be what is meant. For the word stool also refers to faecal material, thus making toadstool mean 'toad excrement'. Now, fungi have been associated with excrement in many parts of the world, as the folk names given to them amply confirm, but it may also be read in another way. Excrement does not always refer solely to faecal matter but has the wider meaning of any substance excreted from the body. That would, of course, include the exuded venom of the toad.

Toads have been widely used in medicine and were believed to have magical powers. This may well suggest that the psychoactive properties of their venom were known to both witches and alchemists. The alchemist Oswald Crollius describes the method for making a prophylactic medicine in the form of an amulet. Firstly the body of a toad must be dried by the heat of the sun and then pulverised using a pestle and mortar (taking care to stop up one's nostrils and turning the head away). Then it must be combined with a number of other ingredients, including 'the Zenith of Maidens' (i.e. the menses of young girls) and rosewater. The resulting paste is then formed into round pentacles and said to be an effective defence against pestilence, poisons and 'astral. diseases' (i.e. disorders caused by the heavenly bodies). A similar but more up-market version of this magical medicine, for 'rich and noble persons', is called the Zenexton and consists of a gold casket containing the powder of a pulverised toad. The name Zenexton (or Xenzethon, as it is sometimes written) was an invention of Paracelsus and is said to derive from the Greek meaning 'slaying strangers'.

These alchemical and medical sources make it clear that toads were routinely used in the sixteenth and seventeenth centuries. But there are other, even earlier, alchemical sources that appear to suggest that the psychoactive properties of toads were known and made use of in the secret traditions of alchemy. To my knowledge no systematic modern research has been undertaken to test European species of toads for their potential hallucinogenic properties, but to judge from the explicit accounts of the alchemists they had already achieved this. Michael Scot, the thirteenth-century alchemist and astrologer wrote in his *Liber Luminus Luminum* that: 'Five toads are shut up in a vessel and made to drink the juices of various herbs with vinegar as the first step in the preparation of a marvelous [sic] powder for the purposes of transformation.' The fifteenth-century alchemist Sir George Ripley wrote a *Vision* in poetic form which has puzzled those who have read it; without knowing that the toad is psychoactive it cannot be understood at all. I reproduce it in full as it is a remarkable little work:

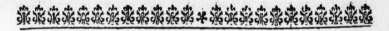

# THE
# VISION OF
## Sr: *GEORGE RIPLEY:*
### Chanon of Bridlington.

Hen busie at my booke I was upon a certeine night,
This Vision here exprest appear'd unto my dim-
(med sight,
A *Toade* full rudde I saw did drinke the juce of
grapes so fast,
Till over charged with the broth, his bowells all to brast;
And after that from poysoned bulke he cast his venome fell,
For greif and paine whereof his Members all began to swell,
With drops of poysoned sweate approaching thus his secret Den,
His cave with blasts of fumous ayre he all be-whyted then;
And from the which in space a golden humour did ensue, (hew:
Whose falling drops from high did staine the soile with ruddy
And when this Corps the force of vitall breath began to lacke,
This dying *Toade* became forthwith like Coale for colour blacke:
Thus drowned in his proper veynes of poysoned flood,
For tearme of eightie dayes and fowre he rotting stood:
By tryall then this venome to expell I did desire,
For which I did committ his carkase to a gentle fire:
Which done, a wonder to the sight, but more to be rehear'st,
The *Toade* with Colours rare through every side was pear'st,
And VVhite appeared when all the sundry hewes were past,
Which after being tincted Rudde, for evermore did last.
Then of the venome handled thus a medicine I did make;
VVhich venome kills and saveth such as venome chance to take.
Glory be to him the graunter of such secret wayes,
Dominion, and Honour, both with Worship, and with Prayse.
### A M E N.

VERSES

Eiraneus Philalethes, a seventeenth-century alchemist, wrote a detailed commentary to the works of Ripley which makes it clear that the *Vision* refers to chemical operations. As Philalethes explains, the 'secret den' of the toad is actually the chemical glass in which the transformation of the creature takes place. He also makes another intriguing comment when he says that the venomous exhalations of Ripley's toad: 'are compared to the Invenomed Fume of Dragons', citing the fourteenth-century French alchemist Nicholas Flamel to support this. The dragons he talks of are most likely to be salamanders or possibly newts, their 'invenomed fume' the psychoactive smoke given off by the burning of their venom. Verses accompanying the Ripley *Scrowle* describe a similar chemical operation to that of the *Vision*, but with a serpent being heated in the vessel rather than a toad. The psychoactive effects of smoking dried snake venom are reported from India (see **Animals**).

(See also **Toadstone**.)

**Sources:** Ashmole 1652, Crollius 1670, Emboden 1975, Gallagher 1994, Morgan 1995, Needham SSC 5/7, Ott 1993, Pegler et al 1995, Philalethes 1678, Rätsch 1992, Ripley 1591, Rudgley 1993, Thorndike 1923–58, Verpoorte et al 1979, Weil and Davis 1994.

## TOADSTONE

The toadstone (also referred to as *craupadina*, *bufonis lapis* and batrachites) is the name given to a wonderful stone said to be found in the head of toads. It has been part of European folklore for at least 600 years. Professor Ray Lankester is cited with approval by the early Egyptologist Wallis Budge as the man who 'solved' the riddle of the toadstone. According to Lankester the toadstones are not stones at all but the teeth of a fish (*Lepidotus*) which were found in rocks. As we shall see, this is very far off the mark. Albertus Magnus is reputed to have said that the stone named borax was found in the heads of toads. The use of the word stone in alchemical writings does not usually refer to gems but rather to solid substances of various kinds; the belief that the toadstone was a precious gem of some kind was a widespread misunderstanding that resulted in a fantastic corpus of spurious identifications.

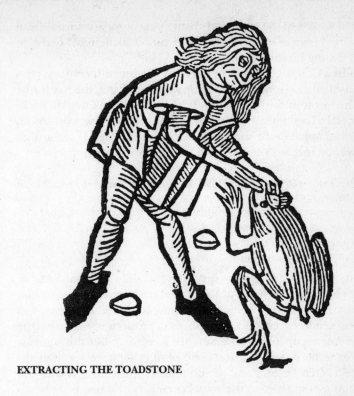

**EXTRACTING THE TOADSTONE**

Alchemists were well aware that the venom of the toad exuded from its head and therefore their assertion that the toadstone was extracted from the head shows that the magical toadstone and the psychoactive venom were one and the same. With the knowledge that the toadstone was either the dried parotoid gland of the toad or the extracted venom many otherwise obscure and absurd descriptions of it become crystal clear. Hermolaus Barbarus wrote that the stone must be snatched away from the toad otherwise it will reabsorb it itself (i.e. the venom will not be forthcoming). John Baptista Porta states that the toad must be aggravated by striking it, otherwise it will not void the stone (a toad treated in this way will release its venom; a similar technique is practised by Haitian sorcerers who use toads in the making of zombi drugs; see **Zombi drug**). Another belief concerning the toadstone was that it would change colour or sweat if its owner were to be bewitched. This is a garbled superstition in which one can see original meaning had been misunderstood – the sweat refers to the exuded venom of the toad, and changes in colour are known from modern chemical experiments (and earlier alchemical texts) to occur during heating of the venom.

Andrea Chiocco, writing in the early seventeenth century, cites and dismisses a contemporary rival, who asserts that the toadstone does not grow in the toad's head but is rather to be found in rocks (echoed by Lankester's later false identification of the toadstone), having an appearance similar to that of small fungi. It seems that one way or another the toad and fungal world are inseparable.

**Sources:** Budge 1978, Crollius 1670, Radford and Radford 1980, Rätsch 1992, Thorndike 1923–58.

## TOBACCO

Whilst tobacco (*Nicotiana* spp.) is certainly a stimulant, in sufficient quantities (such as those used traditionally by American Indians, for which see below) it can have what, for all intents and purposes, may be called hallucinogenic properties. Certainly the South American Indian shamans see it as such, but this appears not just to be due to cultural conditioning (apprentice shamans are instructed beforehand of the nature of the visions they are going to see) but also to the actual chemistry of tobacco. Tobacco contains the harmala alkaloids harman and norharman, and the closely related harmine and harmaline are known hallucinogens. The levels of harman and norharman in cigarette smoke are between forty and 100 times greater than in tobacco leaf, showing that the burning of the plant generates this dramatic increase. The effects of nicotine on the central nervous system are still far from being understood. The hallucinogenic effects of tobacco become far more explicable when it is borne in mind that the strains of tobacco smoked by the American Indians were far more potent than our commercially produced varieties. Furthermore, the amounts consumed by them were often considerably greater than even the most ardent chain-smoker is able to manage.

Petum was a widely used early European word for tobacco and is said to be derived from the Tupi-Guarani Indian word for the plant. The word nicotine is derived from the surname of Jean Nicot de Villemain, who brought back *Nicotiana rustica* to France in 1560. Although he was not the first to do this, he nevertheless

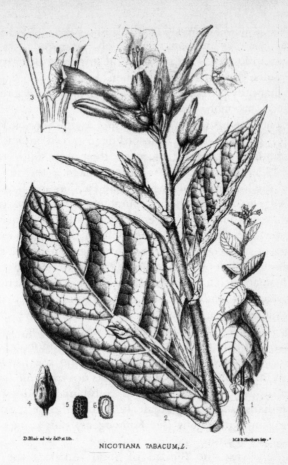

NICOTIANA TABACUM, *L.*

## TOBACCO

got the dubious honour of having this poisonous substance named after him. The word tobacco is first mentioned (in the form *tabaco*) by Gonzalo Fernandez de Oviedo y Valdes (1478–1557) who uses it as a term for the act of smoking and also, in his later writing, for the leaves of the plant itself. The origin of the word tobacco was once believed to derive from a place name (the two candidates being Tabasco in Mexico and Tobago, one of the Lesser Antilles), although this is now rejected as a theory.

It is well known that tobacco is, by nature, an American plant, the use of which, when discovered by the Europeans, was rapidly spread across the globe. Less well known is the fact that there was another region of the world in which wild tobacco not only grew but was used by humans completely independently of any American influence. That region is the arid interior or 'outback' of Australia. Records from Captain Cook's 1770 expedition record that the Aborigines chewed a herb, most likely a reference to tobacco (probably *Nicotiana suaveolens*).

The cultural history of tobacco use begins way back in the prehistory of South America. According to current archaeological understanding, humans first made their way south to Chile around 13,500 years ago. These Palaeoindians, as they are known, reached the lowlands of Patagonia, the Pampas and Gran Chaco by 11,000 years ago. This is the natural home of the tobacco plant, from where it would spread to enchant and addict humankind the world over. According to Johannes Wilbert, the leading expert on the use of tobacco by the South American Indians, these Palaeoindian hunter-gatherers did not make immediate use of the plant. Instead such a use did not emerge until the Indians began to cultivate and tend it in their gardens some 3,000 years later. These pioneer horticulturalists grew some twelve different species, *Nicotiana tabacum* and *N. rustica* being the most significant. Unlike many anthropologists and ethnobotanists who have worked closely with native peoples who use psychoactive plants in their religious life, Wilbert does not trace the origins of shamanism to the use of such substances. He sees the Palaeoindians as following an ascetic path to the spirit world; the shift to using entheogens (see **Entheogens**) only came with the advent of horticulture.

Not only were the Indians of South America the first to domesticate tobacco, they also discovered all the ways of using it, even some which are almost unknown in the West today. As Wilbert says, they: 'chew tobacco quids, drink tobacco juice and syrup, lick tobacco paste, apply tobacco enemas, snuff and smoke. In addition, they administer tobacco products topically to the skin and to the eye.' Their appetite for tobacco is staggering and even the most inveterate chain-smoker pales by comparison. Shamans on the Orinoco have been seen to smoke five or six three-foot cigars in a single ritual session. The toxic effects of tobacco are well understood by the shamans of South America and, as Wilbert says: 'masters take their apprentices after months or even years of progressive nicotine habituation to the very brink of death.' Shamans, whether they use psychoactive substances or not, seek 'near-death' experiences in order to gain spiritual insight into the origins and causes of disease. This is the rationale behind the systematic use of the intoxicating effects of nicotine. The strength of native tobacco and the great quantities of it used can induce hallucinogens which are seen to be of great importance by the tobacco shamans.

South American shamans believe that, whilst the human hunger is for food, the hunger of the spirits is for tobacco. Thus, by taking tobacco in its various forms, the shaman is making direct ar. 1 intimate contact with the spirits. Before the arrival of the Europeans in the New World tobacco use seems to have been restricted to ritual use. The secular use of it was largely due to the influence of Europeans; this holds true for both South and North America.

Despite the prominence of tobacco in world history and the enormous amount of research conducted on the native peoples of North America, there are still some unsolved mysteries concerning its early use in Indian culture. The widespread custom of smoking in other parts of the world does not, of course, always involve the use of tobacco. The smoking of cannabis and opium are two obvious examples of this. Whilst neither of these substances existed in the New World before the European contact period, the continent was not without various other plants suitable for smoking. The spread of tobacco northwards into North America from its southern homeland is a highly complex issue; the exact routes which it took and the time scale in which this culturally dramatic event took place are still obscure. The discovery of pipes, for example, does not simply indicate the presence of tobacco; other plants could have been smoked in this way before tobacco became known in the areas in which such artefacts have been discovered (see **Pipes** for details of the North American Indian pipes which are the major source for the early history of tobacco). The numerous smoking plants that are known to have been smoked by North American Indians on their own or in conjunction with tobacco are detailed elsewhere (see **Kinnikinnik**). Another mystery in the history of tobacco use concerns the chewing of the plant with lime by the Haida and the Tlingit peoples of the north-west coast. Chewing tobacco was a comparatively unusual habit in traditional North American Indian societies and the use of lime even more so. Lime (or similar alkali preparations) is added to a number of other stimulating substances throughout the world as it releases more of the psychoactive properties of the plant in question. Such a use of an alkali is found in the Asian and Oceanic use of betel (see **Betel**), the Australian Aboriginal use of *pituri* (see **Pituri**) and the South American use of coca (see **Coca**). There are those who believe that the chemically highly effective use of lime was discovered in a single place and then the knowledge passed on to other cultures. This kind of argument (known as diffusionism) was once put forward to explain the use of lime among the Haida and Tlingit, the idea being that they borrowed it from the South Americans (presumably by long-distance communication by sea) and, even more improbably that coca-chewing had its ultimate origins in the western pacific use of betel. That the Australian Aborigines used an alkali additive in their *pituri* preparations in near-total isolation from the rest of the world shows quite clearly that such discoveries were made independently.

To return then to the north-west coast. The Haida Indians inhabit the Queen Charlotte Islands off the west coast of Canada and the Tlingit live on the southern coastal mainland of Alaska. Both peoples were chewing tobacco when they were first contacted by Europeans and their respective mythologies attest its cultural importance. Tobacco was apparently the only plant cultivated to any significant degree by these groups before their adoption of some European customs. Both societies lived in a rich environment with access to abundant and varied foods and so had no need to toil away in gardens to supplement their diet. Thus, their motivation for cultivation was not for staple foods but to fulfil their desire for a steady supply of tobacco. Similar motivations for taking up the practice of agriculture have been found elsewhere in the world. The origin of agriculture and the reasons why it occurred are universally seen as among the most critical questions in human history. Why did people give up the millennia-long hunting-and-gathering lifestyle and suddenly start growing and cultivating plants? The standard answer has been that they did so to replace a precarious lifestyle with one based on security, with staple crops as their guarantee. Whilst this was no doubt true in many cases, the motivation seems to have been rather different. In the case of the Haida and Tlingit it is clear that the driving force was the need for tobacco.

The Haida planted their tobacco seeds at the end of April, each separate pod being put in a mound of earth. The tobacco gardens were weeded regularly until September, when the crop was harvested. The leaves were dried by placing them on a timber frame over a fire. When dry they were put in stone mortars and pounded with a pestle. The lime admixture was made by burning shells and then crushing them into powder form. In order to avoid the burning sensations of the lime it was put in the middle of the tobacco quid and not, therefore, in direct contact with the inside of the mouth. Surviving records do not, unfortunately, tell us much about the psychoactive effects of their chewing tobacco, but it has been suggested that because they abandoned the cultivation of their local species (botanists think it was most likely *Nicotiana quadrivalvis*), when they encountered commercially produced trade tobacco it was weaker in its psychoactive effects than the newly available strains. The Tlingit are reported to have sometimes used the inner bark of pine instead of lime but this is highly unlikely to have made the resulting quid stronger in its psychoactive effects. In the extreme north-west of North America (Alaska and the Yukon) both Indians and Eskimos chew tobacco mixed with the ashes of a fungus (see **Fungus**) but this is almost certainly a post-Contact habit.

When Columbus discovered America in 1492 (which had actually been discovered much earlier by the Vikings and, of course, millennia earlier by the first explorers of the New World, the Palaeoindians), members of his expedition became the first Europeans to witness the – to them – curious habit of smoking tobacco. When, in his journal, Columbus describes Indians: 'who always carried a lighted firebrand to light fire, and perfume themselves with certain herbs they carried along with them', he was not writing from his own observations but from the accounts relayed to him by Luis De Torres and another Spaniard who had been sent ashore on 2 November 1492. Jerome Brooks, a historian of tobacco use, has some interesting comments on this passage. He notes that De Torres was a learned man who knew not only his classical sources but also read Hebrew and Arabic. Since the voyagers had thought they would land in Asia, De Torres had been brought along to act as interpreter for Columbus when, as they hoped would happen, they gained an audience with the Great Khan. The phrase 'perfumed themselves' is seen by Brooks to be that of De Torres rather than Columbus. De Torres would have known the work of the Greek historian Herodotus, who describes the ancient Scythian inhalation of cannabis smoke (see

**Cannabis**), and attempted to relate the wholly exotic New World practice of tobacco smoking to this Asian custom. There does not appear to be any evidence that either Columbus or any of his entourage brought back the novel plant to Spain on their triumphant return, although it is possible that some sailors in this or later crews brought it home in small quantities, an occurrence that would have gone unrecorded and therefore is impossible to confirm or deny.

Amerigo Vespucci reached the mainland of South America in 1500 (his claim to have done so earlier is now rejected as a falsehood) and therefore met with tobacco-using peoples, but again there are no records of it being taken back to Europe by him. In 1518 Oviedo, the leader of the Spanish expedition to Mexico, provides us with the earliest description of what we know as a cigarette: 'a little hollow tube, burning at one end, made in such a manner that after being lighted they burn themselves without causing a flame.' Later reports give further details concerning such cigarettes, which were made of reeds and highly ornamented. One of the captains under the command of Cortez saw them for sale in the markets of Mexico – a very early reference to a tobacconist's!

The generally accepted entry of the plant onto European soil occurred when Oviedo brought tobacco leaves back to Spain in 1519. In 1556 André Thevet brought seeds from Brazil to France and initiated its cultivation in Europe. Two years later it was first grown in the Royal garden in Lisbon. With the Europeans entering a whole new phase in their quest for global colonisation, they took tobacco on their travels and instigated its rapid spread across Asia. As this is a largely separate story it is detailed below, and for the moment I shall return to the Europeans' own views on the plant and their interpretation of its use by the Indians who had initiated them into the tobacco cult.

The sixteenth-century physician Nicholas Monardes wrote that the Indian priests made liberal use of tobacco. He cites a case in which such a priest was asked questions which his patients expected him to be able to answer by means of a tobacco-induced trance. After inhaling tobacco the priest 'fell downe uppon the grounde, as a dedde manne, and remainyng so, accordyng to the quantitie of the smoke that he had taken, and when the hearbe had doen his woorke, he did revive and awake, and gave theim their answeres, according to the visions, and illusions whiche he sawe.' He also says that the Indians would chew tobacco and coca (see **Coca**) together, which would make them 'out of their wits' as if drunk. The early black slaves that were sent to the Americas were banned from drinking wine and, according to Monardes, used tobacco in a similar way to the Indians, namely to get intoxicated and enter trance states. Other early accounts paint a similar picture of the native use of tobacco. Edmund Gardiner, writing at the beginning of the seventeenth century, describes native 'enchanters' (i.e. medicine men) as getting drunk on tobacco smoke and then falling into a deep sleep. On awakening they would tell those present of the visions they had seen and interpret their divinatory meaning. Whilst Gardiner, in line with most of his contemporaries, interprets Indian experiences with tobacco as delusions caused by the devil, his and similar accounts make it clear that tobacco was attributed with inebriating and hallucinogenic properties by early Europeans as well as the Indians themselves. The modern smoker experiences neither of these effects, which seem to be caused by more potent strains of the plant, greater quantities consumed and cultural conditioning within a ritual context.

Tobacco was gaining its adherents in Europe but supplies were not always forthcoming. As tobacco was both expensive and scarce the early British pipes were so small they became known as fairy pipes. In Scotland they were called elfin pipes and, apparently, later generations in Ireland saw them as the handiwork of the leprechauns and destroyed them when they came across them. In this early phase of tobacco use it was perceived in numerous conflicting ways as a manna from heaven or the smoke of hell itself, from panacea to poison. The fading echoes of its entheogenic use among the American Indians can be heard in this early phase of Europe's enchantment. Tobacco was certainly the muse of Sir John Beaumont, who described it as 'the philosopher's stone of the alchemists'. He was by his own admission enraptured by 'tabacconalia', as he called it. In an extract from his long (and undistinguished) poem *The Metamorphosis of Tobacco* (1602) he invokes tobacco:

By whom the *Indian* Priests inspired be,
When they presage in barbrous Poetrie:
Infume my braine, make my soules powers subtile,
Give nimble cadence to my harsher stile:

Inspire me with thy flame, which doth excell
The purest streames of the *Castalian* well,
That I on thy ascensive wings may flie
By thine ethereall vapours borne on high,
And with thy feathers added to my quill
May pitch thy tents on the Parnassian hill,
Teach me what power thee on earth did place,
What God was bounteous to the humane race,
On what occasion, and by whom it stood,
That the blest World receiv'd so great a good.

Tobacco was seen by some as a medicinal plant of great value. Because of its association with henbane it was used in similar ways; for example, henbane smoke had long been used to alleviate toothache, and tobacco was said to be even more effective for this. To describe the effects of tobacco use as drunkenness was widespread in Europe. John Gerard, author of a famous herbal, also likened its effects to opium. One of its most vociferous opponents was King James I of England, who attacked tobacco smoking in no uncertain terms in his pamphlet *A Counterblast to Tobacco* (1604), describing it as: 'a custome lathsome to the eye, hateful to the nose, harmeful to the braine, dangerous to the lungs, and the blacke stinking fume thereof, nearest resembling the horrible Stigian smoke of the pit that is bottomlesse.' Yet even the sovereign himself was powerless to prevent the spread of the habit and had to console himself by putting taxes on tobacco.

Another opponent of tobacco was Barnabie Rich, who wrote in 1606: 'I thinke *Flatterie* at this day be in as good requeste as *Tabacco*, two smokie vapours, yet the one purgeth wise-men of their witte, and the other fooles of their money.' An anonymous diatribe of the 1640s describes tobacco as the most pernicious plant of all, with the one exception of hemp. Yet this is not a reference to the psychoactive effects of cannabis but to the use of the plant's fibre in making the hangman's rope (see **Cannabis**) – hemp being seen to attack the throat from without, tobacco from within.

Tobacco smoking was no longer an exotic custom, it had become an integral part of English social life. At the beginning of the seventeenth century it is estimated that there were no fewer than 7,000 shops and other outlets where tobacco could be bought in the London area alone. Tobacco smoking had by now become such a commonplace habit throughout English society that Joverin de Rochefort, a French visitor, wrote in 1671 that in the town of Worcester children were sent to school with a pipe in their satchel. Even the most famous school in all of England was not immune to propagating the habit. A seventeenth-century English diarist by the name of Hearne wrote that during the Great Plague tobacco was considered such a medicinal boon that: 'Even children were obliged to smoak. And I remember that I heard formerly Tom Rogers, who was a yeoman beadle, say that when he was a schoolboy at Eton that year when the Plague raged all the boys of that school were obliged to smoak in the school every morning, and that he was never whipped so much in his life as he was one morning for not smoaking.'

Although the pipe had been the most popular way to use tobacco it was, for a time, to be eclipsed by the habit of snuffing. By the mid-1680s it was integrated into the more exclusive English coffee-houses. In his *History of England* Macaulay haughtily wrote: 'The atmosphere was like that of a perfumer's shop. Tobacco in any other form than that of richly scented snuff was held in abomination. If any clown, ignorant of the usages of the house, called for a pipe, the sneers of the whole assembly and the short answers of the waiters soon convinced him that he had better go elsewhere.' There were opponents to the habit who contemptuously referred to snuff users as 'snivellers'. A mid-eighteenth-century detractor, who described tobacco as a narcotic akin to opium, warned that snuff-taking was liable to cause the loss of the sense of smell, addiction, nasal tumours and cancer. Despite these early health warnings a particular kind of snuff called Spanish *sabillia* was used to treat toothache. More generally the taking of snuff and the inevitable sneeze that it caused were seen as therapeutically clearing the head of 'superfluous vapours'. It was not just in the sphere of medicine that snuff was the subject of controversy. In 1686, during debates concerning the proposed canonisation of a Franciscan monk named Father Joseph Desa of Cupertino, moral concerns were raised about his use of snuff. These objections to his piety were dismissed on the grounds that, rather than his habit being a vice it was, in fact, a means of keeping alert during prayers and suppressing carnal lust. The conclusion was that the use of snuff should not stand in the way of his canonisation.

Snuffs were classified according to their grain – fine (fine grain), demigros (medium grain) and gros (coarse grain). Many snuffs got their particular fragrance from the blending of the tobacco alone, whilst others had numerous odoriferous additives. The various names under which the great diversity of snuff brands were marketed (such as Old Paris, Cuba, Letter F and Dieppe Scented Bergamotte) foreshadows the evocative epithets that were later to be given to cigar and cigarette brands. In fact, the hundreds of different labels and wrappers that snuffs were packaged in represent the first phase of large-scale tobacco advertising. As is the case with tea and coffee, there were snuffs for different times of the day and different occasions. So too there were snuffs for the old, snuffs for the young, snuffs for ladies and so on. To use the wrong snuff at the wrong time or even the right snuff at the wrong time was considered a sign of vulgarity and ignorance. The extravagance of the age is epitomised by the lavish and luxurious consumption of snuff. The bill for the snuff used at the celebrations that accompanied the coronation of George IV came to the then enormous sum of £8,205.15. Lord Petersham, perhaps the greatest snuff connoisseur of them all, owned a snuff box for every day of the year, and, on his death, left behind some £3,000-worth of snuff.

The snuff boxes of the era have become highly collectable objects on account of their intricate craftsmanship and the precious materials of which they were made. Many were decorated with motifs derived from classical legend. Experts consider the French gold snuff boxes to be the best, most other continental examples are seen to be derivative of them; only the English boxes were made in a markedly different style. Glass snuff bottles were also made but never had a comparable role as the snuff boxes, which stood out as socially charged emblems of class. Yet among the Chinese (who had been introduced to snuff by Portuguese merchants and Jesuit missionaries) the glass bottle was the main container used for storing snuff. For the Chinese the use of snuff has many parallels with its role in European societies. It was popular among the class of Chinese officials and, as in Europe, was intimately connected with ostentatious behaviour, snobbery and status. The habit reached its zenith in the middle to late eighteenth century and inspired developments in craftsmanship that even surpass the snuff equipment of the French. The most striking Chinese innovation was in the making of glass snuff bottles with colour decoration painted on the inside of the glass.

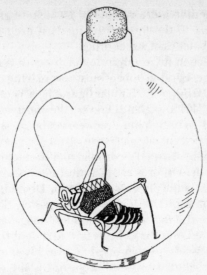

**CHINESE SNUFF BOTTLE**

This was done by the artist holding up the bottle with one hand and painting the design with the other, using a brush that had its tip made at right angles to the handle. In the European case, although the other paraphernalia of the snuff user could not match the snuffbox either socially (as a means of advertising one's wealth and status) or artistically (in terms of refined craftsmanship), it was, nevertheless, essential kit for the aficionado. Although the rasp, pestle and mortar (for use at home), and miniature knife (for removing snuff from under the fingernails) all played their supporting roles in preparing and administering snuff it is the delicate snuff spoon that resonates with twentieth-century sensibilities. For it is an ancestral form of the silver cocaine spoon that was an integral part of the pretentions of the 'glamorous' phase of cocaine use during the 1970s.

There were scares concerning the safety of snuff that also foreshadow later concerns with the quality of cocaine and other street drugs. In 1712 the Dauphine of France was poisoned after taking a pinch from a box of Spanish snuff presented to her. The news spread like wildfire and the Spanish snuff was portrayed as an insidious means of politically motivated assassination blamed on the (long-suffering) Jesuits. Certain other snuffs were apparently not the genuine article, containing no tobacco at all; even worse, its adulterants were rumoured to include ground glass – which, according to the lore of the modern drug scene, is also found in some batches of street drugs.

Snuff use reached its zenith in the eighteenth century. At this time the average London tobacconist was making about 90 per cent of its profit from snuff. Similar figures have been recorded in the accounts of Fribourg and Treyer, the most exclusive snuff shop in London. In its first hundred years of business (from 1720–1820) only 10 per cent of sales were of tobacco and cigars. The patronage of King George IV consolidated the status of the shop as second to none. Other great historical figures who are said to have indulged in snuff include Napoleon, Dryden, Pope, Swift, Burns, Swedenborg, Dr Johnson, Congreve, Sheridan and Gibbon. Despite the fact that the popular image of snuff has it inextricably linked with the delicate and decadent figures of high society, snuff was also widely used by the lower classes. 'Irish Blackguard', distributed by Lundy Foot of Dublin, was the name given to a mixture popular with the Irish working class.

Tobacco was, of course, popular among the leading lights of the arts and sciences. Among reported smokers were Isaac Newton, Jonathan Swift, John Milton, John Keats, William Wordsworth, Samuel Taylor Coleridge, Charles Dickens, William Thackeray, Thomas Hardy, Alfred Tennyson, Ralph Waldo Emerson and Mark Twain. Those who opposed the habit included Rousseau, Voltaire, Goethe, Ruskin and, rather improbably, the inveterate drinker Swinburne.

We have to go back in time to pick up the European introduction of tobacco to Asia (something which now, with full knowledge of its harmful effects, we could compare with the spreading of a plague), which was an element of the interaction between the two continents. Tobacco conquered Asia as it had conquered Europe. So complete was this colonisation by tobacco that the orientalist Berthold Laufer, writing in 1924, claimed that there was only one Asian people that did not use it. This tiny tobacco-free zone was said to be found among the Yami people of Botel Tobago, an island thirty-five miles east of Taiwan (although the name of this island makes one think that this is a leg pull).

Laufer sketched out the three routes by which tobacco diffused through Asia. The first route began in Mexico, from where the Spanish took tobacco (mainly in the form of cigars) to the Philippines in the sixteenth century. Via the Philippines it reached Taiwan, parts of mainland China, Korea, Burma and south India. The beginning of the seventeenth century saw the Portuguese introducing tobacco by way of the maritime routes to many parts of Asia. According to Javanese sources, tobacco had arrived in Java in 1601. By around 1605 it was known in India and eventually filtered through to the more remote tribal areas of the subcontinent, where it was to play an important role in local mythologies. Its arrival in Japan – also around 1605 – was not particularly welcome, according to an account preserved in the diary of Captain Richard Cocks. In an entry dated 7 August 1615, he describes the Emperor ordering the large-scale burning of tobacco. Nevertheless, like James I, the Emperor seems to have been powerless to stop the growth of the habit, as at the same time Kyoto craftsmen were already manufacturing smoking pipes. Interestingly, tobacco chewing did not catch on in Tibet and the Far East (Korea, China and Japan) but was keenly taken up by the Indians and south-east Asians who had long-established traditions of chewing another stimulant, namely betel (see **Betel**). Tobacco and betel are often chewed together, a habit which is also popular in New Guinea. The third and mostly northerly route was across Siberia. When the Russians introduced tobacco into Siberia (although the influence of the Chinese use of tobacco had already entered some parts of north Asia) the local shamans were quick to see its shamanic applications and added it to their traditional practices, despite the fact that to their Russian colonisers it was a drug with no religious connotations.

Despite its overtly secular role in the modern world, tobacco is still referred to by a mixture of personifications, metaphors and folklore. J.M. Barrie, the creator of the eternal youth Peter Pan, had as his own elixir 'My Lady Nicotine', whom he describes with all the epithets worthy of a lover. He felt obliged to abandon his mistress tobacco on the eve of his marriage, lest his wife become jealous of his bachelor vice. In the 1950s Jerome E. Brooks, a historian of tobacco, describes the neophyte smoker becoming an 'incense worshipper paying tribute to the goddess Nicotine'.

There are also a number of superstitions and folk tales surrounding tobacco and its use. Everyone knows that it is supposed to be unlucky to light three cigarettes from one match (for the third person) and almost everyone is aware that the usual explanation for this is that the time it takes from the striking of the match to the third light is just enough time for a sniper to take aim

and fire. This is said to have originated in the trenches during the
First World War, but Boer War veterans remember it from their
day. It seems that it actually stems from a much earlier belief
(traced back to the seventeenth century but most likely to be even
earlier) that it is a bad omen to light three candles or lamps with a
single taper. This belief may have been transferred to the cigarette
as electric lights tended to restrict the instances in which the old
form of the superstition could be put to use, thus the superstition
survived by moving with the times. Another piece of folklore that
has sprung up around the cigarette concerns the packet of the
Marlboro brand which, if one has the eyes to see – and an active
imagination – can be seen as being invested with hidden messages
from the extreme right wing. Immediately suggestive are the very
colours of the packet (red, white and black – exactly the same
colours used in the Nazi swastika symbol); then, if the packet is
opened out flat, the triangular interfaces between the red and
white parts of the box are revealed as Ks, signifying the Ku Klux
Klan. If this were not evidence enough (for the highly gullible),
then if one reads the word Marlboro on the pack backwards and
upside down it spells out the anti-Semitic 'horrible Jew'. The best
thing that can be said about this 'reading' is that, for creativity, it
beats most of the daydreams conjured up by bored drinkers sitting
around in bars picking apart their cigarette packets.

In the botanical order of things, tobacco lies midway between
the innocent potato and tomato on the one hand and a sinister
cluster of hallucinogenic weeds on the other. The social standing
of tobacco has swung from one extreme to the other throughout
European history. Often, even in recent times, smoking has been
widely accepted as an innocuous or even positive pastime. It has
been in times of social upheaval that the cigarette has really come
into its own. During the World Wars tobacco was seen as an
indispensable part of the soldier's staple diet, helping him combat
the combined assaults of cold, hunger, fear and boredom. The
morale of the troops often depended on the uninterrupted supply
of cigarettes to the front line. Smoking provided a solace that food
simply could not. In times of mass poverty and unemployment we
might expect that smoking would decline for economic reasons.
This would make sense if we acted in such a utilitarian fashion as
some would have us believe, but human nature is altogether too
capricious to function in such a straightforward way.

In the current social climate, tobacco-smoking is one of the most exemplary acts of political incorrectness (and this, in itself, might suggest that it is due for a short-lived revival, for there is no better way to get people to do something – particularly the young – than admonish them for even contemplating it) and medical opinion has swung the pendulum firmly (and probably permanently) back towards the negative pole. Tobacco is now seen as one of the most virulent of poisonous plants, surpassing its relatives (such as the old witches' herbs henbane and belladonna) by its sheer popularity and ubiquity. The clear-cut liberal argument to the anti-smoking lobby, namely that it is a citizen's own private business if he or she wishes to smoke such a dangerous but licit substance, has collapsed in the wake of the discovery of the phenomenon of passive smoking, which makes the habit interfere with the rights of other citizens.

In recognition of its awesome properties, native Americans traditionally restricted their use of tobacco by smoking only in the context of sacred ceremonies. Our secular society, with no recourse to such means, has sought to limit it via medical repudiation: a message that seems slowly to be getting through. Yet the genie of tobacco shows no signs of disappearing overnight in a puff of smoke. With more deaths to its name than all the illicit narcotics put together, there can be no doubt that tobacco is the most dangerous drug in the world.

**Sources:** Anon 1641, Beaumont 1602, Brooks 1953, Dixon 1933, Evans 1921, Feinhandler, Fleming and Monahon 1979, Gardiner 1610, Gerard 1597, Heiser 1969, Heizer 1940, Hill 1761, James I King of England 1604, Janiger and Dobkin de Rios 1976, Knight 1975, Laufer 1924a, Laufer 1924b, Mehra 1979, Monardes 1577, Norton and Norton 1938, Penn 1901, Radford and Radford 1980, Rich 1606, Salmon 1710, Turner and Taylor 1972, Wilbert 1987, Wilbert 1991, Wilbert 1993.

## TREE DATURAS see Brugmansia

## TROPANE ALKALOIDS

Whilst they are typically associated with the family of plants called the Solanaceae (for members of this family containing this psychoactive alkaloid group see **Belladonna**, **Brugmansia**, **Datura**, **Henbane**, **Mandrake**, **Pituri**, and **Scopolia**), they are also found elsewhere in the plant kingdom. All the plants above have been used for both their psychoactive effects and as medicines. Often they have been added to alcoholic drinks to increase their potency, such as the making of henbane beer in Europe and *Brugmansia* drinks in South America. The tropane alkaloids have also played their role in warfare and criminal activities – mandrake, henbane, belladonna and *Datura* have all been used for these nefarious ends.

(See also **Scopolamine**.)

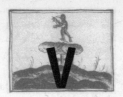

## VIROLA

There are about sixty species of tree belonging to the genus *Virola* that grow in the tropical zone of the Americas. Many of them (*V. theiodora*, *V.* spp.) have been used for the red resin in the inner bark, which has powerful hallucinogenic effects. The psychoactive constituents are tryptamine and ß-carboline alkaloids, particularly DMT and 5-Meo-DMT. The effects of using *Virola* begin with a phase of excitable behaviour which is then followed by numbness and loss of muscular co-ordination, nausea, hallucinations and an eventual succumbing to a narcotic sleep.

This psychoactive substance is used by a number of Indian groups in Colombia, Brazil, Venezuela, Ecuador and Peru. In Colombia it is known as *yákee* or *yáto* and its use is generally restricted to shamans. In Brazil it may be used by all men and is known as *paricá*, *ebene* and *epéna* (all three names being general terms for snuff and not just restricted to those made from *Virola* species) and *nyakwana*. It is most commonly made into the form of a snuff by drying the collected bark, then making it into a powder, often with other plants mixed in. The Makú Indians of Colombia do not make a snuff but simply consume the resin without preparation directly from the bark. Some shamans of the Peruvian Amazon make the resin into pellets and eat it in order to contact spirits in the form of 'the little people' (it is striking how often 'the little people' are seen under the influence of different psychoactive substances in diverse parts of the world; see, for example, **Fly-Agaric**). There are also vague reports of *Virola* bark being smoked. Richard Schultes has described the cultural and mythological importance of this entheogen among a Colombian people:

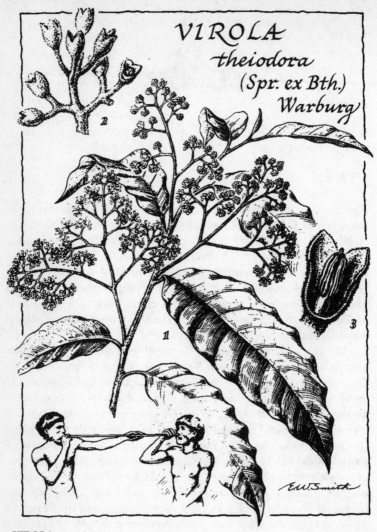

*VIROLA theiodora (Spr. ex Bth.) Warburg*

**VIROLA**

At the beginning of time, Father Sun practised incest with his daughter who acquired *Viho* by scratching her father's penis. Thus the Tukano received this sacred snuff from the sun's semen, and since it is still hallowed, it is kept in containers called *muhipu-nuri* or 'penis of the sun'. This hallucinogen enables the Tukano to consult the spirit world, especially

*Viho-mahse*, the 'snuff-person' who, from his dwelling in the Milky Way, tends to all human affairs. Shamans may not contact other spiritual forces directly but only through the good graces of *Viho-mahse*. Consequently, the snuff represents one of the most important tools of the *payé* or medicine man.

**Sources:** Bennett and Alarcón 1994, De Smet 1985a, Ott 1993, Schultes and Hofmann 1980a, Schultes and Hofmann 1980b.

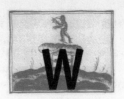

## WATER LILIES

In Europe the water lily (*Nymphaea* spp.) was known by a number of names including the Water Rose, Clavis Veneris, Clava Herculis and Digitus; to the apothecaries it was Nenuphar. Oils and decoctions of it were used as soporifics and anaphrodisiacs, these two qualities being combined to suppress nocturnal pollution (wet dreams) and other dreams of a sexual nature (this is, of course, the exact opposite use of the plant to that of the Ancient Egyptians; for which see below). It was believed that too regular use of the water lily could cause impotency. William Bulleyn includes in a book of compound medicines an entry on *Oleum Nimphæatum album* (i.e. an oil of the white or yellow water lily), which he describes in the medical terminology of the time: 'this oyle hath almost the vertues of the oile [sic] Poppie, but because it is not so cold, it doth not so much dul ye senses.' In other words, the water lily was seen as analogous to opium in its effects but not as potent. John Hartman, writing in the seventeenth century, describes a medical preparation in which opium powder is dissolved in an infusion of water lilies, thus combining the psychoactive effects of the two. Water lilies occasionally feature among the ingredients of the witches' ointments (see **Witches' Ointments**) yet are also known to have been used by nuns and monks to suppress sexual desires!

Although there are reports of the narcotic and sedative effects of this and other genera of water lilies being used in other parts of the world, it is among the ancient Maya and Egyptians that these plants seem to have had a significant cultural role. Among the ancient Maya of the New World works of art depicting mushrooms, amphibians and water lilies (*Nymphaea ampla*) are relatively common. These depictions have led the anthropologist

Marlene Dobkin de Rios to propose that they were portrayed so prominently in Maya iconography because of their psychoactive qualities and that they were used as entheogens. It has also been suggested that the Aztec plant known as *quetzalxochiatl* (meaning 'precious water flower') refers to the water lily *N. ampla*. The distinguished botanist William Emboden has written a number of articles in which he has suggested that not only did the Maya use water lilies for their psychoactive effects, but so too did the ancient Egyptians.

Alkaloids extracted from *N. ampla* are very close in chemical structure to apomorphine, which is a synthetic derivative of morphine. This confirms the opinions of early European physicians that the effects of opium and the water lily were of the same kind. Emboden tried the Old World water lily (*N. caerulea*) for himself and found the extracts of the flower to cause visual and auditory hallucinations. By a striking coincidence, as the Maya related their water lily to two other psychoactive substances (the toad and the mushroom), the ancient Egyptian iconography portrays the water lily in a close relationship with two known psychoactive plants – the opium poppy and the mandrake. These three plants seem to have been used in both medical and magical ways and Emboden has suggested that they would have been imbibed from ritual vessels which are commonly referred to by Egyptologists as 'unguent jars'. Until these vessels are subjected to various scientific procedures which would identify the nature of any remains of what they contained, one can only speculate. Bearing in mind that over the last thirty years the full extent of the ritualistic use of psychoactive substances in other parts of the ancient world has come to be accepted (e.g. the renewed interest in the Indo-Iranian hallucinogen *soma/haoma*; see **Soma**; the prominence of opium cults in the ancient Mediterranean and the use of the hallucinogenic fungus ergot in Greece; see **Ergot**) it is becoming increasingly difficult to imagine that the ancient Egyptians made no use of such substances. Most Egyptologists seem to have little interest in pursuing such lines of research and until colloborations between botanical experts and Egyptologists come about it seems likely to be an aspect of ancient Egypt that will continue to be a mystery.

In response to Emboden's researches on the use of the water lily by both the ancient Egyptians and the Maya, Thor Heyerdahl, the famous veteran of numerous ocean crossings in replicas of ancient boats, wrote that this curious parallel use of a psychoactive substance *may* be a cultural practice that diffused from the Old World to the New. Although his critics have often lampooned Heyerdahl for his heretical ideas, he is clearly a sincere and learned scholar. One suspects that his spectacular *Ra* and *Kon-Tiki* expeditions, which showed that the major oceans could be navigated successfully within the technological capacities of the ancient world, caused a great deal of envy among desk-bound experts who had dismissed out of hand the possibility that such voyages could have been made by the ancients.

**Sources:** Bulleyn 1562, Coles 1657, Crollius 1670, Dobkin de Rios 1974, Emboden 1978, Emboden 1979, Emboden 1981, Heyerdahl 1982, Manniche 1989, Ott 1993, Rätsch 1992, Rudgley 1993, Salmon 1693.

## WATER PIPE see **Pipe**

## WITCHES' OINTMENTS

Largely due to the fact that most of the records we have concerning the practices and beliefs of the European witches are from hostile sources, such as the Inquisition and the witch finders, they have long been portrayed as evil conspirators and collaborators with the demonic world. However, much of the so-called evidence for the nefarious activities of the witches – such as cannibalism, incestuous orgies and other abominations (such charges have a long and ignoble history; the early Christians, among others, were accused of the same) – is now accepted by historians to have taken place not in the actual secretive meetings of witches but in the depraved minds of their interrogators, who extracted what they wished to hear from their (mainly female) victims by a variety of means ranging from mild suggestion to the most extreme forms of torture. It seems that witchcraft was not so much anti-Christian as pre-Christian in its beliefs. Central to the shamanistic ceremonial life of the witches was the preparation and use of the so-called flying ointments. These salves, or ointments (usually described as green or greenish in colour), when rubbed on the naked body of the witch were said to enable her to fly. In the mountains of Afghanistan the use of a similar ointment, containing the hallucinogenic fly-agaric mushroom, is reported from recent history. In Uzbekistan and other parts of Central Asia adjacent to Afghanistan, cannabis extracts are rubbed on the skin in the form of a kind of massage oil. The topical administration of psychoactive substances was also practised by the Aztecs whose ointments included tobacco, poisonous insects and hallucinogenic plants among the ingredients.

The making of such ointments is known to be very old. Ovid in his *Metamorphoses* (XV:356) describes Scythian women using magical salves in order to transform into birds, a distinctly shamanic activity. Pamphile, a malevolent sorceress in the *Golden Ass* of Apuleius (written in the second century AD), turns into an owl with the help of a flying ointment. The flight of the witch was not, of course, literal but was rather a hallucinatory experience induced by psychoactive substances in the ointment. Yet so vivid and so powerful were the sensations caused by the drugs that many seemed to believe the experience to be actual flight and transportation of the physical body. Travelling on a broomstick, or by transforming into a bird or other creature, the witch would find her way to the sabbats – the name given to the nocturnal gatherings of witches, demons and other spirits, at which frenzied dancing and sexual orgies took place.

In many accounts the witch is said to have applied the flying ointment all over her body, but some modern researchers have questioned how effectively the drugs could have permeated the skin and so intoxicated the user (although the experiments of Peukert, cited below, suggest that this is adequate). Nevertheless, it has been suggested that the psychoactive effects would have been intensified if the ointment were introduced through the sensitive vaginal membranes by means of an anointed staff or broomstick. Not only does this help to explain how the ointment worked on a chemical level but also explains the frequent sexual fantasies of the sabbat. Another common experience of the witches, at least according to their accounts before their inquisitors, was that when they had sexual intercourse with the 'devil' his penis was painfully cold. This may refer to the insertion of the broom, accompanied by rapid changes in body temperature caused by the initial effects of the drugs. Whilst the vaginal method of administering the hallucinogenic ointments may well have been a common means, it is also possible that anal administration was practised. Many of the heretical enemies of the

Church were accused of propagating anal intercourse – the Manichaeans, the Albigensians, the Cathars and the Bogomils among them. In fact, the English word 'buggery' derives from *Bulgarus* (Bulgaria), the home of the Bogomils. Certainly the use of enemas or clysters (glysters) for administering medicines (including henbane) was known in Europe long before medieval times. The insertion of hallucinogenic substances by way of an enema is a fairly common practice in native South American cultures.

There are numerous accounts of the use of flying ointments in the annals of witchcraft, but only a fraction of these give more than a hint of what ingredients actually made up the ointments themselves. It seems likely that witches, like present-day shamans, kept their own recipes secret, not only for fear of persecution but also to enhance their own status and reputation among their own kind. A number of reliable formulae for the composition of flying ointments do remain. Among a welter of bizarre and often sinister admixtures, such as human fat, cat's brains and bat's blood, there are a few particular plants which recur in the brews again and again and which are also known to have hallucinogenic properties. So, chemically speaking, the visions and sensations of the witches' flights were induced by a small number of key plants, most of them closely related members of the potato family, the Solanaceae. The most important were the 'infernal trinity' of saturnian herbs; see **Henbane**, **Belladonna**, **Mandrake** and **Saturnian/Saturnine herbs**. Other hallucinogenic and narcotic plants that made up the ointments include thorn-apple (see **Datura**), black hellebore, sweet flag (see **Acorus Calamus**), **Opium** and **Cannabis**.

Wolf's bane or aconite is almost invariably included in the recipe of the ointments and this plant is supposed to make the user feel that they have fur or feathers. This may go towards explaining the bird transformations alluded to above, as well as the legend of the werewolf. As a number of early observers were aware that the witches' flights were caused by psychoactive substances (see below), so the idea that lycanthropy (the apparent transformation of a human into a wolf) was an effect caused by drugs is no modern discovery. In 1599 Chauvincourt wrote that such metamorphoses were illusions caused by: 'unguents, powders, potions, and noxious herbs, which are able to dazzle all who come under their baneful and magic influence.' Jean de

Nynauld, writing at the beginning of the seventeenth century, not only concurred with Chauvincourt on the hallucinogenic origins of werewolf transformations but also gave details of the specific type of ointment used to turn into an animal. The ointment included amongst its ingredients parts of snakes, toads, hedgehogs and other animals mixed with plants and human blood. There has been little investigation of the human and animal ingredients of the ointments and it has been generally presumed that their inclusion in the brews was for their 'magical', not chemical, effects. However, with the comparatively recent discovery of the possible extent of psychoactive fauna (see **Animals**), the idea that some animal parts may have been used for chemical effects needs investigating. The toad was one of the most important of the witches' familiars and the now well-established fact of the hallucinogenic properties of certain species makes it the prime candidate (see **Toad**).

Alfonso Tostado, the Bishop of Avila and the greatest Spanish theologian of his time, gave the opinion in 1436 that the witches' sabbat was a delusion caused by the drugs in the witches' ointments. The enlightened Spanish doctor Andrés Fernández de Laguna (1499–1560), physician to Emperor Charles V and Philip II, believed that the users of the ointments were suffering from a kind of mental illness. De Laguna undertook his own experimental work on the effects of such ointments by obtaining a supply of a salve from a friend who was a constable. He did not use the ointment on himself but:

> In the city of Metz I had the wife of the public executioner anointed with it from head to foot. She through jealousy of her husband had completely lost power of sleep and had become half insane in consequence ... no sooner did I anoint her than she opened her eyes wide like a rabbit, and soon they looked like those of a cooked hare when she fell into such a profound sleep that I thought I should never be able to awake her ... after a lapse of thirty-six hours, I restored her to her senses and sanity. Her first words were 'why did you awaken me ... at such an inauspicious moment? Why I was surrounded by all the delights of the world.' Then turning to her husband (he was beside her, she stinking like a corpse) and smiling at him she said 'Skinflint! I want you to know that I have put the horns on you [i.e. she

had made him a cuckold], and with a younger and lustier
lover than you.'

What is made clear from this account is that the ointment
certainly worked, even though it does not seem to have been
administered into the vagina. De Laguna is of the opinion that the
commonly reported sensation of excessive cold attributed to the
devil's penis is actually due to the physiological effects of the
ointment, which makes the user feel cold to the marrow of their
bones.

Such experimental attitudes to the ointments, if not exactly
commonplace, were certainly more frequent than might be
supposed for an era too often portrayed as entirely dominated by
superstition and bigotry. The French philosopher and
astronomer Pierre Gassendi (1592–1655) massaged some
unwitting peasants with a psychoactive salve, who promptly fell
into a deep sleep; on awakening they reported that they had
visited the sabbat. John Baptista Porta, in his sixteenth-century
work *Natural Magick*, reports on the strange behaviour of some
men (the ointments were not exclusively a feminine preserve)
who were under the influence of such a powerful witches' potion.
He describes one case in which a man thought himself changed
into a goose and would eat grass and beat the ground with his
teeth in imitation of a beak, singing whilst clapping his hands as if
they were wings. Another believed he was a fish and would swim
on the ground diving and surfacing as he went. Such bizarre and
ludicrous behaviour is reminiscent of the accidental mass *Datura*
intoxication experienced at Jamestown (see **Datura**). Whilst the
individuals described by Porta may simply have been using the
drugs in a recreational fashion it is possible that they may have
been seeking magical transformation into an animal spirit, a
practice of shamans throughout the world.

Francis Bacon (1561–1626), one of the founders of modern
science, notes that the 'imaginings'(i.e. hallucinations) of both
the ancient witches of Thessaly in northern Greece and their later
European counterparts were caused not by incantations or
ceremonies but by ointments which are 'opiate and soporiferous'.
He said that these were such 'potent medicines' that if they were
taken internally the result would be fatal. He also recognised that
only some of the ingredients were actually psychoactive.
According to Bacon, the 'soporiferous medicines' included

henbane, hemlock, mandrake, moon shade, tobacco, opium, saffron and poplar leaves.

Sometimes observers who were aware that the flights of the witches were caused by psychoactive substances tried to rationalise with the users of the ointments, successfully in a case described by Johannes Nider in a book published in 1692:

> I shall ... show how so many people are deceived in their sleep, that upon wakening they altogether believe that they have actually seen what has happened only in the inner part of the mind. I heard my teacher give this account: a certain priest of our order entered a village where he came upon a woman so out of her senses that she believed herself to be transported through the air during the night with Diana [the pagan goddess] and other women. When he attempted to remove this heresy from her by means of wholesome discourse she steadfastly maintained her belief. The priest then asked her: 'Allow me to be present when you depart on the next occasion.' She answered: 'I agree to it and you will observe my departure in the presence (if you wish) of suitable witnesses.' Therefore, when the day for the departure arrived, which the old woman had previously determined, the priest showed up with trustworthy townsmen to convince this fanatic of her madness. The woman, having placed a large bowl, which was used for kneading dough, on top of a stool, stepped into the bowl and sat herself down. Then, rubbing ointment on herself to the accompaniment of magic incantations she lay her head back and immediately fell asleep. With the labour of the devil she dreamed of Mistress Venus and other superstitions so vividly that, crying out with a shout and striking her hands about, she jarred the bowl in which she was sitting and, falling down from the stool seriously injured herself about the head. As she lay there awakened, the priest cried out to her that she had not moved: 'For Heaven's sake, where are you? You were not with Diana and as will be attested by these present, you never left this bowl.' Thus, by this act and by thoughtful exhortations he drew out this belief from her abominable soul.

There do not seem to be accounts of accidental self-poisoning by witches using these ointments, which is quite striking bearing in mind the great number of potentially toxic plant extracts contained in them. This may suggest that the recipes were handed down so that the health risks were minimised. Karl Kiesewetter, who seems to have been the first modern investigator to try out the ointment recipes on himself, accidentally died as a consequence of administering a lethal preparation. Professor Will-Erich Peukert, a scholar of folklore from Göttingen in Germany, concocted a flying ointment based on a mixture of belladonna, henbane and datura, and, along with some colleagues, he experimented with it by rubbing it on the forehead and armpits. They fell into a twenty-four-hour sleep in which they experienced wild dreams. Terrible faces floated before their eyes. The initial hallucinations were followed by sensations of flying for miles through the air, periodically falling at great speeds before soaring off again. In the last phantasmagorical phase of their trip they saw images of an orgiastic feast with grotesque sexual excesses. Whilst the contents of their hallucinations can be put down to their desire to re-live the witches' sabbat, the rapid soaring and descending sensations are clearly fundamental effects of the ointments.

An eccentric English experiment is rather tame by comparison. In 1939 Gerald Gardner, the founder of the modern witchcraft or Wicca movement, was initiated into a coven that used to perform its rituals in the New Forest in the south of England. The members of the coven made an ointment from bear's fat, not for the purpose of flying but to keep themselves warm in the forest at night, whilst performing their rituals 'sky-clad', that is to say naked. The ointment does not seem to have been particularly successful as on one cold night in 1940, whilst the witches were performing a ritual designed to thwart Hitler's planned invasion of Britain, several of the older members died, apparently of pneumonia, thus giving their lives, albeit in the most bizarre of ways, for the war effort. It is, however, unlikely that the RAF shall ever have to share the honour of winning the Battle of Britain with these patriotic but earthbound witches.

There are good reasons to believe that the witches' ointments demonstrate that psychoactive preparations were very significant in European cultures. That there are numerous accounts of their use in a number of European countries and that the use of such salves is about 2,000 years old (if not longer) suggests that they may have played a central role in the pre-Christian religions of

Europe. The considerable number of plants (and animals) used shows a complex and sophisticated tradition at work, and in this sense the witches' preparations can be compared with the shamanistic use of hallucinogens in other regions of the world, such as Mexico and the Amazon. The psychoactive substances taken by the witches became degraded to satanic plants under the ascetic rule of the Church (for an apparently exceptional case of such an ointment being used in conjunction with Christian ritual see **Henbane**). The subsequent names given to such plants in folk botany bear witness to the relegation of these plants from entheogens to demonic drugs.

Would-be witches and werewolves are cautioned against experimenting with any of the recipes detailed above; the cautionary tale of Karl Kiesewetter should be sufficient deterrent. Many of the plants used in such ointments are poisonous and their consumption can be fatal. Regular use of psychoactive species of the *Solanaceae* family can cause damage to the mind, largely due to the presence of the alkaloid scopolamine in these plants (see **Scopolamine**).

The use of psychoactive substances by the witches was not limited to ointments; there are also accounts suggesting that, like the sorcerers of Haiti (see **Zombi Drug**) they used both poisonous powders and antidotes to the same. Francesco-Maria Guazzo, a fanatical friar of the early seventeenth century, reports in his *Compendium Maleficarum* ('Handbook of Witches') the tale of a woman who sought revenge on a baker who had refused her credit. She called on the devil who:

> eager for any chance of doing ill, gave her some herbs wrapped in a paper, telling her to scatter them in the place most often used by the baker and his family. She at once took them and spread them in the doorway by which they had to go to the village, and the baker, and after him his wife and children, walked over them and were all afflicted with the same sickness. And they did not recover until the witch, moved by pity, obtained from the demon another herb to restore them. This she hid secretly in their beds, as she had been told to do, and they were soon all restored from sickness to their former health.

Guazzo fails to explain why the devil who is so eager to cause sickness should be equally willing to supply an antidote to restore the health of his victims!

**Sources:** Bacon 1627, Benet 1975, Emboden 1975, Gerard 1597, Guazzo 1929, Hansen 1978, Harner 1973, Lea 1907, Moreau de Tours 1973, Ott 1993, Rätsch 1992, Robbins 1959, Rothman 1972, Rudgley 1993, Rudgley 1995, Schultes and Hofmann 1980b, Scot 1665, Sherratt 1996a.

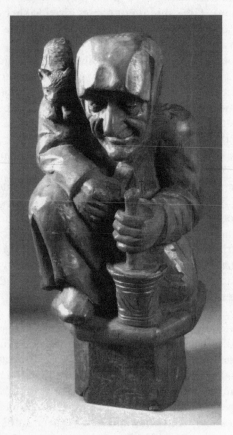

**WITCH, WITH CAT AND PESTLE AND MORTAR**

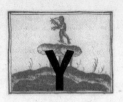

**YAJÉ** see **Ayahuasca**

**YOHIMBE**

The inner bark of the West African *yohimbe* tree (*Corynanthe yohimbe*) has a long history of use as an aphrodisiac in the region. The bark was made into a beverage and drunk to promote virility and sexual desire. It was reportedly used in vast quantities to allow orgies to continue unabated for days on end, although such stories must be treated with some scepticism. What is more certain is that there is a chemical basis for its erotic reputation. The alkaloid *yohimbine* has the effect of strengthening and prolonging erections and, in higher doses, can cause minor hallucinogenic effects. In twentieth-century Europe *yohimbine* has been widely used as a sexual stimulant and recently the bark has been used in the sexual rites of Western occultists.

**Sources:** Rätsch 1992, Thorwald 1962.

**YOHIMBINE** see **Yohimbe**

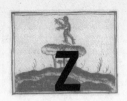

## ZOMBI DRUG

The zombies, or living dead, of Haiti have long enthralled not only the natives of the island but also Westerners who have, in the main, seen it as a sensational but unfounded piece of folklore. As a consequence the Western rendition of the zombi figure has taken its place alongside the vampire, werewolf and mummy and appeared in numerous horror movies. The Haitian view of zombies is very different: as Wade Davis has put it, Haitians are not afraid of zombies but of becoming one themselves. Not all Western attitudes to zombi lore were entirely spurious. Nathan Kline, a pioneer in the use of tranquillisers and an eminent figure in the medical world, had worked for more than thirty years in Haiti. He was convinced that he had come across a genuine case of zombification in the person of one Clairvius Narcisse, a man who had dramatically returned to his village after being missing for eighteen years, for which time he had been working as a slave after being turned into a zombi. By 1982 Kline was determined to get to the bottom of the zombi phenomenon and suspected that the explanation was to be found in the form of a drug. He discussed his interest in trying to solve this mystery with Richard Schultes, the then Director of the Botanical Museum of Harvard University, who had extensive field experience in South America. Schultes suggested to Kline that one of his students, a remarkable young ethnobiologist named Wade Davis, would be the man for the job. Davis was offered the job which he eagerly accepted. He succeeded in obtaining the formula of the zombi drug from four separate places in Haiti and brought back actual samples of the substance in the form of a very dark grey powder.

Although some of the constituents of the zombi poison varied from place to place (including tarantulas and various reptile parts), certain plant, animal and human substances were found to be present in all cases. The most significant among the plant additives were the ground-up seeds of the *concombre zombi* ('zombi cucumber', the Haitian name for the hallucinogenic plants *Datura stramonium* and *D. metel*). All preparations of the drug reported by Davis also contained burnt and ground human remains, a certain species of tree frog, the marine toad (*Bufo marinus*), a polychaete worm (such worms were used by early Greek doctors for removing hair but, as Dioscorides notes, touching the worm causes highly unpleasant itching; the reason the zombi makers included it in their preparations was to aggravate the toad into releasing its venom) and one or more species of puffer fish. Although Davis originally suspected that *Datura* was the ingredient causing the symptoms of zombification it actually turned out to be the neurotoxins of the puffer fish that induced the profound paralysis and anaesthesia. This is corroborated by medical evidence from Japan. The puffer fish is a dangerous, but highly prized, delicacy eaten by Japanese gastronomes. Those who have been accidentally poisoned in this way report strikingly similar symptoms to those associated with zombification. The resurrection of the victims of the zombi maker is done by giving them *Datura*, after which they are led away to be sold off as slave labourers, often on the sugar plantations.

On his return from Haiti, in addition to publishing a number of scholarly papers and an academic monograph on his fieldwork, Davis also wrote a more popular book, entitled *The Serpent and the Rainbow*. A film of the same name, directed by Wes Craven of

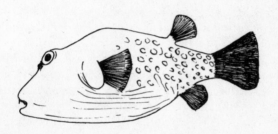

**PUFFER FISH**

*Nightmare on Elm Street* fame, followed soon afterwards and mixed real events with a liberal dose of Hollywood horror. The film, whilst entertaining enough, was criticised by Haitian scholars for reinforcing the facile view of Haitian voodoo that Davis himself had sought to challenge. The sensational nature of Davis' findings caused something of a furore in medical and academic circles. William H. Anderson, of the Massachusetts General Hospital in Boston, did not accept that there was sufficient proof that the zombi poisons actually contained the puffer-fish toxin (tetrodotoxin), and found the scientific analyses of the powders brought back from Haiti insubstantial. He also questioned the ethical nature of some of Davis' fieldwork, particularly those instances where Davis was present at graveyards during the digging-up of corpses by his sorcerer-informant. In his own defence Davis makes it clear that he did not instigate any of these acts of necromancy and that they would have taken place without his presence anyway.

Anderson was not the only critic of Davis' work and certainly not the most vociferous. C.Y. Yao went so far as to call the whole thing a 'scientific fraud', an accusation which Davis attributed to 'old-fashioned jealousy'. Yao and his colleague Takeshi Yasumoto dismissed Davis' claim that tetrodotoxin was the causal agent in the process of zombification largely on the grounds that the way the zombi drug was made meant that no active tetrodotoxin could be present in the finished product and thus could not have been responsible for the effects it was said to have caused.

**Sources:** Anderson 1988, Booth 1988, Davis 1983, Davis 1985, Davis 1988, Davis 1989, Yasumoto and Kao 1986.

# BIBLIOGRAPHY

Abel, E.L., 1980. *Marihuana: The First Twelve Thousand Years*, Plenum Press, New York and London.

Abu-Rabia, A., 1983. *Folk Medicine Among the Bedouin Tribes in the Negev*, Social Studies Center, Ben-Gurion University, Israel.

Adovasio, J.M. and Fry, G.F., 1976. 'Prehistoric Psychotropic Drug Use in Northeastern Mexico and Trans-Pecos Texas', EB 30/1, 94–96.

Ager, T.A. and Ager, L.P., 1980. 'Ethnobotany of the Eskimos of Nelson Island, Alaska', ARCT 17/1, 27–48.

Agrippa, H.C., 1651. *Three Books of Occult Philosophy*, trans. J. French, Moule, London.

Aiston, G., 1937. 'The Aboriginal Narcotic Pitcheri', OCE 7, 372–77.

Anderson, W.H., 1988. 'Tetrodotoxin and the Zombi Phenomenon', JEp 23/1, 121–126.

Andrews, G. and Solomon, D. (eds.), 1975. *The Coca Leaf and Cocaine Papers*, Harcourt Brace Jovanovich, New York.

Anon., 1641. *Tobacco Battered; and the Pipes Shattered*, 'Mount Helicon'.

Anon., 1963. *Narcotic Drugs Under International Control: Multilingual List*, United Nations.

Anon., 1978. *Terminology of Drugs and Narcotics*, European Parliament, Directorate for Translation and Terminology Services.

Anon., 1993. *Coca, Cocaine and the War on Drugs*, Catholic Institute for International Relations, London.

Antonil [Pseudonym of Anthony Henman], 1978. *Mama Coca*, Hassle Free Press, London.

Artaud, A., 1976. *The Peyote Dance*, trans. Helen Weaver, Farrar Strauss and Giroux, New York.

Ashmole, E., 1652. *Theatrum Chemicum Britannicum*, Nathaniel Brooks, London.

Bacon, F., 1627. *Sylva Sylvarum: or A Naturall Historie in Ten Centuries*, William Lee, London.

Balfour, H., 1922. 'Earth Smoking-Pipes from South Africa and Central Asia', MAN May 1922, 65–69.

Balick, M.J. and Cox, P.A., 1996. *Plants, People, and Culture: The Science of*

*Ethnobotany*, Scientific American Library, New York.

Barger, G., 1931. *Ergot and Ergotism*, Gurney and Jackson, London.

Beaumont, J. Sir, 1602. *The Metamorphosis of Tobacco*, John Flasket, London.

Beck, J. and Rosenbaum, M., 1994. *Pursuit of Ecstasy: The MDMA Experience*, State University of New York Press, Albany.

Belardi, W., 1979. *The Pahlavi Book of the Righteous Viraz I* (Chapters 1–2), University Department of Linguistics and Italo-Iranian Culture Centre, Rome.

Benet, S., 1975. 'Early Diffusion and Folk Uses of Hemp', 39–49 in V. Rubin (ed.) *Cannabis in Culture*.

Bennett, B.C. and Alarcón, R., 1994. '*Osteophloeum platyspermum* and *Virola duckei* (Myristicaceae): Newly Reported as Hallucinogens from Amazonian Ecuador', EB 48/2, 152–158.

Bennett, J., 1991. *Lilies of the Hearth: The Historical Relationship Between Women and Plants*, Camden House, Ontario, Canada.

Beran, H., 1988. *Betel-Chewing Equipment of East New Guinea*, Shire Ethnography No.8, Shire, Aylesbury.

Beschner, G.M. and Feldman, H.W., 1979. 'Introduction', 1–17 in H.W. Feldman et al., *Angel Dust*.

Beverley, R., 1705. *The History and Present State of Virginia in Four Parts*, R. Parker, London.

Bisset, N.G. et al., 1994. 'Was Opium known in 18th Dynasty Ancient Egypt? An Examination of Materials from the Tomb of the Chief Royal Architect Kha', JEp 41/1–2, 99–114.

Blackburn, T., 1976. 'A Query Regarding the Possible Hallucinogenic Effects of Ant Ingestion in South-Central California', JCA 3/2.

Blackwood, B., 1940. 'Use of Plants Among the Kukukuku of South-East Central New Guinea', 111–126 in *Proceedings of the Sixth Pacific Science Congress* (Vol. 4), California.

Blofeld, J., 1985. *The Chinese Art of Tea*, Allen and Unwin, London.

Bocek, B.R., 1984. 'Ethnobotany of Costanoan Indians, California, Based on Collections by John P. Harrington', EB 38/2, 240–255.

Booth, W., 1988. 'Voodoo Science', SCI 240, 274–277.

Bourke, J.G., 1891. *Scatalogic Rites of All Nations*, Lowdermilk, Washington D.C.

Boyce, M., 1975. *A History of Zoroastrianism* (Vol. 1: The Early Period), Brill, Leiden.

Boyd, C.E. and Dering, J.P., 1996. 'Medicinal and Hallucinogenic Plants Identified in the Sediments and Pictographs of the Lower Pecos, Texas Archaic', AQ 70, 256–75.

Brady, M., 1992. *Heavy Metal: The Social Meaning of Petrol Sniffing in Australia*, Aboriginal Studies Press, Canberra.

Braun, S., 1996. *Buzz: The Science and Lore of Alcohol and Caffeine*, Oxford University Press, New York.

Braunschweig, H., 1527. *The Vertuose Boke*, Laurence Andrew, London.

Brekhman, I.I. and Sam, Y.A., 1979. 'Ethnopharmacological Investigations of Some Psychoactive Drugs used by Siberian and Far-Eastern Minor Nationalities of USSR', 415 in Efron et al., 1979.

Britton, E.B., 1984. 'A Pointer to a New Hallucinogen of Insect Origin', JEp 12/3, 331–33.

Brooks, J.E., 1953. *The Mighty Leaf: Tobacco Through the Ages*, Alvin Redman, London.

Brownrigg, H., 1991. *Betel Cutters from the Samuel Eilenberg Collection*, Edition Hansjörg Mayer, Stuttgart.

Brunton, R., 1989. *The Abandoned Narcotic: Kava and Cultural Instability in Melanesia*, Cambridge University Press, Cambridge.

Budge, E.A.W., 1978. *Amulets and Superstitions*, Dover, New York.

Bulleyn, W., 1562. *Bulwarke of Defence against all Sicknes*, John Kyngston, London.

Burroughs, W.S., 1959. *The Naked Lunch*, Olympia Press, Paris.

Burton-Bradley, B.G., 1972. 'Betel Chewing', 66–67 in P. Ryan (ed.) *The Encyclopedia of Papua and New Guinea Vol.1*, Melbourne University Press, Carlton, Victoria.

Bye, R.A., 1979. 'Hallucinogenic Plants of the Tarahumara', JEp 1/1, 23–48.

Camporesi, P., 1989. *Bread of Dreams: Food and Fantasy in Early Modern Europe*, trans. D. Gentilcore, Polity Press, Cambridge.

Camporesi, P., 1994. *Exotic Brew: The Art of Living in the Age of Enlightenment*, trans. C. Woodall, Polity Press, Cambridge.

Carmichael, M., 1996. 'Wonderland Revisited', LM 28, 19–28.

Carmichael, M., 1997. Personal communication.

Carroll, M., 1985. *PCP: The Dangerous Angel*, EOPD, Chelsea House, New York.

Carroll, M. and Gallo, G., 1985. *Methaqualone: The Quest for Oblivion*, EOPD, Burke, London.

Cipriani, L., 1966. *The Andaman Islanders*, Weidenfeld and Nicolson, London.

Cleckner, P.J., 1979. 'Freaks and Cognoscenti: PCP Use in Miami', 183–210 in H.W. Feldman et al., *Angel Dust*.

Coles, W., 1657. *Adam in Eden: Or Natures Paradise, The History of Plants . . .*, Nathaniel Brooke, London.

Collin de Plancy, 1825–26. *Dictionnaire Infernal*, Paris.

Cooke, M.C., 1860. *The Seven Sisters of Sleep: Popular History of the Seven Prevailing Narcotics of the World*, James Blackwood, London.

Cooper, J.M., 1949. 'Stimulants and Narcotics', 525–58 in *Handbook of South American Indians Volume 5, The Comparative Ethnology of South*

*American Indians*, Bureau of American Ethnology, Bulletin 143, Government Printing Office, Washington DC.

Corbett, L., et al., 1978. 'Hallucinogenic N-Methylated Indolealkylamines in the Cerebrospinal Fluid of Psychiatric and Control Populations', BJP 132, 139–44.

Crollius, O., 1670. *Bazilica Chymica*, John Starkey, London.

Crowley, A., 1955. *777 Revised*, Neptune Press, London.

Courtwright, D.T., 1995. 'The Rise and Fall and Rise of Cocaine in the United States' in J. Goodman et al., *Consuming Habits: Drugs in History and Anthropology*.

Culpeper, N., 1805. *The English Physician and Complete Herbal*, Lewis and Roden, London.

Cunnison, I., 1958. 'Giraffe Hunting among the Humr Tribe', SNR 39, 49–60.

Dalgarno, P.J. and Shewan, D., 1995. 'Illicit Use of Ketamine in Scotland', JPD 28/2, 191–93.

Davis, E.W., 1983. 'The Ethnobiology of the Haitian Zombi', JEp 9/1, 85–104.

Davis, E.W., 1985. *The Serpent and the Rainbow*, Warner, New York.

Davis, E.W., 1988. *Passage of Darkness: The Ethnobotany of the Haitian Zombie*, University of North Carolina Press, Chapel Hill, North Carolina.

Davis, E.W., 1989. 'Untitled Letter to the Editors', JEp 25/1, 119–22.

Davis, E.W. and Yost, J.A., 1983. 'Novel Hallucinogens From Eastern Ecuador', BMLHU 29/3, 291–95.

De Smet, P.A.G.M., 1983. 'A Multidisciplinary Overview of Intoxicating Enema Rituals in the Western Hemisphere', JEp 9/2–3, 129–66.

De Smet, P.A.G.M., 1985a. 'A Multidisciplinary Overview of Intoxicating Snuff Rituals in the Western Hemisphere', JEp 13/1, 3–49.

De Smet, P.A.G.M., 1985b. *Ritual Enemas and Snuffs in the Americas*, Latin American Studies 33, Foris, Dordrecht, Holland.

De Smet, P.A.G.M., 1996. 'Some Ethnopharmacological Notes on African Hallucinogens', JEp 50/3, 141–46.

Devereux, P., 1992. 'An Apparently Nutmeg-Induced Experience of Magical Flight', YESC 1, 189–91.

Ditton, J. and Hammersley, R., et al., 1996. *A Very Greedy Drug: Cocaine in Context*, Harwood Academic, Amsterdam.

Dixon, R.B., 1933. 'Tobacco Chewing on the Northwest Coast', AA 35, 146–50.

Dobkin de Rios, M., 1973. 'Curing with *Ayahuasca* in an Urban Slum', 67–85 in M.J. Harner (ed.), *Hallucinogens and Shamanism*.

Dobkin de Rios, M., 1974. 'The Influence of Psychotropic Flora and Fauna on Maya Religion', CA 15/2, 147–64.

Dobkin de Rios, M., 1984. *Hallucinogens: Cross-Cultural Perspectives*,

University of New Mexico, Albuquerque.

Dronfield, J., 1995. 'Migraine, Light and Hallucinogens: The Neurocognitive Basis of Irish Megalithic Art', OJA 14/3, 261–75.

Du Toit, B.M., 1975. 'Dagga: The History and Ethnographic Setting of *Cannabis sativa* in Southern Africa', 81–116 in V. Rubin (ed.) *Cannabis in Culture*.

Dunn, E., 1973. 'Russian Use of *Amanita muscaria*: A Footnote to Wasson's *Soma*', CA 14/4, 488–92.

Efron, D.H., Holmstedt, B., and Kline, N.S., (eds.), 1979. *Ethnopharmacologic Search for Psychoactive Drugs*, Raven Press, New York.

Ellis, E.S., 1946. *Ancient Anodynes: Primitive Anaesthesia and Allied Conditions*, Heinemann, London.

Ellis, H., 1898. 'Mescal: A New Artificial Paradise', CR 73, 130–41.

Emboden, W.A., 1974. *Bizarre Plants: Magical, Monstrous, Mythical*, Studio Vista, London.

Emboden, W.A., 1975. 'The Compelling Toad', TER 13/4, 27–32.

Emboden, W.A., 1976. 'Plant Hypnotics Among the North American Indians', 159–67 in W.D. Hand (ed.) *American Folk Medicine: A Symposium*, University of California Press, Berkeley.

Emboden, W.A., 1978. 'The Sacred Narcotic Lily of the Nile: Nymphaea Caerulea', EB 32/4, 395–407.

Emboden, W.A., 1979. *Narcotic Plants: Hallucinogens, Stimulants, Inebriants, and Hypnotics, Their Origins and Uses*, Studio Vista, London.

Emboden, W.A., 1981. 'Transcultural Use of Narcotic Water Lilies in Ancient Egyptian and Maya Drug Ritual', JEp 3, 39–83.

Emboden, W.A., 1997. Personal communication.

Erickson, H.T., Corrêa, M.P.F., and Escobar, J.R., 1984. 'Guaraná (*Paullinia cupana*) as a Commercial Crop in Brazilian Amazonia', EB 38/3, 273–86.

Evans, A.C. and Raistrick, D., 1987. 'Phenomenology of Intoxication with Toluene-based Adhesives and Butane Gas', BJP 150, 769–73.

Evans, G., 1921. *The Old Snuff House of Fribourg and Treyer*, privately published, London.

Evans, J., 1989. 'Report', E-I 20, 153–54.

Evans, W.C., 1979. 'Tropane alkaloids of the Solanaceae', 241–54 in J.G. Hawkes et al, *The Biology and Taxonomy of the Solanaceae*.

Feinhandler, S.J., Fleming, H.C., and Monahon, J.M., 1979. 'Pre-Columbian Tobaccos in the Pacific', EB 33/2, 213–26.

Feldman, H.W., 1979. 'PCP Use in Four Cities: An Overview', 29–51 in H.W. Feldman et al, *Angel Dust*.

Feldman, H.W., Agar, M.H., and Beschner, G.M., (eds.), 1979. *Angel Dust: An Ethnographic Study of PCP Users*, Lexington Books, Lexington, Mass.

Fernandez, J.W., 1972. '*Tabernanthe iboga*: Narcotic Ecstasis and the

Work of the Ancestors', 237–60 in P.T. Furst (ed.), *Flesh of the Gods.*

Fernandez, J.W., 1982. *Bwiti: An Ethnography of the Religious Imagination in Africa,* Princeton University Press, Princeton.

Fieve, R.R., 1994. *Prozac,* Thorsons, London.

Flattery, D.S. and Schwartz, M., 1989. *Haoma and Harmaline: The Botanical Identity of the Indo-Iranian Sacred Hallucinogen 'Soma' and Its Legacy in Religion, Language, and Middle Eastern Folklore,* University of California Press, Berkeley.

Fleisher, A. and Fleisher, Z., 1994. 'The Fragrance of Biblical Mandrake', EB 48/3, 243–51.

Frontinus, S.J., 1925. *The Stratagems / The Aqueducts of Rome,* trans. C.E. Bennett, (Loeb) Heinemann, London.

Furst, P.T., 1988. *Mushrooms: Psychedelic Fungi,* EOPD, Burke, London.

Furst, P.T. (ed.), 1972. *Flesh of the Gods: The Ritual Use of Hallucinogens,* Allen and Unwin, London.

Gallagher, L., 1994. 'Smoking Toad', *New York Times Magazine,* 5 June, 48–49.

Gardiner, E., 1610. *The Triall of Tobacco,* Mathew Lownes, London.

Gerard, J., 1597. *The Herball or Generall Historie of Plantes,* John Norton, London.

Gernet, A. von., 1995. 'Nicotian Dreams: The Prehistory and Early History of Tobacco in Eastern North America', 67–87 in J. Goodman et al., *Consuming Habits: Drugs in History and Anthropology.*

Glick, L.B., 1967. 'Medicine as an Ethnographic Category: The Gimi of the New Guinea Highlands', ETHN 6/1, 31–56.

Godwin, H., 1967. 'The Ancient Cultivation of Hemp', AQ 41, 42–49 and 137–38.

Goodman, J. 1995. 'Excitantia: Or, how Enlightenment Europe took to soft drugs' in J. Goodman et al., *Consuming Habits: Drugs in History and Anthropology,* Routledge, London.

Goodman, J., Lovejoy, P.E., and Sherratt, A. (eds.), 1995. *Consuming Habits: Drugs in History and Anthropology,* Routledge, London.

Goodman, S.M. and Hobbs, J.J., 1988. 'The Ethnobotany of the Egyptian Eastern Desert: A Comparison of Common Plant Usage Between Two Culturally Distinct Bedouin Groups', JEp 23/1, 73–89.

Grant, K., 1972. *The Magical Revival,* Muller, London.

Graves, R., 1976. *The White Goddess: A Historical Grammar of Poetic Myth,* Octagon, New York.

*The Grete Herball,* 1526, Peter Treveris, London.

Grillot de Givry, 1931. *Witchcraft, Magic and Alchemy,* London.

Grinspoon, L. and Bakalar, J.B., 1985. *Cocaine: A Drug and Its Social Evolution,* Revised Edition, Basic Books, New York.

Guazzo, F.M., 1929. *Compendium Maleficarum,* trans. M. Summers, London.

Gunther, R.T., 1959. *The Greek Herbal of Dioscorides,* Hafner, New York.

Habermehl, G.G., 1981. *Venomous Animals and Their Toxins*, Springer-Verlag, New York.

Haddon, A.C. and Seligmann, C.G., 1904. 'The Training of a Magician in Mabuiag', 321–23 in *Reports of the Cambridge Anthropological Expedition to Torres Straits* (Vol. V), Cambridge University Press, Cambridge.

Haining, P., 1972. 'The Ointments and Drugs of Black Magic', 67–77 in *The Warlock's Book: Secrets of the Ancient Grimoires*, W.H. Allen, London.

Hajicek-Dobberstein, S., 1995. 'Soma Siddhas and Alchemical Enlightenment: Psychedelic Mushrooms in Buddhist Tradition', JEp 48/2, 99–118.

Halifax, J., 1979. *Shamanic Voices: A Survey of Visionary Narratives*, Arkana, Harmondsworth.

Hansen, H.A., 1978. *The Witch's Garden*, trans. Muriel Crofts, Unity Press-Michael Kesend, Santa Cruz.

Harner, M.J., 1973. 'The Role of Hallucinogenic Plants in European Witchcraft', 12–50 in M.J. Harner (ed.) *Hallucinogens and Shamanism*.

Harner, M.J.(ed.), 1973. *Hallucinogens and Shamanism*, Oxford University Press, Oxford.

Hart, J.A., 1979. 'The Ethnobotany of the Flathead Indians of Western Montana', BMLHU 27/10.

Hassan, I., 1967. 'Some Folk Uses of *Peganum harmala* in India and Pakistan', EB 21/3, 284.

Hawkes, J.G., Lester, R.N. and Skelding, A.D., 1979. *The Biology and Taxonomy of the Solanaceae*, Linnean Society Symposium Series No. 7, Academic Press, London.

Heim, R. and Wasson, R.G., 1965. 'The "Mushroom Madness" of the Kuma', BLMHU 21/1, 1–36.

Heiser, C.B., 1969. *Nightshades: The Paradoxical Plants*, W.H.Freeman, San Francisco.

Heizer, R.F., 1940. 'The Botanical Identification of Northwest Coast Tobacco', AA 42, 704–06.

Helfrich, P. and Banner, A.H., 1960. 'Hallucinatory Mullet Poisoning: A Preliminary Report' (Contribution No. 126 of the Hawaii Marine Laboratory), JTMH 63/4, 86–89.

Helmont, J.B. van., 1662. *Oriatrike or, Physick Refined*, Lodowich Lloyd, London.

Helmont, J.B. van., 1688. *One Hundred and Fifty Three Chymical Aphorisms*, William Cooper/D. Newman, London.

Henningfield, J.E., 1986. *Barbiturates: Sleeping Potion or Intoxicant*, EOPD, Burke, London.

Herodotus, 1880. *Histories*, trans. G. Rawlinson, John Murray, London.

Heyerdahl, T., 1982. 'Letter to the Editors', JEp 5, 113–14.

Hill, J., 1761. *Cautions Against the Immoderate Use of Snuff*, R. Baldwin/J. Jackson, London.

Hoffer, A. and Osmond, H., 1967. *The Hallucinogens*, Academic Press, London.

Hofmann, A., 1980. *LSD: My Problem Child*, trans. J. Ott, McGraw-Hill, New York.

Holzer, H.(ed.), 1974. *Encyclopaedia of Witchcraft and Demonology*, London.

Huxley, A., 1954. *The Doors of Perception*, Harper, New York.

Huxley, A., 1956. *Heaven and Hell*, Chatto and Windus, London.

Hyndman, D.C., 1984. 'Ethnobotany of Wopkaimin *Pandanus*: Significant Papua New Guinea Plant Resource', EB 38/3, 287–303.

James I, King of England, 1604. *A Counterblaste to Tobacco*, R.B., London.

James, J. and Andresen, E., 1979. 'Sea-Tac and PCP', 109–58 in H.W. Feldman et al., *Angel Dust*.

James, W. 1992. Personal communication.

Janiger, O. and Dobkin de Rios, M., 1976. 'Nicotiana an Hallucinogen?', EB 30, 149–51.

Jansen, K.L.R. and Prast, C.J., 1988. 'Ethnopharmacology of Kratom and the *Mitragyna* Alkaloids', JEp 23/1, 115–19.

Johnston, T.F., 1972. '*Datura fastuosa*: Its Use in Tsonga Girls' Initiation', EB 26/4, 340–51.

Josephus, 1961. *The Jewish War* (Books IV–VII), trans. H.St.J. Thackeray, (Loeb) Heinemann, London.

Julian (Emperor), 1953. *Works* (Vol. III), trans. W.C. Wright, (Loeb) Heinemann, London.

Kalix, P., 1991. 'The pharmacology of psychoactive alkaloids from *Ephedra* and *Catha*', JEp 32/1–3, 201–8.

Kaplan, R.W., 1975. 'The Sacred Mushroom in Scandinavia', MAN (new series) 10, 72–79.

Karageorghis, V., 1976. 'A Twelfth-Century B.C. Opium Pipe from Kition', AQ 50, 125–29.

Keewaydinoquay, 1978. *Puhpohwee for the People: A Narrative Account of Some Uses of Fungi Among the Ahnishinaubeg*, Ethnomycological Studies No.5, Botanical Museum of Harvard University, Cambridge, MA.

Kenk, V.C., 1963. 'The Importance of Plants in Heraldry', EB 17/3, 169–79.

King, J.C.H., 1977. *Smoking Pipes of the North American Indians*, British Museum, London.

Klein, R., 1995. *Cigarettes are Sublime*, Picador, London.

Knight, V.J., 1975. 'Some Observations Concerning Plant Materials and Aboriginal Smoking in Eastern North America', JALA 21/2, 120–44.

Kohn, M., 1987. *Narcomania: On Heroin*, Faber and Faber, London.

Kohn, M., 1992. *Dope Girls: The Birth of the British Drug Underground*,

Lawrence and Wishart, London.

Kramer, P.D., 1994. *Listening to Prozac*, Fourth Estate, London.

Kroeger, P., 1993a. '*Piptoporus betulinus* in the Fraser Valley', MYCO, MLIV, 5.

Kroeger, P., 1993b. '"Chew-ash"; Unusual Use of a Fungus in the Yukon', MYCO, MLV, 2–5.

Krikorian, A.D., 1984. 'Kat and Its Use: An Historical Perspective', JEp 12/2, 115–78.

La Barre, W., 1980. *Culture in Context, Section One: Psychotropics*, Duke University Press, Durham, North Carolina.

La Barre, W., 1989. *The Peyote Cult* (5th edition), University of Oklahoma Press, Norman and London.

Lange, W.R. and Fralich, J., 1989. 'Nitrite Inhalants: promising and discouraging news', BJA 84/2, 121–23.

Laufer, B., 1924a. *Tobacco and Its Use in Asia*, Anthropology Leaflet 18, Field Museum of Natural History, Chicago.

Laufer, B., 1924b. *Introduction of Tobacco into Europe*, Anthropology Leaflet 19, Field Museum of Natural History, Chicago.

Lea, H.C., 1907. *A History of the Inquisition in Spain* (Vol. IV), Macmillan, London.

Leary, T., 1970. *The Politics of Ecstasy*, MacGibbon and Kee, London.

Lebot, V., Merlin, M. and Lindstrom, L., 1992. *Kava: The Pacific Drug*, Yale University Press, New Haven.

Lenson, D., 1995. *On Drugs*, University of Minnesota Press, Minneapolis.

Lewin, L., 1964. *Phantastica: Narcotic and Stimulating Drugs, Their Use and Abuse*, Routledge and Kegan Paul, London.

Li, H-L., 1974a. 'The Origin and Use of Cannabis in Eastern Asia Linguistic-Cultural Implications', EB 28/3, 293–301.

Li, H-L., 1974b. 'An Archaeological and Historical Account of Cannabis in China', EB 28/4, 437–48.

Li, H-L., 1977. 'Hallucinogenic Plants in Chinese Herbals', BMLHU 25/6, 161–81.

Lietava, J., 1992. 'Medicinal plants in a Middle Paleolithic grave Shanidar IV ?', JEp 35/3, 263–66.

Lindstrom, L., 1987. *Drugs in Western Pacific Societies: Relations of Substance*, ASAO Monograph 11, University Press of America, Lanham, New York.

Litzinger, W.J., 1981. 'Ceramic Evidence for Prehistoric *Datura* Use in North America', JEp 4, 57–74.

Lockwood, T.E., 1979. 'The Ethnobotany of *Brugmansia*', JEp 1/ 2, 147–64.

Love, B., 1995. *The Encyclopedia of Unusual Sex Practices*, Abacus, London.

Lukas, S.E., 1985. *Amphetamines: Danger in the Fast Lane*, EOPD, Burke, London.

Mabey, R., 1996. *Flora Britannica*, Sinclair-Stevenson, London.

Mackenzie, D.N., 1971. *A Concise Pahlavi Dictionary*, Oxford University Press, London.

MacLaren, D., 1873. *Nugae Canorae Medicae: Lays by the Poet Laureate of the New Town Dispensary*, Edmonston and Douglas, Edinburgh.

Macmillan, H., 1861. *Footnotes From the Page of Nature or First Forms of Vegetation*, Macmillan, London.

Manandhar, N.P., 1995. 'An Inventory of Some Herbal Drugs of Myagdi District, Nepal', EB 49/4, 371–79.

Manniche, L., 1989. *An Ancient Egyptian Herbal*, University of Texas Press, Austin.

Martin, M.A., 1975. 'Ethnobotanical Aspects of Cannabis in Southeast Asia', 63–75 in V. Rubin (ed.) *Cannabis in Culture*.

Martin, R.T., 1970. 'The Role of Coca in the History, Religion, and Medicine of South American Indians', EB 24/4, 422–38.

McKenna, T., 1992. *Food of the Gods: The Search for the Original Tree of Knowledge*, Rider, London.

McMeekin, D., 1992. 'Representations on Pre-Columbian Spindle Whorls of the Floral and Fruit Structure of Economic Plants', EB 46/2, 171–80.

Mehra, K.L., 1979. 'Ethnobotany of Old World Solanaceae', 161–70 in J.G. Hawkes et al., *The Biology and Taxonomy of the Solanaceae*.

Merlin, M.D., 1972. *Man and Marijuana: Some Aspects of Their Ancient Relationship*, Associated University Presses, Cranbury, N.J.

Merlin, M.D., 1984. *On the Trail of the Ancient Opium Poppy*, Associated University Presses, London.

Merrill, W.L. 1977. *An Investigation of Ethnographic and Archaeological Specimens of Mescalbeans* (Sophora secundiflora) *in American Museums*, Research Reports in Ethnobotany 1, Museum of Anthropology, University of Michigan, Ann Arbor.

Merrillees, R.S., 1962. 'Opium Trade in the Bronze Age Levant', AQ 36, 287–92.

Monardes, N., 1577. *Joyfull Newes out of the Newe Founde Worlde . . .*, trans. John Frampton, Willyam Norton, London.

Monter, E.W., 1976. *Witchcraft in France and Switzerland*, London.

Moreau de Tours, J.J., 1973. *Hashish and Mental Illness*, trans. G.J. Barnett, Raven Press, New York.

Morgan, A., 1995. *Toads and Toadstools: The Natural History, Folklore, and Cultural Oddities of a Strange Association*, Celestial Arts, Berkeley.

Morgan, G.R., 1980. *The Ethnobotany of Sweet Flag Among North American Indians*, BMLHU 28/3, 235–46.

Mortimer, W.G., 1974. *History of Coca: 'The Divine Plant' of the Incas*, Fitz Hugh Ludlow, Memorial Library Edition, San Francisco.

Motley, T.J., 1994. *The Ethnobotany of Sweet Flag, Acorus calamus* (Araceae), EB 48/4, 397–412.

Munro, R. et al., 1879. 'Notice of the Excavation of a Crannog at Lochlee, Tarbolton, Ayrshire', PSAS 1 (N.S.), 175–252.

Myerhoff, B.G., 1974. *Peyote Hunt: The Sacred Journey of the Huichol Indians*, Cornell University Press, Ithaca and London.

Needham, J., 1954–. *Science and Civilisation in China*, Cambridge University Press, Cambridge.

Nelson, E.W., 1899. 'The Eskimo About Bering Strait', 19–518 in *Eighteenth Annual Report of the Bureau of American Ethnology: Part One*, Washington D.C.

Norton, R. and Norton, M., 1938. *A History of Gold Snuff Boxes*, S.J. Phillips, London.

Opie, I. and Tatem, M., 1992. *A Dictionary of Superstitions*, Oxford University Press, Oxford.

Ott, J., 1993. *Pharmacotheon: Entheogenic Drugs, Their Plant Sources and History*, Natural Products Co., Kennewick, WA.

Ott, J., 1994. *Ayahuasca Analogues: Pangæan Entheogens*, Natural Products Co., Kennewick, WA.

Ott, J., 1995. *The Age of Entheogens/The Angel's Dictionary*, Natural Products Co., Kennewick, WA.

Ott, J., 1996. 'Entheogens II: On Entheology and Entheobotany', JPD 28/2, 205–9.

Paracelsus, 1656. *Dispensatory and Chirurgery*, Philip Chetwind, London.

Parssinen, T.M., 1983. *Secret Passions, Secret Remedies: Narcotic Drugs in British Society 1820–1930*, Institute for the Study of Human Issues, Philadelphia.

Pegler, D.N., Laessøe, T., and Spooner, B.M., 1995. *British Puffballs, Earthstars and Stinkhorns: An Account of the British Gasteroid Fungi*, Royal Botanic Gardens, Kew.

Penn, W.A., 1901. *The Soverane Herbe: A History of Tobacco*, Grant Richards, London.

Peterson, N., 1979. 'Aboriginal Uses of Australian Solanaceae', 171–89 in J.G. Hawkes et al., *The Biology and Taxonomy of the Solanaceae*.

Philalethes, E., 1678. *Ripley Reviv'd: Or, an Exposition upon Sir George Ripley's Hermetico-Poetical Works*, William Cooper, London.

Poole, F.J.P., 1987. 'Ritual rank, the self, and ancestral power: liturgy and substance in a Papua New Guinea society', 149–96 in L. Lindstrom (ed.) *Drugs in Pacific Societies*.

Pope, H.G., 1969. '*Tabernanthe iboga*: An African Narcotic Plant of Social Importance', EB 23/2, 174–84.

Powell, J.M., 1976. 'Ethnobotany', 106–183 in K. Paijmans (ed.), *New Guinea Vegetation*, Elsevier, Oxford.

Prance, G.T., 1970. 'Notes on the Use of Plant Hallucinogens in Amazonian Brazil', EB 24/1, 62–68.

Prance, G.T., 1972. 'Ethnobotanical Notes from Amazonian Brazil', EB 26/3, 221–37.

Radford, E. and Radford, M.A., 1980. *The Encyclopedia of Superstitions*, (edited and revised by C. Hole), Helicon, Oxford.

Ramsbottom, J., 1953. *Mushrooms and Toadstools: A Study of the Activities of Fungi*, Collins, London.

Ratner, M.S. (ed.), 1993. *Crack Pipe as Pimp: An Ethnographic Investigation of Sex-for-Crack Exchanges*, Lexington, New York.

Rätsch, C., 1992. *The Dictionary of Sacred and Magical Plants*, Prism Press, Bridport.

Reay, M., 1960. ' "Mushroom Madness" in the New Guinea Highlands', OCE 31, 137–39.

Reichel-Dolmatoff, G., 1975. *The Shaman and the Jaguar: A Study of Narcotic Drugs Among the Indians of Colombia*, Temple University Press, Philadelphia.

Reichel-Dolmatoff, G., 1978. *Beyond the Milky Way: Hallucinatory Imagery of the Tukano Indians*, UCLA, Latin American Center Publications, University of California, Los Angeles.

Reichel-Dolmatoff, G., 1987. *Shamanism and Art of the Eastern Tukanoan Indians*, Brill, Leiden.

Reichel-Dolmatoff, G., 1989. *Desana Texts and Contexts*, Acta Ethnologica Et Linguistica 62, Series Americana 12, Wien-Fohrenau.

Reis, S. Von, 1979. 'Vilca and Its Use', 307–14 in Efron et al.(eds.), *Ethnopharmacologic Search for Psychoactive Drugs*.

Rich, B., 1606. *Faultes, Faults, And nothing else but Faultes*, Jeffrey Chorleton, London.

Richardson, P.M., 1988. *Flowering Plants: Magic in Bloom*, EOPD, Burke, London.

Riedlinger, T.J.(ed.), 1990. *The Sacred Mushroom Seeker: Essays for R. Gordon Wasson*, Ethnomycological Studies No.11, Dioscorides Press, Portland, Oregon.

Ripley, G., 1591. *The Compound of Alchymy*, Thomas Orwin, London.

Robbins, R.H., 1959. *The Encyclopedia of Witchcraft and Demonology*, Nevill, London.

Ross, W.A., 1936. 'Ethnological Notes on Mt. Hagen Tribes', ANTH 31, 341–63.

Roth, H.L., 1899. *The Aborigines of Tasmania*, Second Edition, F. King, Halifax, England.

Rothman, T., 1972. 'De Laguna's Commentaries on Hallucinogenic Drugs and Witchcraft in Dioscorides' Materia Medica', BHM 46, 562–67.

Rubin, V., (ed.), 1975. *Cannabis and Culture*, Mouton, The Hague.

Ruck, C.A.P. et al., 1979. 'Entheogens', JPD 11/1-2, 145–46.

Rudgley, R., 1993. *The Alchemy of Culture: Intoxicants in Culture*, British Museum Press, London.

Rudgley, R.I., 1995. 'The Archaic Use of Hallucinogens in Europe: An

Archaeology of Altered States', ADD 90/2, 163–64.

Russell, J., 1993. 'Fuel of the forgotten deaths', NS 6 Feb., 21–23.

Saar, M., 1991a. 'Ethnomycological Data from Siberia and North-East Asia on the Effect of *Amanita muscaria*', JEp 31, 157–73.

Saar, M., 1991b. 'Fungi in Khanty Folk Medicine', JEp 31, 175–79.

Safford, W.E., 1922. 'Daturas of the Old World and New: An Account of Their Narcotic Properties and Their Use in Oracular and Initiatory Ceremonies', 537–67 in Annual Report of the Smithsonian Institution 1920, Washington DC.

Salmon, W., 1693. *Selapsium – The Compleat English Physician: Or, The Druggist's Shop Opened*, Matthew Gilliflower/George Sawbridge, London.

Salmon, W., 1707. *Medicina Practica: Or, The Practical Physician*, Edmund Curll, London.

Salmon, W., 1710. *Botanologica, The English Herbal: Or, History of Plants*, 2 vols., Rhodes/Taylor, London.

Sanford, J.H., 1972. 'Japan's "Laughing Mushrooms" ', EB 26, 174–81.

Sarianidi, V., 1994. 'Temples of Bronze Age Margiana: Traditions of Ritual Architecture', AQ 68, 388–97.

Saunders, N., 1995. *Ecstasy and the Dance Culture*, Nicholas Saunders, London.

Schenk, G., 1956. *The Book of Poisons*, trans. M. Bullock, Weidenfeld and Nicolson, London.

Schultes, R.E., 1940. 'Teonanacatl: The Narcotic Mushroom of the Aztecs', AA 42, 429–43.

Schultes, R.E., 1977. 'The Botanical and Chemical Distribution of Hallucinogens', 25–55 in B.M. Du Toit (ed.), *Drugs, Rituals and Altered States of Consciousness*, Balkema, Rotterdam.

Schultes, R.E. and Hofmann, A., 1980a. *The Botany and Chemistry of Hallucinogens*, Second Edition, Charles C. Thomas, Springfield, Illinois.

Schultes, R.E. and Hofmann, A., 1980b. *Plants of the Gods: Origins of Hallucinogen Use*, Hutchinson, London.

Scot, R., 1665. *The Discovery of Witchcraft*, A. Clark/Dixy Page, London.

Seymour, J.D., 1913. *Irish Witchcraft and Demonology*, Dublin.

Sharon, D.G. and Donnan, C.B., 1977. 'The Magic Cactus: Ethnoarchaeological Continuity in Peru', ARCH 30/6, 374–81.

Sharp, C.W. and Rosenberg, N.L., 1992. 'Volatile Substances', 303–27 in J.H. Lowinson et al., (eds.), *Substance Abuse: A Comprehensive Textbook*, Second Edition, Williams and Williams, Baltimore.

Sherratt, A.G., 1987. 'Cups that Cheered', 81–106 in W.H. Waldren and R.C. Kennard (eds.), *Bell-Beakers of the West Mediterranean*, British Archaeological Reports, International Series 331, Oxford.

Sherratt, A.G., 1991. 'Sacred and Profane Substances: The Ritual Use of

Narcotics in Later Neolithic Europe', 50–64 in P. Garwood et al.(eds.), *Sacred and Profane: Proceedings of a Conference on Archaeology, Ritual and Religion*, Oxford University Committee for Archaeology, Monograph 32, Oxford.

Sherratt, A.G., 1994. 'Alice in Wonderland', OXM 110, 8–10.

Sherratt, A.G., 1996a. *With Baleful Weeds and Precious-Juicéd Flowers: Grooved Ware, Grape-Cups and Prehistoric Pharmacognosy*, unpublished manuscript.

Sherratt, A.G., 1996b. *Cash-Crops Before Cash: Hunting, Farming, Manufacture and Trade in Early Eurasia*, unpublished manuscript.

Smith, W.D., 1995. 'From Coffeehouse to Parlour' in J. Goodman et al., *Consuming Habits: Drugs in History and Anthropology*, Routledge, London.

Stearn, W.T., 1975. 'Typification of *Cannabis sativa* L.', 13–20 in V. Rubin (ed.), *Cannabis in Culture*.

Stevens, J., 1989. *Storming Heaven: LSD and the American Dream*, Paladin, London.

Stevenson, M.C., 1915. 'Ethnobotany of the Zuñi Indians', 31–102 in Thirtieth Annual Report of the Bureau of American Ethnology, Washington DC.

Störck, A., 1763. *An Essay on the Internal Use of Thorn-Apple, Henbane, and Monkshood*, Becket and De Hondt, London.

Strong, S., 1995. *Whitewash: Pablo Escobar and the Cocaine Wars*, Macmillan, London.

Theophrastus, 1916. *Enquiry Into Plants* (2 Vols.), trans. A. Hort, (Loeb) Heinemann, London.

Thieret, J.W., 1957. 'Economic Botany of the Cycads', EB 12/1, 3–41.

Thompson, C.J.S., 1934. *The Mystic Mandrake*, Rider, London.

Thorndike, L., 1923–58. *A History of Magic and Experimental Science*, 8 vols., Macmillan, New York/Columbia University Press, New York.

Thorwald, J., 1962. *Science and Secrets of Early Medicine*, Thames and Hudson, London.

Torres, C.M. et al., 1991. 'Snuff Powders from Pre-Hispanic San Pedro de Atacama: Chemical and Contextual Analysis', CA 32/5, 640–49.

Tucker, L.S., 1910. 'The Divining Basket of the Ovimbundu', JAI 70, 171–201.

Turner, N.J. and R.L. Taylor, 1972. 'A Review of the Northwest Coast Tobacco Mystery', SYE 5, 249–57.

Turner, W., 1568. *Herball, Three Partes*, Arnold Birchman, London.

Tyler, A., 1995. *Street Drugs*, Second Revised Edition, Hodder and Stoughton, London.

Tyler, V.E., 1966. 'The Physiological Properties and Chemical Constituents of Some Habit-Forming Plants', LL 29/4, 275–92.

Vahman, F., 1986. *Arda Wiraz Namag: The Iranian 'Divina Commedia'*, Scandinavian Institute of Asian Studies, Monograph Series No. 53, Curzon Press, London.

Verpoorte, R., Phan-Quoc-Kinh and A. Baerheim Svendsen, 1979. 'Chemical Constituents of Vietnamese Toad Venom Collected from *Bufo melanostictus* Schneider', JEp 1 /2, 197–202.

Waite, A.E., 1990. *The Book of Ceremonial Magic: A Complete Grimoire*, Carol, New York.

Waller, M.B., 1993. *Crack-Affected Children: A Teacher's Guide*, Corwin, Newbury Park, California.

Wasson, R.G., 1968. *Soma: Divine Mushroom of Immortality*, Ethnomycological Studies No.1, Harcourt Brace Jovanovich, New York.

Wasson, R.G., 1979. 'Traditional Use in North America of *Amanita muscaria* for Divinatory Purposes', JPD 11/1–2, 25–28.

Wasson, R.G. et al., 1974. *María Sabina and Her Mazatec Mushroom Velada*, Ethnomycological Studies No.3, Harcourt Brace Jovanovich, New York.

Wasson, R.G., Hofmann, A. and Ruck, C.A.P., 1978. *The Road to Eleusis: Unveiling the Secrets of the Mysteries*, Ethnomycological Studies No.4, Harcourt Brace Jovanovich, New York.

Wasson, R.G. and Wasson, V.P., 1957. *Mushrooms, Russia and History*, (Two vols.), Pantheon, New York.

Watson, P., 1983. *This Precious Foliage: A Study of the Aboriginal Psycho-active Drug Pituri*, Oceania Monograph 26, University of Sydney, Sydney.

Watling, R., 1975. 'Prehistoric Puff-balls', BBMS 9/2, 112–14.

Watling, R. and Seaward, M.R.D., 1976. 'Some Observations on Puff-balls from British Archaeological Sites', JAS 3, 165–72.

Watt, J.M. and Breyer-Brandwijk, M.G., 1962. *The Medicinal and Poisonous Plants of Southern and Eastern Africa*, Second Edition, E&S Livingstone, Edinburgh and London.

Weil, A.T., 1977. 'The Use of Psychoactive Mushrooms in the Pacific Northwest: An Ethnopharmacologic Report', BMLHU 25/5, 131–49.

Weil, A.T., 1979. 'Nutmeg as a Psychoactive Drug', 188-201 in Efron et al., (eds), *Ethnopharmacologic Search for Psychoactive Drugs*.

Weil, A.T. and Davis, W., 1994. '*Bufo alvarius*: A Potent Hallucinogen of Animal Origin', JEp 41/1–2, 1–8.

Weir, S., 1985. *Qat in Yemen: Consumption and Social Change*, British Museum Publications, London.

Whiting, M.G., 1963. 'Toxicity of Cycads', EB 17/4, 271–302.

Wilbert, J., 1987. *Tobacco and Shamanism in South America*, Yale University Press, New Haven.

Wilbert, J., 1991. 'Does Pharmacology Corroborate the Nicotine Therapy and Practices of South American Shamanism?', JEp 32/1–3, 179–86.

Wilbert, J., 1993. *Mystic Endowment: Religious Ethnography of the Warao Indians,* Harvard University Press, Cambridge, Mass.

Wilcox, J.A., 1995. 'Psychoactive Properties of Pergolide Mesylate', JPD 27/2, 181–82.

Williams, T.I., 1947. *Drugs From Plants,* Sigma, London.

Winkelman, M. and Dobkin de Rios, M., 1989. 'Psychoactive Properties of !Kung Bushmen Medicine Plants', JPD, 51–59.

Wissler, C. and Duvall, D.C., 1909. 'Mythology of the Blackfoot Indians', APAMNH 2, Part 1.

Withington, E.T., 1917. 'Dr. John Weyer and the Witch Mania', 189–224 in C. Singer (ed.), *Studies in the History and Method of Science,* Clarendon Press, Oxford.

Wurtzel, E., 1994. *Prozac Nation: Young and Depressed in America,* Quartet, London.

Yasumoto, T. and Kao, C.Y., 1986. 'Tetrodotoxin and the Haitian Zombie', TOX 24/8, 747–49.

Yefimenko, A.A., 1995. Personal communication.

Zackon, F., 1988. *Heroin: The Street Narcotic,* EOPD, Burke, London.

Zaehner, R.C., 1957. *Mysticism Sacred and Profane,* Clarendon Press, Oxford.

Zaehner, R.C., 1972. *Drugs, Mysticism and Make-Believe,* Collins, London.

Zzaro, J., 1977. *Heroin: Lifting the Lid Off the $Billion Dollar Death Racket,* Stockwell, Ifracombe, Devon.

## ABBREVIATIONS OF JOURNALS, PERIODICALS AND SERIES

AA: American Anthropologist
ADD: Addiction
ANTH: Anthropos
APAMNH: Anthropological Papers of the American Museum of Natural History
AQ: Antiquity
ARCH: Archaeology
ARCT: Arctic Anthropology
BBMS: Bulletin of the British Mycological Society
BHM: Bulletin of the History of Medicine
BJA: British Journal of Addiction
BJP: British Journal of Psychiatry
BMLHU: Botanical Museum Leaflets of Harvard University
CA: Current Anthropology
CR: Contemporary Review
EB: Economic Botany
E-I: Eretz-Israel

EOPD: Encyclopedia of Psychoactive Drugs
ETHN: Ethnology
JAI: Journal of the Anthropological Institute
JALA: Journal of Alabama Archaeology
JAS: Journal of Archaeological Science
JCA: Journal of California Anthropology
JEp: Journal of Ethnopharmacology
JPD: Journal of Psychedelic Drugs (later renamed Journal of Psychoactive Drugs)
JTMH: Journal of Tropical Medicine and Hygiene
LL: Lloydia
LM: London Miscellany
MAN: Man (The Journal of the Royal Anthropological Institute)
MYCO: Mycofile (The Newsletter of the Vancouver Mycological Society)
NS: New Scientist
OCE: Oceania
OJA: Oxford Journal of Archaeology
OXM: Oxford Magazine
PSAS: Proceedings of the Society of Antiquaries of Scotland
SCC: Science and Civilisation in China
SCI: Science
SNR: Sudan Notes and Records (incorporating Proceedings of the Philosophical Society of Sudan)
SYE: Syesis
TER: Terra
TOX: Toxicon
YESC: Yearbook for Ethnomedicine and the Study of Consciousness

# PICTURE CREDIT LIST

1. **ACORUS CALAMUS** drawing by Juliet Henry.
2. **AFRICA, PSYCHOACTIVE PLANTS OF** caption: *Devil's Foot Root*, drawing by Juliet Henry.
3. **ANIMALS** caption: *Goatfish*, drawing by Juliet Henry.
4. **BELLADONNA** from: Natural History Museum Botany Library Plate Collection (hereafter NHMBLPC) Folder 114: Atropa.
5. **CANNABIS** from: NHMBLPC Folder 153 (153/5).
6. **COCAINE** caption: *Advertisement for Vin Mariani* from: McKenna 1992, fig. 23, p. 213. Originally from the Fitz Hugh Ludlow Library.
7. **DATURA** from: NHMBLPC Folder 114: Datura.
8. **DATURA** caption: *Prehistoric Incense Burner From North America in Shape of Datura Fruit*, drawing by Juliet Henry.
9. **DATURA** caption: *Pre-Colombian Spindle Whorl in Form of Datura Flower, Quimbaya culture, Colombia*, drawing by Juliet Henry.
10. **ERGOT** caption: *Saint Anthony Besieged by Demonic Apparitions* from: Schultes and Hofmann 1980b, p. 104. Original is an engraving by Martin Schongauer ca. 1471–1473.
11. **ETHER** from: Victor Robinson (1947) *Victory over Pain: A History of Anesthesia*, Sigma, London, p. 157. Original from *Punch* magazine 1847.
12. **ETHER** from: Robinson 1947, p. 155. Original from a French cartoon 1847.
13. **FLY-AGARIC** caption: *Prehistoric Siberian Rock Art Depicting Fly-Agaric People* from: N.N. Dikov (1972) 'Les Pétroglyphes de Pegtymel et Leur Appartenance Ethnique' 245–261 in *Inter-Nord* 12 (fig. 12).
14. **FUNGI** caption: *Demon of the Mushroom from the Florentine Codex* from: Schultes and Hofmann 1980b, p. 146. Original drawing in the Florentine Codex of Bernardino de Sahagun.
15. **FUNGI** caption: *Bronze Age Razor from Scandinavia with 'Mushroom' motif*.
16. **HENBANE** from: NHMBLPC Folder 114: Hyoscyamus.
17. **HEROIN** caption: *Morphine Addict* from: Science Photo Library, W2, ref. No. M370/177USA 06N.

18. **MANDRAKE** caption: *Female and Male Mandrakes.* Science Photo Library. Original drawing in Meydenbach's *Hortus Sanitatus* of 1491.

19. **MANDRAKE** caption: *The Hand of Glory* from: Waite 1990, p. 311. Originally in *Petit Albert*, an anonymous work of 19th century. Numerous editions.

20. **OPIUM** caption: *Prehistoric Opium Pipe from Cyprus,* drawing by Juliet Henry.

21. **OPIUM** caption: *Chinese Opium Den* from: Science Photo Library, ref. No. M370/175USA02S.

22. **PIPES** caption: *Blackfoot Medicine Pipe* from: R.H. Lowie (1982) *Indians of the Plains,* University of Nebraska Press, Lincoln and London, fig. 15, p. 28.

23. **PIPES** caption: *The Method of Smoking an Earth-Pipe,* drawing by Juliet Henry.

24. **PSILOCYBE** from: Schultes and Hofmann 1980b, p. 144.

25. **PUFFBALLS** caption: *Lycoperdon mixtecorum* (*left*) *and Lycoperdon marginatum* (*right*), drawing by Juliet Henry.

26. **SCOPOLIA** from: NHMBLPC Folder 114: Scopolia.

27. **TOAD** caption: *Bufo alvarius* from: *Wall Street Journal,* 3rd July 1994.

28. **TOAD** from: Ashmole 1652, p. 374.

29. **TOADSTONE** caption: *Extracting the Toadstone* from: Grillot de Givry 1931, fig. 321, p. 345. Original in Johannes de Cuba's 'Hortus Sanitatis', Paris ca. 1498.

30. **TOBACCO** from: NHMBLPC Folder 114: Nicotiana.

31. **TOBACCO** caption: *Chinese Snuff Bottle,* drawing by Juliet Henry.

32. **VIROLA** from: Schultes and Hofmann 1980a, fig. 49, p. 129.

33. **WITCHES' OINTMENTS** caption: *Witch, with Cat and Pestle and Mortar.* Early twentieth-century French wooden carving (Science and Society Picture Library, Science Museum).

34. **ZOMBI DRUG** caption: *Puffer Fish,* drawing by Juliet Henry.

# INDEX

Bold page numbers refer to main entries. Numbers in *italic* refer to the illustrations